Medical Sciences at a Glance

This title is also available as an e-book.
For more details, please see
www.wiley.com/buy/9781118360927
or scan this QR code:

Medical Sciences at a Glance

Edited by

Michael D Randall

Professor of Pharmacology
School of Life Sciences
University of Nottingham
Nottingham, UK

WILEY Blackwell

This edition first published 2014 © John Wiley & Sons, Ltd

Registered Office
John Wiley & Sons Ltd, The Atrium, Southern Gate, Chichester, West Sussex, PO19 8SQ, UK

Editorial Offices
350 Main Street, Malden, MA 02148-5020, USA
9600 Garsington Road, Oxford, OX4 2DQ, UK
The Atrium, Southern Gate, Chichester, West Sussex, PO19 8SQ, UK

For details of our global editorial offices, for customer services, and for information about how to apply for permission to reuse the copyright material in this book please see our website at www.wiley.com/wiley-blackwell.

The right of Michael D Randall to be identified as the author(s) of the editorial material in this work has been asserted in accordance with the UK Copyright, Designs and Patents Act 1988.

Library of Congress Cataloging-in-Publication Data

Medical sciences at a glance / edited by Michael D. Randall.
    p. ; cm. – (At a glance series)
  Includes bibliographical references and index.
  ISBN 978-1-118-36092-7 (pbk. : alk. paper) – ISBN 978-1-118-36093-4 –
ISBN 978-1-118-36094-1 – ISBN 978-1-118-36095-8 (emobi) – ISBN 978-1-118-36096-5 (epub) –
ISBN 978-1-118-36097-2 (epdf)
  I. Randall, Michael D., editor of compilation.   II. Series: At a glance series (Oxford, England)
  [DNLM: 1. Medicine. WB 100]
  R706
  610–dc23
                         2013026509

A catalogue record for this book is available from the British Library.

Cover image: iStock © BlackJack3D
Cover design by Meaden Creative

Set in 9/11.5 pt Times Roman by Toppan Best-set Premedia Limited
Printed and bound in Malaysia by Vivar Printing Sdn Bhd

1 2014

Contents

Preface

The *At a Glance* series provides brief summaries of the medical curriculum for medical, pharmacy and nursing students. Recent changes in curricula at medical schools have reduced the emphasis on students learning large amounts of factual detail and now focus more on core knowledge. Courses have also moved away from the traditional discipline-based approach of studying anatomy, physiology, biochemistry, pathology and pharmacology as distinct preclinical subjects, and many courses are now integrated. This provides a seamless study of the key physiological systems. The purpose of *Medical Sciences at a Glance* is to reflect the modernisation of medical courses and, as such, provides a single text to support students.

To understand and practise medicine the student needs to have a grasp of underlying biomedical sciences, and this book is intended for the early years' students. It should also help as a refresher of the medical sciences as students enter clinical phases of their courses, as a thorough knowledge of the medical sciences inevitably underpins clinical practice. For example, to understand the ECG in clinical practice one needs to understand the relevant anatomy, the underlying electrical events and the cardiac cycle.

By providing the background in biomedical sciences this edition feeds directly into *Medicine at a Glance* (Edited by Patrick Davey).

The aim of this book is to set out core material on which students can build a framework of learning and understanding. By using this book students should be able to define what they need to know and use the material as key summary points. It is all too easy for students to attempt to learn all lecture material superficially, but the key to medical studies is to *understand* the core material. We also feel that *Medical Sciences at a Glance* would be of use to students on the newer problem-based learning courses by setting a background against which students can define their own learning needs.

We hope that this text will help support early years' students getting to grips with physiological systems. We have deliberately limited the clinical content as this is the domain of the sister publication *Medicine at a Glance*, but have inevitably used some examples of diseases and treatment to place biomedical sciences in context.

The authors of *Medical Sciences at a Glance* are all from the University of Nottingham and all currently teach the relevant medical sciences to medical, science and pharmacy students.

Michael D Randall

Contributors

Dr Jane Arnold
University Teacher
School of Life Sciences
University of Nottingham

Dr Stuart Brown
Director of Biomedical Sciences Teaching
School of Life Sciences
University of Nottingham

Dr Steven Burr
Formerly University Teacher
School of Biomedical Sciences
University of Nottingham Medical School
Now Associate Professor in Physiology
Medical School
University of Plymouth

Dr Sue Chan
Lecturer in Cell Signalling
School of Life Sciences
University of Nottingham

Dr Chien-Yi Chang
Research Fellow
School of Life Sciences
University of Nottingham

Dr Fergus Doherty
Lecturer in Biochemistry
School of Life Sciences
University of Nottingham

Dr Lucy Fairclough
Lecturer in Immunology
School of Life Sciences
University of Nottingham

Dr James Lazenby
Research Fellow
School of Life Sciences
University of Nottingham

Dr Siobhan Loughna
Lecturer in Anatomy
School of Life Sciences
University of Nottingham

Dr Deborah Merrick
Lecturer in Anatomy
School of Life Sciences
University of Nottingham

Dr Ian Todd
Associate Professor and Reader in Cellular Immunology
School of Life Sciences
University of Nottingham

Prof Michael D Randall
Professor of Pharmacology
School of Life Sciences
University of Nottingham

Dr Sebastiaan Winkler
Associate Professor in Gene Expression
School of Pharmacy
University of Nottingham

Abbreviations

5-HT	5-hydroxytryptamine
AI	angiotensin I
AII	angiotensin II
AC	adenylyl cyclase
AcCoA	acetyl coenzyme A
ACE	angiotensin-converting enzyme
ACh	acetylcholine
AChE	acetylcholinesterase
ACTH	adrenocorticotropic hormone
ADCC	antibody-dependent cellular cytotoxicity
ADH	antidiuretic hormone
ADP	adenosine diphosphate
AIDS	acquired immune deficiency syndrome
ALT	alanine aminotransferase
AMP	adenosine monophosphate (AMP)
ANP	atrial natriuretic peptide
AP	action potential
APCs	antigen-presenting cells
AST:	aspartate aminotransferase
AT_1	angiotensin II receptor type 1
AV	atrioventricular
AVP	arginine vasopressin
BNP	b-type natriuretic peptide
BPH	benign prostatic hypertrophy
BSE	bovine spongiform encephalopathy
CABG	coronary artery bypass graft
CAH	congenital adrenal hyperplasia
cAMP	cyclic adenosine monophosphate
CCK	cholecystokinin
CCRs	central chemoreceptors
cGMP	cyclic guanosine monophosphate
CHF	chronic heart failure
CJD	Creutzfeldt–Jakob disease
CML	chronic myeloid leukaemia
CNS	central nervous system
CO	cardiac output
COMT	catechol-O-methyltransferase
COPD	chronic obstructive pulmonary disease
Cox	cyclooxygenase
CRH	Corticotropin-releasing hormone
CSF	colony-stimulating factors (e.g. G-CSF, granulocyte CSF)
CSF	cerebrospinal fluid
CTLR	C-type lectin receptors
CYP450	cytochrome P450
D	dopamine receptor
DCT	distal convoluted tubule
DHAE	dehydroepiandrosterone
DHAP	dihydroxyacetone phosphate
DHFR	dihydrofolate reductase
DM	diabetes mellitus
DPP-IV	dipeptidyl peptidase IV
DVT	deep vein thrombosis
dUMP	deoxy uridine monophosphate
ECF-like	enterochromaffin-like cells
ECG	electrocardiogram
EDHF	endothelium-derived hyperpolarising factor
EDV	end diastolic volume
EGF	epidermal growth factor
EPO	erythropoietin
EPPs	excitatory postsynaptic potentials
ER	endoplasmic reticulum
ERV	expiratory reserve volume
ESV	end systolic volume
ETC	electron transport chain
F	Faraday's constant
FCR	Fc receptors
FDC	follicular dendritic cells
FEV_1	forced expiratory volume in the first second
FSH	follicle-stimulating hormone
FVC	forced vital capacity
G-CSF	granulocyte colony-stimulating factor
GFR	glomerular filtration rate
GLP-1	glucagon-like peptide 1
GLUTs	glucose transporters
GLUT2	glucose transporter 2
GLUT5	glucose transporter 5
GnRH	gonadotrophin-releasing hormone
GPCR	G-protein-coupled receptors
GTN	glyceryl trinitrate
HAART	highly active antiretroviral therapy
Hb	haemoglobin
hCG	human chorionic gonadotrophin
HDL	high-density lipoprotein
HER2	human growth factor receptor-2
HIV	human immunodeficiency virus
HLA	human leucocyte antigens
HMG-CoA reductase	hydroxyl-methylglutaryl coenzyme A reductase

hnRNA	heterogeneous nuclear RNA	P_ACO_2	arterial carbon dioxide
IC	immune complex	PCV	packed cell volume
IF	intrinsic factor	PCRs	peripheral chemoreceptors
I_f	'funny' current	PCT	proximal convoluted tubule
IFN	interferon	PDE	phosphodiesterase
IHD	ischaemic heart disease	PDH	pyruvate dehydrogenase
IMM	inner mitochondrial membrane	PE	phosphatidyl-ethanolamine
INR	international normalised ratio	PEF	peak expiratory flow
IPSP	inhibitory postsynaptic potential	PEFR	peak expiratory flow rate
		PFK-1	phosphofructokinase-1
IRV	inspiratory reserve volume	PGI_2	prostacyclin
JVP	jugular venous pressure	PI	phosphatidyl-inositol
K_d	dissociation constant	PIF	peak inspiratory flow
KIRs	killer cell immunoglobulin-like receptor	PL	phospholipase
		PPAR-γ	peroxisome proliferator-activated receptor-gamma
KLRs	killer cell lectin-like receptor	PPI	proton pump inhibitor
K_M	Michaelis-Menten constant	PRR	pathogen recognition receptor
LDL	low-density lipoprotein		
LH	luteinising hormone	PS	phosphatidyl-serine
LPS	lipopolysaccharide	PTH	parathyroid hormone
LTA	lipoteichoic acid	R	gas constant
LTD	long-term depression	RAAS	renin-angiotensin-aldosterone system
LT	long-term potentiation		
M-receptors	muscarinic receptors	RBC	red blood cell
MAO	monoamine oxidase	RER	rough endoplasmic reticulum
MAP	mean arterial pressure	RhD	rhesus antigen
MCV	mean corpuscular volume	RLRs	RIG-like helicase receptors
MDR1	multidrug resistance 1	rRNA	ribosomal RNA
mEPP	miniature end plate potential	SAN	sinoatrial node
MG	myasthenia gravis	SCID	severe combined immunodeficiencies
MHC	major histocompatibility complex		
		SCN	suprachiasmatic nucleus
MI	myocardial infarction	SIADH	syndrome of inappropriate antidiuretic hormone secretion
mRNA	messenger RNA		
MT	melatonin receptor		
NA	noradrenaline	sIg	surface immunoglobulin
nAChR	nicotinic acetylcholine receptor	SGLT1	the sodium-glucose transporter protein 1
NADP	nicotinamide adenine dinucleotide phosphate	SSRI	serotonin-selective reuptake inhibitor
NCR	natural cytotoxicity receptor	TAG	triacylglycerol
NLR	NOD-like receptor	Tc	T cytotoxic
NK	natural killer	TCA	tricyclic antidepressant
NMDA	N-methyl-D-aspartate	TCA cycle	tricarboxylic acid or Krebs cycle
NMJ	neuromuscular junction		
NO	nitric oxide	TCR	T cell receptor
NSAIDs	non-steroidal anti-inflammatory drugs	TIA	transient ischaemic attack
		Th	T helper
NTS	nucleus tractus solitarius (nucleus of the solitary tract)	TLC	total lung capacity
		TLR	toll-like receptors
PAMP	pathogen-associated molecular pattern	TNF-α	tumour necrosis factor-alpha
		TPR	total peripheral resistance
P_AO_2	arterial oxygen	tRNA	transfer RNA
PC	phosphatidyl-choline	TSG	tumour suppressor gene

V	rate of reaction	**V$_m$**	resting membrane potential
VC	vital capacity	**V$_{max}$**	maximum rate of reaction
VEGF	vascular endothelial growth factor	**VOCs**	voltage-operated channels
		V/Q	ventilation-perfusion
VIP	vasoactive intestinal polypeptide	**vWF**	Von Willebrand's factor
		UCP1	uncoupling protein 1
VLDL	very low-density lipoprotein	**UTI**	urinary tract infection

How to use your textbook

Features contained within your textbook

Each topic is presented in a double-page spread with clear, easy-to-follow diagrams supported by succinct explanatory text.

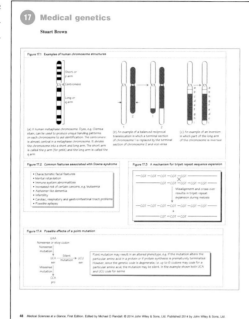

Your textbook is full of photographs, illustrations and tables.

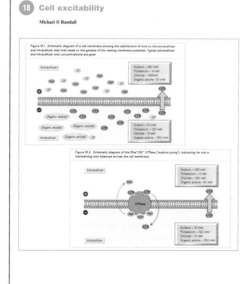

The anytime, anywhere textbook

Wiley E-Text

Your book is also available to purchase as a Wiley E-Text: Powered by VitalSource version – a digital, interactive version of this book which you own as soon as you download it.

Your Wiley E-Text allows you to:

Search: Save time by finding terms and topics instantly in your book, your notes, even your whole library (once you've downloaded more textbooks)

Note and Highlight: Colour code, highlight and make digital notes right in the text so you can find them quickly and easily

Organise: Keep books, notes and class materials organised in folders inside the application

Share: Exchange notes and highlights with friends, classmates and study groups

Upgrade: Your textbook can be transferred when you need to change or upgrade computers

Link: Link directly from the page of your interactive textbook to all of the material contained on the companion website

The Wiley E-Text version will also allow you to copy and paste any photograph or illustration into assignments, presentations and your own notes.

To access your Wiley E-Text:

• Visit www.vitalsource.com/software/bookshelf/downloads to download the Bookshelf application to your computer, laptop, tablet or mobile device.
• Open the Bookshelf application on your computer and register for an account.
• Follow the registration process.

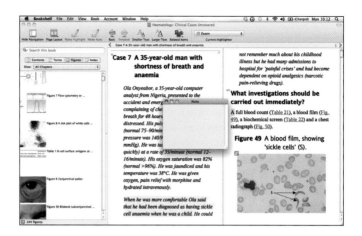

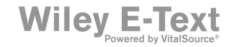

The VitalSource Bookshelf can now be used to view your Wiley E-Text on iOS, Android and Kindle Fire!

• **For iOS:** Visit the app store to download the VitalSource Bookshelf: http://bit.ly/17ib3XS
• **For Android:** Visit the Google Play Market to download the VitalSource Bookshelf: http://bit.ly/ZMEGvo
• **For Kindle Fire, Kindle Fire 2 or Kindle Fire HD:** Simply install the VitalSource Bookshelf onto your Fire (see how at http://bit.ly/11BVFn9). You can now sign in with the email address and password you used when you created your VitalSource Bookshelf Account.

   Full E-Text support for mobile devices is available at: http://support.vitalsource.com

CourseSmart

CourseSmart gives you instant access (via computer or mobile device) to this Wiley-Blackwell e-book and its extra electronic functionality, at 40% off the recommended retail print price. See all the benefits at: www.coursesmart.com/students

Instructors . . . receive your own digital desk copies!

CourseSmart also offers instructors an immediate, efficient and environmentally-friendly way to review this book for your course.

For more information visit www.coursesmart.com/instructors.

With CourseSmart, you can create lecture notes quickly with copy and paste, and share pages and notes with your students. Access your CourseSmart digital book from your computer or mobile device instantly for evaluation, class preparation and as a teaching tool in the classroom.

Simply sign in at http://instructors.coursesmart.com/bookshelf to download your Bookshelf and get started. To request your desk copy, hit 'Request Online Copy' on your search results or book product page.

We hope you enjoy using your new book. Good luck with your studies!

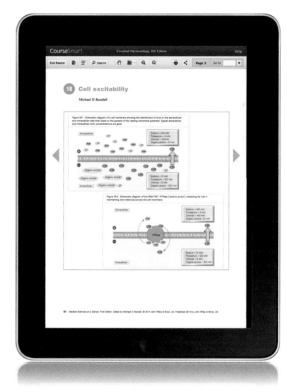

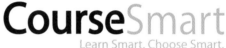

About the companion website

Don't forget to visit the companion website for this book:

 www.ataglanceseries.com/medicalsciences

There you will find valuable material designed to enhance your learning, including:
- Interactive multiple-choice questions
- Key summary points for each chapter

1 Cells

Sebastiaan Winkler

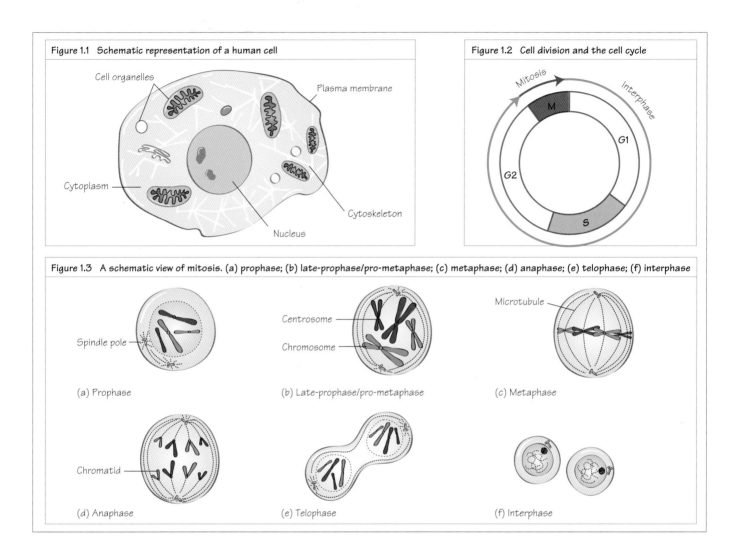

Figure 1.1 Schematic representation of a human cell

Cell organelles
Plasma membrane
Cytoplasm
Nucleus
Cytoskeleton

Figure 1.2 Cell division and the cell cycle

Mitosis
Interphase
M
G1
G2
S

Figure 1.3 A schematic view of mitosis. (a) prophase; (b) late-prophase/pro-metaphase; (c) metaphase; (d) anaphase; (e) telophase; (f) interphase

Spindle pole
Centrosome
Chromosome
Microtubule

(a) Prophase
(b) Late-prophase/pro-metaphase
(c) Metaphase

Chromatid

(d) Anaphase
(e) Telophase
(f) Interphase

 Medical Sciences at a Glance, First Edition. Edited by Michael D Randall. © 2014 John Wiley & Sons, Ltd. Published 2014 by John Wiley & Sons, Ltd.

A cell is the smallest functional and structural unit capable of replicating itself. As such, a cell is considered the basic unit of life. The boundary of a cell is the **plasma membrane** (see Chapter 2), while the **cytoskeleton** provides structural support (Figure 1.1). Cells of the human body have a characteristic nuclear compartment, which contains the genetic material, and are thus classified as **eukaryotic** cells as opposed to **prokaryotic** bacterial cells, which do not contain a nucleus. Cellular structures with specific functions, **organelles**, are discussed in Chapter 3.

Tissues

There are more than 200 different types of cells in the human body. These types are highly specialised (**differentiated**) to carry out specific functions. Groups of cells carrying out a similar function and forming a structure are called **tissue**. Different tissues combine to form organs. There are four main types of tissue.

• **Epithelial** tissue is found at the boundaries of structures in the body. The basal (**basolateral**) side faces the underlying tissue, which provides nutrients and support, while the **apical** side is exposed to a different environment. For instance, the apical side of intestinal epithelium faces the inside of the intestine and is exposed to constituents from (digested) food; the apical side of stomach epithelium is exposed to the acidic environment inside the stomach; lung and skin are exposed to air. Secreting glands are also formed by epithelial tissue. There are distinct types of epithelial structures:
  – **stratified** epithelium: formed by layers of epithelial cells;
  – **simple** epithelium: formed by a single layer of cells;
  – **squamous** epithelium: formed by cells which are wider than tall;
  – **columnar** epithelium: formed by cells which are taller than wide.
• Stratified squamous epithelium can be **keratinised**, forming a hard and dry layer as found in the skin, nails and hair, or **non-keratinised**, which is found in soft tissue such as the inside of the mouth. An example of simple columnar epithelium is the lining of the stomach.
• **Connective** tissue provides structure and rigidity. It is characterised by a large space between cells, which is filled with fibrous material that is part of the **extracellular matrix**. **Fibroblasts** are the most common cell type in connective tissue. **Adipose** tissue stores energy in the form of fat, but is also important for the protection and insulation of organs and is now recognised as having an endocrine role. Other types of connective tissue include blood, cartilage and bone.
• **Muscle** cells (**myocytes**) are characterised by their ability to contract when they receive appropriate signals. There are three different types of muscle tissue: skeletal muscle is directly attached to bones; cardiac muscle is the muscle of the heart; smooth muscle lines blood vessels and organs of the body.
• **Nerve cells** can sense stimuli and transfer electrical signals to chemical signals, which are sensed by surrounding cells. Nerve cells can have long extensions that are involved in the sensing and transmittance of signals (Chapters 18 and 19).

Cell division

The mass and volume of tissues can increase by **cell growth**, the increase of cell mass and volume by taking up nutrients and synthesising new cell structures, and **cell proliferation**, the increase of cell numbers by cell division. There are two types of cell division.
• **Mitosis**, in which each daughter cell acquires the same amount of genetic material as the parental cell.
• **Meiosis**, in which each daughter cell acquires half the amount of genetic material of the parental cell, only occurs in specialised germ tissue.

When cells receive signals to divide they progress through the cell cycle (Figure 1.2). In adult tissue, most cells reside in the **interphase**. The interphase can be further divided into three phases. In the **G1 phase** (first gap phase), cells prepare for the duplication of the genetic material. When cells start duplicating their DNA, they progress through the **S phase** (synthesis phase). Following the **G2 phase** (second gap), cells undergo mitosis (**M phase**). Compared with the interphase, the mitotic phase is very short. Mitosis (Figure 1.3) can be separated into the following distinct stages.
• **Prophase**: the DNA/chromatin condenses and the characteristic chromosomes become visible. The **mitotic spindle** starts to form outside the nucleus.
• In the **late prophase/pro-metaphase**, the nuclear membrane starts to degrade and the mitotic spindle body moves into the nuclear region. Regions in the chromosomes, **centrosomes**, are attached to the mitotic spindle.
• **Metaphase**: the chromosomes are aligned in the centre plane between the spindle poles.
• **Anaphase**: the chromatids of the sister chromosomes start to separate while the spindle poles move further apart.
• **Telophase**: the chromatids reach the spindle poles, which starts to disappear. The chromatids decondense and a nuclear membrane is formed around the chromatids.
During mitosis, the division of the cytoplasm between the two daughter cells is called **cytokinesis**. Cytokinesis starts during prophase, but is not completed until after the end of telophase when the two daughter cells have formed.

Stem cells

Stem cells are undifferentiated cells with two characteristics.
• **Self-renewal**: the ability to repeatedly divide while maintaining an undifferentiated state. Stem cells undergo **asymmetric cell division**: one of the daughter cells retains stem cell characteristics while the other daughter cell undergoes differentiation.
• The ability to differentiate into specialised cell types.
Stem cells are **pluripotent** if they retain the ability to differentiate into all cell types and tissues. For example, **embryonic stem cells** are pluripotent stem cells derived from early-stage embryos. **Adult stem cells** are not pluripotent, but are more specialised and can only form one or several tissues. For example, adult haematological stem cells isolated from the bone marrow can differentiate into the various cell types found in blood. Other adult stem cells are more specialised, e.g. skin stem cells found in the epidermis, which can only differentiate into skin cells. **Induced pluripotent** stem cells are derived from differentiated tissue that is genetically reprogrammed to return to their undifferentiated state.

② Organisation of cell membranes

Sebastiaan Winkler

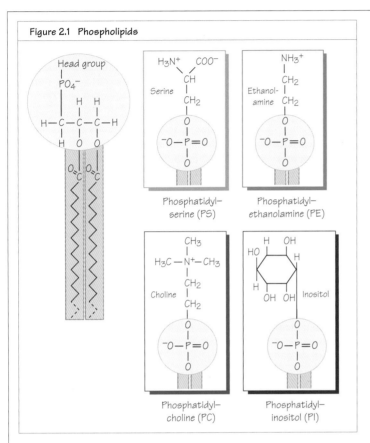

Figure 2.1 Phospholipids

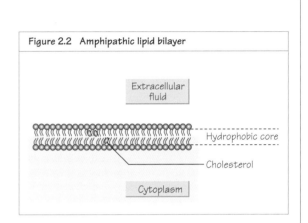

Figure 2.2 Amphipathic lipid bilayer

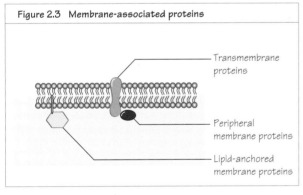

Figure 2.3 Membrane-associated proteins

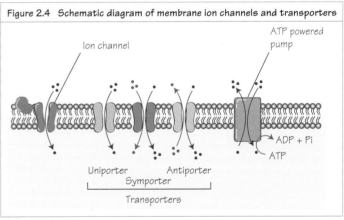

Figure 2.4 Schematic diagram of membrane ion channels and transporters

Medical Sciences at a Glance, First Edition. Edited by Michael D Randall. © 2014 John Wiley & Sons, Ltd. Published 2014 by John Wiley & Sons, Ltd.

Cell membranes

Cell membranes are large cellular structures that constitute the boundary of a cell or a cell organelle. In contrast to proteins or nucleic acids, membranes are not made up of polymers, but a large number of diverse, relatively small molecules that form non-covalent interactions.

Phospholipids

The principal building blocks of cell membranes are a variety of compounds that are collectively known as **phospholipids**. Phospholipids are composed of three different parts: the backbone, a **polar head group** and a **fatty acid chain** (Figure 2.1). Different combinations of backbone, head groups and fatty acids result in a wide variety of phospholipids. In mammalian cells, glycerol is the backbone of the most abundant class of phospholipids, termed **phosphoglycerides**, although **sphingolipids** are also abundant. Backbone moieties have three hydroxyl groups, which are available for the conjugation of the polar head group, and two fatty acid chains. The polar head group is linked to the backbone via a phosphoester bond. In addition, two fatty acids are conjugated to the remaining hydroxyl groups of the backbone. The fatty acids can be broadly divided into two groups. The **saturated fatty acids** do not contain double bonds and always contains an even number of carbon atoms (usually 16–20). Due to the free rotation of the single carbon–carbon bonds, these lipid chains can adopt linear configurations. By contrast, the **unsaturated fatty acids** contain one or more double bonds. When the groups that lie on either side of the double bond are on opposite sides of the double bond (trans configuration) they are called **trans fatty acids** (Chapter 5). Like unsaturated fatty acids, trans fatty acids can adopt (near) linear configurations. However, when the groups next to the double bond are on the same side of the double bond (cis configuration) the fatty acids adopt very different shapes. The **cis fatty acids** have characteristic bends and cannot adopt linear configurations (Chapter 5).

A characteristic feature of the phospholipids is that they are **amphipathic**: they are both **hydrophilic** (due to the polar head group) and **lipophilic** (due to their fatty acid chain).

The lipid bilayer

Due to their amphipathic nature, phospholipids spontaneously organise in such a way that they form two sheets, with the polar head groups facing the aqueous exterior and the fatty acid chains forming a hydrophobic core (Figure 2.2). This structure is termed the **lipid bilayer**. Phospholipids can diffuse freely in the lipid bilayer, which behaves as a two-dimensional fluid. The lipid bilayer is **asymmetrical**, because phospholipids on one side of the bilayer do not freely flip to the other side. Thus, on the outside of cell membranes, phospholipids with PC head groups are enriched, while the cytoplasmic side is enriched with PE and PS lipids. The composition of the lipid bilayer is not homogeneous. The properties of cell membranes is influenced by the properties of the locally enriched phospholipids, e.g. the length of fatty acid chains influences the thickness of the lipid bilayer, and the presence of phospholipids containing cis fatty acids reduces the density of phospholipids in the lipid bilayer.

Sterols are another class of lipid components. **Cholesterol** is the most abundant sterol found in cell membranes (Chapter 5). Cholesterol impacts on the fluidity of the membrane: low concentrations of cholesterol can increase fluidity, whereas high concentrations of cholesterol can have the opposite effect.

Membrane proteins

Proteins are a third group of molecules found in cell membranes. There are three classes of membrane proteins (Figure 2.3).

- **Transmembrane proteins**: these traverse the lipid bilayer. In human cells, most integral membrane proteins contain a number of membrane-spanning **alpha helices**. In addition, the proteins may have extracellular and cytosolic domains. Examples of transmembrane proteins are **receptors**, proteins that mediate cell-cell interactions and transport proteins.
- **Lipid-anchored membrane proteins**: these contain lipid modifications, such as prenyl groups or fatty acids, that function as membrane anchors. Examples are proteins that mediate signals received by receptor proteins.
- **Peripheral (accessory) membrane proteins**: these proteins are not anchored in the membrane, but interact strongly with transmembrane proteins or proteins anchored in the lipid bilayer. As a consequence, these proteins do not diffuse freely in the cytoplasm. Similar to lipid-anchored membrane proteins, examples include proteins that mediate receptor signalling.

Membrane proteins do not diffuse freely in the lipid bilayer. Additional polar and non-polar interactions with phospholipids and cholesterol, as well as other membrane proteins, result in order around membrane proteins. These areas, which are more structured and packed compared with the lipid bilayer, are termed **lipid rafts**. Lipid rafts can diffuse freely in the lipid bilayer.

Transport across membranes

The lipid bilayer is a **semi-permeable** barrier that prevents the free diffusion of molecules. Gases, such as O_2, N_2 and CO_2, as well as small polar molecules, can diffuse through the membrane. In contrast, the lipid bilayer is impermeable to large polar molecules or charged molecules. Three types of membrane proteins facilitate and control the transport of ions and small molecules, including sugars and amino acids, across cell membranes (Figure 2.4).

- **Ion channels** facilitate the transport of small ions. The movement of ions is driven by a differential concentration on either side of the membrane.
- **Transporters** allow the transport of specific molecules and can be divided into three groups:
  - **uniporter**: facilitates the transport of specific molecules down its concentration gradient, for example the GLUT1 glucose transporter;
  - **symporter**: facilitates the transport of a specific molecules *against* its concentration gradient driven by the co-transport of one or more ions down their concentration gradient;
  - **antiporter**: facilitates the transport of a specific molecules *against* its concentration gradient driven by the movement in the opposite direction of one or more ions down their concentration gradient.
- **ATP-powered pumps** allow the transport of ions or specific small molecules against their electrochemical gradient by using energy released by the hydrolysis of ATP. Examples are the $3Na^+/2K^+$ ion pump (Chapter 18) and the H^+/K^+ gastric proton pump (Chapter 41).

3 Cell organelles

Sebastiaan Winkler

Figure 3.1 Schematic representation of the location of cellular organelles and junction complexes in a eukaryotic cell

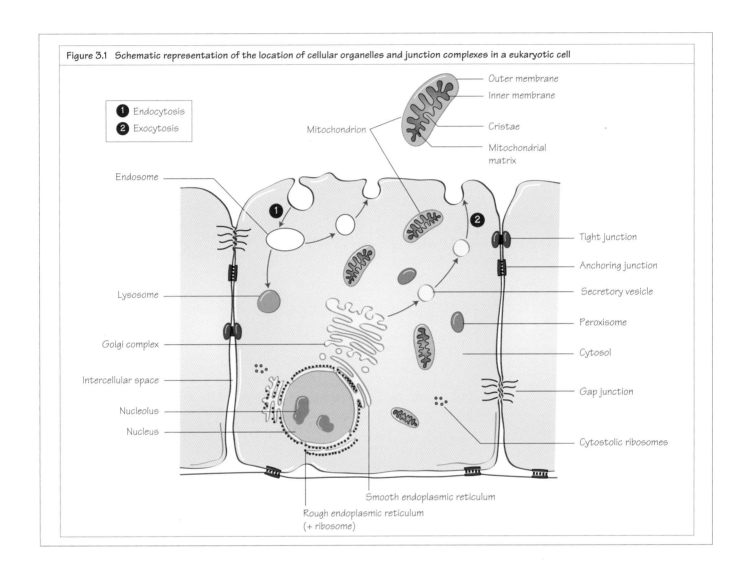

Medical Sciences at a Glance, First Edition. Edited by Michael D Randall. © 2014 John Wiley & Sons, Ltd. Published 2014 by John Wiley & Sons, Ltd.

Organelles (Figure 3.1) are most commonly defined as specialised structures within a cell that are enclosed by a membrane. The most prominent organelle of eukaryotic cells is the **nucleus**, which stores the maternally and paternally inherited **DNA**. The DNA in the nucleus is bound to proteins (**histones**) to form **chromatin** fibres, which help package the DNA into the nucleus. The DNA is used as a template for **messenger RNA** in a process called **transcription** (Chapter 16). The nucleus is separated from the **cytoplasm** by the **nuclear envelope**, a double membrane structure. Transport of proteins and nucleic acids (ribonucleic acid, **RNA**) between the nucleus and the cytoplasm is facilitated by the **nuclear pore complex**. The **nucleoskeleton** provides structure and rigidity to the nuclear compartment. One or several clearly distinct regions (**nucleoli**) are visible within the nucleus using light microscopy. The nucleoli are sites of ribosomal RNA production.

Mitochondria are the major sites of O_2 consumption. The majority of **ATP** (adenosine triphosphate), a central source of energy in cells, is produced by mitochondria. The outer membrane is smooth, while the inner membrane forms characteristic folds (**cristae**). While the initial stage of glycolysis, in which glucose is converted into pyruvate, takes place in the cytosol, mitochondrial enzymes associated with the cristae and present in the **mitochondrial matrix** transfer energy present in pyruvate and fats to ATP via the **tricarboxylic acid (TCA) cycle** and the **electron transport chain** (Chapter 10). Mitochondria contain specialised enzymes encoded by **mitochondrial DNA**, which resides in the mitochondrial matrix. Because mitochondria in the embryo are derived from the egg cell, mitochondrial DNA is **maternally inherited**.

The **endoplasmic reticulum (ER)** is membrane-containing structure surrounding the nucleus and attached to the nuclear envelope. Based on its appearance on electron micrographs, the endoplasmic reticulum is divided into the **smooth endoplasmic reticulum** and **rough endoplasmic reticulum**. The smooth endoplasmic reticulum is associated with phospholipid biosynthesis, storage of Ca^{2+} ions and other processes. The **rough endoplasmic reticulum** is associated with many **ribosomes**. Whereas **ribosomes** present in the cytosol produce soluble proteins that will function in the cytosol, ribosomes associated with the RER are involved in the synthesis of three classes of proteins.

• **Membrane proteins**, which contain hydrophobic regions and are inserted into the ER membrane during translation.

• Soluble proteins that contain a sorting signal resulting in the release of the protein into the **lumen** of the ER. These proteins will eventually be secreted into the extracellular space (**secretory proteins**).

• Proteins of other organelles.

Many proteins undergo **post-translational modifications** in the lumen of the ER. Branched sugar chains are attached to serine and asparagine residues (**glycosylation**). The formation of the covalent bond between two cysteine residues (**disulfide bond**) also occurs in the lumen of the ER.

Proteins synthesised by the RER are transported in **transport vesicles** to the **Golgi complex**, a network of membrane-enclosed compartments. Both proteins inserted in the ER membrane as well as proteins present in the lumen of the ER are transported in this manner to the **cis-Golgi** network. The proteins in the Golgi continue to be transported in membrane-enclosed vesicles to the **trans-Golgi** network. At least two processes are carried out in the Golgi network.

• **Glycosylation** initiated in the ER is modified and completed in the Golgi complex, where both addition and removal of sugar moieties take place.

• **Protein sorting**: membrane and soluble proteins are sorted into membrane-enclosed vesicles. During **exocytosis**, these vesicles will travel from the trans-Golgi network and fuse with the plasma membrane, resulting in the release of secretory proteins and the delivery of trans-membrane proteins to the plasma membrane. Vesicles with specific signals will not travel to the plasma membrane, but target specific organelles. The signals required for sorting to specific organelles may be sugar moieties (lysosome) or short amino acid sequences (peroxisome).

Endosomes are formed from **endocytic vesicles**, which are pinched off from the plasma membrane facilitating transport from the plasma membrane into the cell (**endocytosis**). Often, membrane receptors bound to their ligands are involved. The lumen of endosomes gradually becomes more acidic and the contents of endosomes are finally delivered to lysosomes.

The **lysosome** is a membrane-enclosed organelle specialised in the degradation and recycling of proteins, lipids, polysaccharides and nucleic acids. Many lysosomal enzymes catalyse hydrolysis reactions. The products of these reactions, such as simple sugars and amino acids, are re-used in the cytosol.

Peroxisomes are enclosed by membranes and consume significant amounts of O_2, which is used to form hydrogen peroxide (H_2O_2). The enzyme catalase uses H_2O_2 for oxidative degradation of diverse substrates, including large fatty acids and ethanol. Peroxisomes are also important for the synthesis of the main phospholipid components of myelin. This role of peroxisomes is especially relevant for the function of nerve cells.

The system containing the numerous vesicles involved in transport between the ER, Golgi, endosomes, lysosomes and peroxisomes is collectively referred to as the **membrane trafficking network**.

In addition, there are a number of structures that are not enclosed by membranes, but which have clearly identified roles. These structures are sometimes classified as non-membrane organelles.

• The **cytoskeleton**: structural support is provided by a network of filaments. This results in a shape characteristic for a specific cell type. The main kinds of filaments are:

   – **actin filaments** play a particularly important role in cellular movement (**motility**);

   – **microtubules** are formed by tubulin and are important for cell movement as well as the movement of vesicles inside the cell;

   – **intermediate filaments** are made from a collection of different proteins. These filaments are important for the basic shape of cells and provide mechanical strength.

• **Cell junctions** are involved in the organisation of cells in tissues. The main types are:

   – **desmosomes**, which are multi-protein complexes that join cells (e.g. connect epithelial cells) and lead to integrity. Hemidesmosomes adhere the basal membranes of epithelial cells to the basement membrane;

   – **tight junctions**, which prevent passage of small molecules and fluid between cells;

   – **anchoring junctions**, which are linked to cytoskeletal structures (mostly intermediate filaments) and provide rigidity in a group of cells;

   – **gap junctions**, which provide channels between cells thereby facilitating movement of small molecules between neighbouring cells.

4 Protein biochemistry

Fergus Doherty

Figure 4.1 The hierachy of protein structure

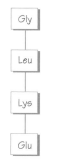 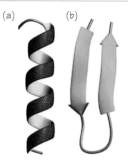 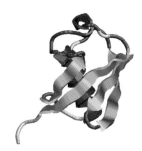 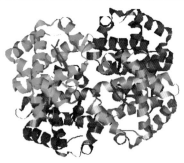

Primary structure
The linear sequence of amino acids joined by peptide bonds

Secondary structure
Regions of regular polypeptide structure: α-helix (a), β-sheet (b) and β-turn

Tertiary structure
How secondary structure is arranged in space. Soluble, globular proteins generally hide hydrophobic residues in the interior

Quaternary structure
This is only found in proteins of more than one polypeptide chain (subunit) and describes how these are arranged

---

Figure 4.2 Protein secondary structure

(a) The right-handed α-helix with 3.6 residues per turn and an H-bond between every fourth residue. Side chains protrude from the helix
(b) A type 1 β-turn, there are two types of these turns

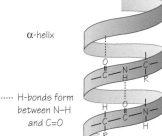 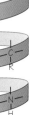 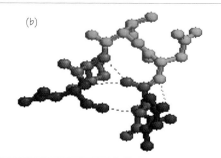

α-helix

┈┈┈┈ H-bonds form between N–H and C=O

Figure 4.3 A slice through the soluble, globular protein, haemoglobin

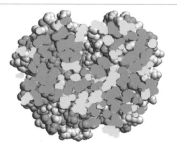

Shows hydrophobic amino acids (green) largely in the interior of the protein away from the aqueous environment

Figure 4.4 Membrane proteins that span the lipid bilayer

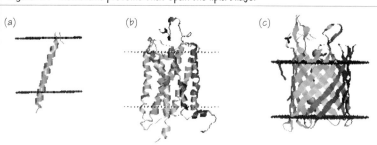

Membrane spanning regions may be single (a) or many (b) α-helices of about 20 residues. Some membrane proteins (e.g. the porins) consist of 'barrel' structures composed of β-strands (c)

 Medical Sciences at a Glance, First Edition. Edited by Michael D Randall. © 2014 John Wiley & Sons, Ltd. Published 2014 by John Wiley & Sons, Ltd.

Proteins are polymers of the 20 common L-amino acids and constitute about 16% of the body weight of the average adult. Proteins have a wide range of functions in the human body, including as enzymes, motors, transporters, receptors and other signalling factors; components of the immune system; as well as structural components of cells and the extracellular matrix. Proteins do not serve as a primary energy store, although during starvation protein is degraded, especially in skeletal muscle, to release amino acids, the carbon skeletons of which can be used for **gluconeogenesis** in the liver (Chapter 12).

Structure

L-amino acids are combined in proteins by the formation of a bond between the carbon atom of the α-carboxyl group of one amino acid and the nitrogen of the α-amino group of the next. This is the **peptide bond**. A small number of amino acids (residues) joined in this way are called a peptide, a larger number a polypeptide. The electrons of the double bond of the carbonyl group are delocalised, giving the C–N peptide bond a partial double bond character, which restricts rotation about this bond and influences how polypeptides fold in space. The sequence of amino acids joined by peptides in a polypeptide, the primary sequence or structure, is determined by the sequence of the gene coding for that polypeptide, and in turn determines how the polypeptide folds in three-dimensional space (Figure 4.1). **Primary sequence** is always written from the free amino terminus on the left to the free carboxyl terminus on the right, which is the direction of protein synthesis. The structure of polypeptides exhibits a hierarchy, with the primary structure being the first level.

The next level of polypeptide or protein structure is the **secondary structure** (Figure 4.2), which describes some of the folding of the polypeptide in 3D space. Regions of polypeptides can adopt three types of secondary structure determined by the amino acid sequence. The **α-helix** (Figure 4.2a) has a right-handed thread with 3.6 amino acids per turn and is stabilised by hydrogen bonds between every fourth amino acid formed by the carbonyl and NH groups of peptide bonds. Amino acid side chains point out from the helix. **β-strands** are pleated structures that hydrogen bond together to **form β-sheets** with amino acids side chains positioned above or below the plane of the sheet, while the strands can run in the same (parallel) or opposite (anti-parallel) directions. Secondary structure also includes **β-turns** (Figure 4.2b), consisting of about 4–7 amino acids, which introduce a turn into the backbone of the polypeptide (e.g. between two anti-parallel β-strands). Polypeptides can also include regions lacking in the clearly defined secondary structures described, such as various loops, random coils, or disordered regions. An example of a polypeptide containing mostly α-helix is **myoglobin**, while some **membrane channel proteins** contain extensive β-sheets that form a barrel-like structure.

Tertiary structure describes how secondary structures are arranged in space with respect to each other and the overall 'fold' of the polypeptide, and is stabilised mainly by hydrophobic interactions. Soluble proteins (Figure 4.3) generally fold to hide hydrophobic amino acid side chains in the interior away from water, while polypeptides resident in membranes (Figure 4.4) tend to have hydrophobic amino acids in the membrane-spanning regions, with side chains facing the interior of the membrane. Many polypeptides fold to create distinct domains, which are associated with a particular function, for example binding ATP, and similar domains can be found in different polypeptides with this function. The final level of protein structure is **quaternary** and describes how many polypeptide chains are grouped together in the functional protein, held together largely by non-covalent interactions, although inter-chain disulfide bonds between cysteine residues can play a role. Individual polypeptides in proteins are called subunits; although many proteins will have only one subunit many have two, four, or more.

Life cycle

Proteins are synthesised (**translated**) from amino acids on ribosomes using the information transcribed from DNA on to mRNA (Chapters 15 and 16). Following translation, covalent modification may occur (proteolytic processing, formation of disulfide bonds, or modification of some amino acid side chains, e.g. hydroxylation of proline in collagen). Some proteins will be secreted from the cell (e.g. extracellular matrix proteins). Intracellular proteins are subjected to degradation to amino acids at various rates, depending on the protein, so different proteins have different half-lives. Degradation is carried out by the **ubiquitin-proteasome system**, which regulates the concentration of many regulatory proteins, or in lysosomes. Proteins that have become damaged or fail to fold correctly are rapidly degraded to prevent their accumulation. The accumulation of undegraded 'abnormal' proteins can be lead to disease, for example prion proteins in the transmissible encephalopathies (BSE in cows, CJD in humans) and amyloid in Alzheimer's disease.

5 Lipid biochemistry

Jane Arnold

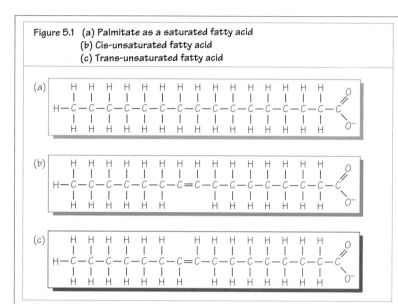

Figure 5.1 (a) Palmitate as a saturated fatty acid
(b) Cis-unsaturated fatty acid
(c) Trans-unsaturated fatty acid

Figure 5.2 Triacylglycerol (TAG)

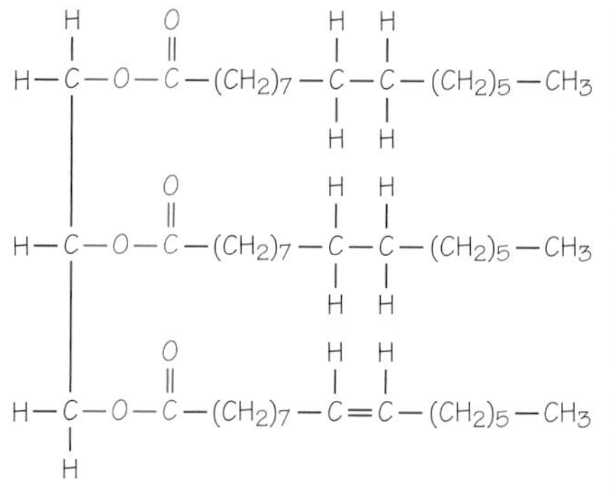

Figure 5.3 Cholesterol and an esterified cholesterol with RO-added

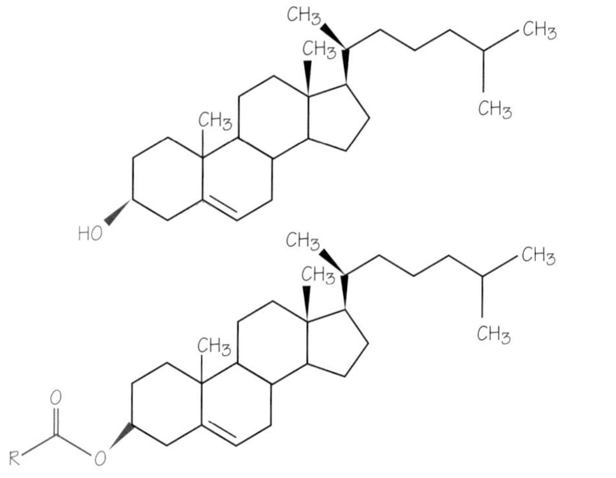

Table 5.1 Different fatty acids

Saturated		
Fatty acid	Formula	symbol
Palmitate	$CH_3(CH_2)_{14}COO^-$	16:0
Stearate	$CH_3(CH_2)_{16}COO^-$	18:0
Arachidate	$CH_3(CH_2)_{18}COO^-$	20:0
Unsaturated		
Fatty acid	Formula	
Palmitoleate	$CH_3(CH_2)_5CH=CH(CH_2)_7COO^-$	16:1
Oleate	$CH_3(CH_2)_7CH=CH(CH_2)_7COO^-$	18:1
Linoleate	$CH_3(CH_2)_4CH=CHCH_2CH=CH(CH_2)_7COO^-$	18:2
Linolenate	$CH_3CH_2CH=CHCH_2CH=CHCH_2CH=CH(CH_2)_7COO^-$	18:3
Arachidonate	$CH_3(CH_2)_4(CH=CHCH_2)_4(CH_2)_2COO^-$	20:4

Lipids are defined as organic molecules that share the property of being water insoluble but are highly soluble in organic solvents. They are structurally diverse and have many different functions, including:

- components of cell membranes (Chapter 2)
- fuel molecules (Chapter 11)
- signalling molecules.

Some of the most important biological lipids include fatty acids, triglycerides and cholesterol.

Fatty acids
Structure
Fatty acids are composed of a long hydrocarbon chain with a terminal carboxylic acid. They normally contain between 14 and 24

 Medical Sciences at a Glance, First Edition. Edited by Michael D Randall. © 2014 John Wiley & Sons, Ltd. Published 2014 by John Wiley & Sons, Ltd.

carbon atoms and have the general formula $CH_3(CH_2)_nCOOH$ (Figure 5.1a). They exist in a **saturated** (no double bonds in hydrocarbon chain), **monounsaturated** (one double bond) and **polyunsaturated** (two or more double bonds) form. Most of the double bonds in naturally occurring unsaturated fatty acids exist in a **cis configuration** (same side of the double bond) (Figure 5.1b). A **trans configuration** (opposite sides of the double bond) can also occur (Figure 5.1c). The addition of the double bond causes a bend or kink in the hydrocarbon chain, which impacts on the packing of these molecules and causes a reduction in the melting point of the molecule. For example, stearate, an 18C saturated fatty acid has a melting point of 69°C, while oleate, a monosaturated 18C fatty acid, has a melting point of 13°C. This is important when considering the role of fatty acids in cell membrane structure (Chapter 2). The chain length also affects the melting point; the longer the chain length, the higher the melting point.

Nomenclature
The naming of fatty acids is slightly confusing, as while systematic names exist, naturally occurring fatty acids are generally called by their common names. A numbering system is also used, whereby the left-hand number depicts the number of carbon atoms and the right hand number reflects the number of double bonds in the hydrocarbon chain. Table 5.1 lists some of the naturally occurring common fatty acids. Normally the name of the fatty acid ends in '**oic acid**', but most fatty acids are ionised at physiological pH (COO^- instead of $COOH$) and end in '**ate**'. For example, palmitic acid ($CH_3(CH_2)_{14}COOH$) will occur physiologically as palmitate ($CH_3(CH_2)_{14}COO^-$).

Sources
Most fatty acids are ingested in the diet in the form of triglycerides. However, there is a *de novo* pathway of fatty acid synthesis in the liver where **acetyl coenzyme A** (**acetylCoA**) is used as the building block to produce long-chain fatty acids. Two important fatty acids, however, cannot be synthesised in the body and must be taken in the diet. These are linoleate and linolenate (Table 5.1), which are collectively called the omega fatty acids. Linoleate (omega 6) is a precursor to a family of signalling molecules known as prostaglandins, while linolenate (omega 3) is an important constituent of some specialised membranes (e.g retinal cell membranes).

The majority of trans fatty acids are produced as a product of hydrogenation of vegetable oils (e.g. in margarine production). Ingestion of trans fatty acids is of concern as they have been linked to an increased risk of coronary heart disease.

Functions
Component of cell membranes – fatty acids and modified forms of fatty acids are an important component of the lipid bilayer of membranes (Chapter 2).

In metabolism – fatty acids can either be obtained from the diet or can be synthesised from AcCoA. These can then be stored as triglycerides in adipose tissue (see below). The energy stored in these molecules can then be released by beta oxidation to produce large quantities of ATP (see Chapter 11).

In cell signalling – fatty acids are used in a number of ways in cell signalling.
• Linoleate is metabolised to arachidonic acid, which is an important precursor in prostaglandin synthesis.

• Some derivatives of fatty acids (e.g inositol phosphate) are important in signal transduction pathways.
• Some fatty acids can be attached to proteins (post-translational modification) to activate specific proteins.

Triglycerides
Triglycerides are a major fuel source for the body and are commonly referred to as fats (if solid at room temperature) or oils (if liquid at room temperature). **Triacylglycerol** (TAG) contains a glycerol backbone to which three fatty acids chains are attached by an ester linkage. The three fatty acids can be identical (simple TAG) or different (mixed TAG) (see Figure 5.2). As both the chain length and level of saturation affect the melting point of the fatty acid, the composition of the fatty acids in the TAG will determine whether the TAG is a fat (longer chain lengths and/or saturated C-bonds, e.g. lard) or an oil (shorter chain lengths and/or mono- or polyunsaturated, e.g. one of the major TAGS of olive oil contains two oleic and one palmitic acid).

TAGS can be obtained through the diet or made from de *novo* fatty acids and will be stored in the cytoplasm of adipose cells. As these molecules are hydrophobic, they contain very little water and so are an efficient way of storing energy. They can be mobilised to break down and produce ATP under the appropriate hormonal signals (see Chapter 10).

Cholesterol
Despite elevated plasma cholesterol being linked to increased risk of coronary heart disease, cholesterol performs some essential functions in the body.

Structure
Cholesterol is structurally very different to the other lipids already discussed. It is a 27-carbon molecule containing four fused hydrocarbon rings. A branched eight-carbon chain is attached to the C17 of the D ring (Figure 5.3). Cholesterol is the major sterol in animal cells.

Cholesterol also exists in an esterified form where the OH at C3 is esterified with a long-chain fatty acid. This makes the cholesterol molecule even more hydrophobic.

Sources
Cholesterol can be taken up from the diet but there is an active *de novo* synthesis pathway in the liver.

Lipoproteins and cholesterol transport
• **Low-density lipoprotein** (**LDL**) ('bad cholesterol') is cholesterol rich and is taken up by the liver and tissues, and this involves the LDL receptor. LDL provides cholesterol for cell membranes, steroid synthesis and the production of bile acids. Its uptake into arterial walls is associated with atherogenesis.
• **High-density lipoprotein** (**HDL**) ('good cholesterol') takes up cholesterol from cellular breakdown and prevents its deposition.

Functions
• Component of cell membranes (Chapter 2).
• Precursor to bile acids.
• Precursor to steroid hormones.
• Precursor to vitamin D.

6 Carbohydrate biochemistry

Fergus Doherty

Figure 6.1 Simple carbohydrates

CHO
H — C — OH
CH₂OH

D-glyceraldehyde

CHO
HO — C — H
CH₂OH

L-glyceraldehyde

CH₂OH
C = O
CH₂OH

Dihydroxyacetone

The simplest carbohydrates are the trioses glyceraldehyde (an aldose) and dihydroxyacetone (a ketose). Glyceraldehyde has an asymmetric carbon at position two, which means there are two optically active mirror images molecules possible (enantiomers), D- and L-glyceraldehyde

---

Figure 6.2 Glucose

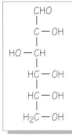

D-glucose

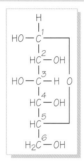

D-glucopyranose

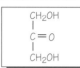

α D-glucopyranose

Glucose, the most abundant carbohydrate in humans, is a six-carbon (hexose) monosaccharide with an aldehyde group (aldose) at carbon atom 1. Carbon 4 is asymmetric so there are two enantiomers of glucose, D- and L-glucose. D-glucose is the metabolically active enantiomer in humans. Glucose readily forms six-membered oxygen-containing ring structures (a pyranose) in solution. This produces an anomeric carbon at position 1, so two forms α and β exist. α D-glucopyranose is the building block for glycogen

---

Figure 6.3 Glycogen

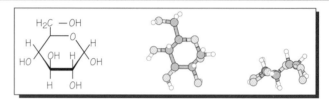

Branching enzyme

α1-6 glycosidic links at branch points

α1-4 glycosidic links in linear chain

Glycogenin

UDP

Glycogen synthase

UDP-glucose

Hexokinase/glucokinase

UTP + glucose-1-phosphate ◄—— Glucose-6-phosphate ◄—— Glucose

Glycogen is the storage form of glucose in animals and is a highly branched polymer of α-D-glucopyranose units joined by α1-4 glycosidic bonds to form linear chains, with α1-6 glycosidic bonds forming branch points every 5–8 glucose units. Glycogen is built up on a glycogen fragment ('seed') or on the protein glycogenin by the enzyme glycogen synthase, which transfers glucose from UDP-glucose to the end of a glycogen chain to form the α1-4 glycosidic bond. Branching enzyme transfers a string of glucose units from the end of a chain to an internal glucose to form the α1-6 branch point

---

Carbohydrates (CHOs) are probably the most abundant organic molecules in living organisms and serve a variety of roles. Carbohydrates provide about 55% of dietary calories for a healthy human, so they are our major fuel. Humans store some carbohydrate, in the form of glycogen, in tissues such as skeletal muscle and liver. Carbohydrates are also found as structural components of membranes, mostly attached to membrane proteins, and the carbohydrates on these proteins can have a role in cell-to-cell signalling.

Carbohydrate structure

As their name implies, carbohydrates are molecules made up of 'hydrated carbon', containing many hydroxyl groups, plus an aldehyde or a keto group, and can be represented by the simple empirical formula CH_2O_n. Simple carbohydrates (or **monosaccharides**) consist of a single carbohydrate unit, the smallest of which is glyceraldehyde. This has three carbons and is therefore classed as a triose. Typically, carbohydrates in humans range from three to nine (**nonose**) carbon atoms, with many abundant and important carbohydrates containing six carbons (**hexoses**). Monosaccharides with an aldehyde group are classed as aldoses (e.g. glyceraldehyde), while those with keto groups are ketoses (e.g. dihydroxyacetone).

Glyceraldehyde (Figure 6.1) has an asymmetric carbon atom at position 2 (the four groups attached to it are different) and therefore can exist in two conformations that are mirror images of each other (**enantiomers**). These are known as the D and L forms. The majority of carbohydrates in humans are in the **D-form**. Enzymes are stereospecific and will only act on the correct enantiomer of a carbohydrate.

Glucose

The most abundant carbohydrate in the human body is glucose, with the empirical formula $C_6H_{12}O_6$, which can be represented as a linear chain of carbon atoms with an aldehyde group at one end (designated carbon atom 1) and hydroxyl groups attached to the other carbons (Figure 6.2). Other **hexoses** share the same empirical formula as glucose but differ in the arrangement of the various hydroxyl and aldehyde groups and are therefore isomers. Epimers differ in the arrangement of groups around a single carbon, e.g. glucose and mannose. In solution, monosaccharides rapidly cyclise by reaction of the aldehyde (e.g. C6 in an aldohexose) or keto (e.g. C5 in ketohexose) to form ring structures resembling a chair. A pyranose is a six-membered ring and a furanose a five-membered ring. Formation of a ring creates an anomeric carbon (which carried the aldehyde or keto group), and two isomers (diastereomers) are possible, α and β. Glucose exists in both forms in solution, but these rapidly interconvert; however, enzymes are specific for a particular diastereomer. Glucose also exists as enantiomers, but it is the D form that is metabolically active in humans.

Polysaccharides

Monosaccharide units can be joined together to form polymers of various lengths, e.g **disaccharides** such as lactose in milk (galactose and glucose) and sucrose in fruit (glucose and fructose). Larger polymers are called oligosaccharides and very large polymers are called polysaccharides. Monosaccharide units are joined together via **glyco-sidic bonds**, named after the carbon atoms involved and the configuration of the **anomeric carbon**, e.g α1-4 in the polymer of glucose known as glycogen.

Glycogen

Glucose cannot be stored in cells as it is osmotically active, and at high intracellular concentrations would lead to osmotic lysis. The supply of glucose in the diet is intermittent, so to overcome these problems glucose is stored as an insoluble polysaccharide known as glycogen. Glycogen is composed of linear chains of α1-4 linked glucose units with an α1-6 linked branch point every 8–10 glucose units. To this branch is added more α1-4 linked glucose units, creating a very large (molecular weight approximately 10^8 Daltons), highly branched structure.

Skeletal muscle, which comprises a large proportion of the body weight of a human, is approximately 2% by weight glycogen, and liver is about 10% by weight glycogen. Glycogen is found in cytoplasmic granules associated with the enzymes of glycogen metabolism. Synthesis of glycogen occurs when glucose is abundant, after feeding, and starts with glucose-6-phosphate, which is formed when glucose enters the cell and can be converted to glucose-1-phosphate. This is followed by the transfer of the glucose moiety to UTP (a high-energy phosphate compound) to form UDP-glucose, which serves as the donor of glucose for elongation of the glycogen chain by glycogen synthase from a small glycogen 'seed' (Figure 6.3). Alternatively, the glycogen may be built on a protein, **glycogenin**. A separate branching enzyme transfers 5–8 glucosyl residues from the end of the chain to a branch point. The highly branched structure of glycogen allows for its rapid breakdown when glucose is needed (e.g. during fasting or exercise).

Structural carbohydrates

As well as being important fuels, carbohydrates serve as structural components of the body. **Glycosaminoglycans** are long unbranched chains of monosaccharide units, including monosaccharide units with amino groups (e.g. glucosamine or galactosamine). These are often further modified by N-acetylation or sulfation. Glycosaminoglycans associate with small amounts of protein and are found in the extracellular matrix where, with their affinity for water, they form a jelly-like substance. Glycosaminoglycans can also act like lubricants and are known as **mucopolysaccharides**. Inherited deficiencies in the lysosomal enzymes that degrade glycosaminoglycans/mucopolysaccharides result in accumulation of these molecules, leading to skeletal muscle problems and mental retardation.

Many secreted or cell-surface proteins are modified (glycosylated) by the addition of relatively small, branched, heterogeneous carbohydrate chains. Glycosylated proteins at the cell surface can act as important signal molecules between adjacent cells and between cells and the extracellular matrix. Glycosylation of proteins occurs in the endoplasmic reticulum and Golgi apparatus.

Prolonged, high levels of glucose in the circulation, for instance in uncontrolled diabetes, leads to non-enzymatic modification of protein by glucose (glycation). High levels of glycation of blood proteins is a major contributor to diabetic pathology and is associated with increased morbidity.

7 Basic mechanisms of drug action

Michael D Randall

Figure 7.1 A schematic diagram of a G-protein coupled receptor

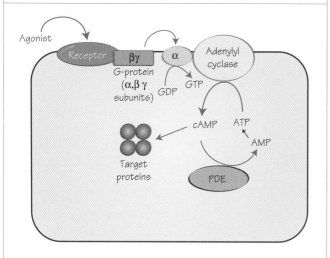

A G-protein coupled receptor (such as the β-adrenoceptor) in which agonist binding leads to the exchange of GDP with GTP on the α-subunit of the G-protein which disassociates from the βγ subunits and activates the adenylyl cyclase, leading to an increase in cAMP. The cAMP interacts with target proteins and is also broken down (and recycled) by the phosphodiesterase (PDE) enzyme

Figure 7.2 A schematic diagram of 3 different receptor-transduction mechanisms

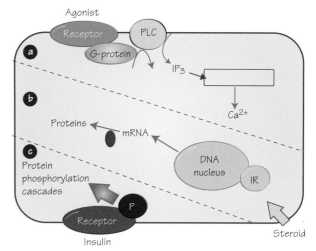

a) G-protein coupling of receptor to phospholipase C activation (PLC), leading to the release of inositol 1,4,5-trisphosphate (IP_3) and calcium release b) an intracellular receptor (IR) which regulates DNA transcription and protein synthesis c) a catalytic receptor (such as the insulin receptor) which undergoes autophosphorylation (P), which initiates an intracellular cascade

Figure 7.3 A ligand-gated ion channel

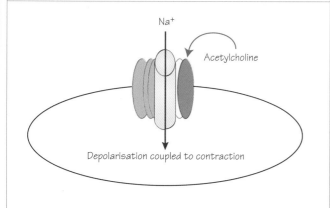

This case shows the nicotinic receptor at the neuromuscular junction, which is opened by acetylcholine binding, which leads to cellular depolarisation

Figure 7.4 A log concentration-response curve

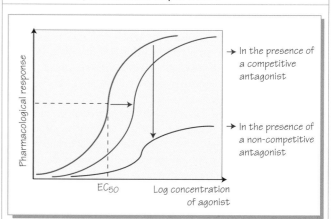

A log concentration-response curve to an agonist, which undergoes a rightward parallel shift in the presence of a competitive antagonist and suppression of the maximal response in the presence of a non-competitive antagonist

Drugs interact with their specific target, which may be coupled to a second messenger and/or effector system, leading to a cellular response.

Pharmacological targets
Receptors
Receptors are proteins that are targets for drug action and are located in the membrane or intracellularly. Many receptor classes have subtypes with different locations and physiological roles. For example, **noradrenaline** acts at:

- α_1-adrenoceptors (e.g. vascular smooth muscle)
- α_2-adrenoceptors (e.g. CNS, presynaptically)
- β_1-adrenoceptors (e.g. heart)
- β_2-adrenoceptors (e.g. airways).

 Medical Sciences at a Glance, First Edition. Edited by Michael D Randall. © 2014 John Wiley & Sons, Ltd. Published 2014 by John Wiley & Sons, Ltd.

Acetylcholine acts at **nicotinic (N)** receptor subtypes at autonomic ganglia and neuromuscular junctions, and in the parasympathetic nervous system at **muscarinic (M)** receptors.

7-transmembrane receptors: many receptors are transmembraneous and are coupled to G-proteins (**G-protein-coupled receptors**, GPCR). For example, β-adrenoceptors following activation are coupled via a **G-protein**, which leads to activation of **adenylyl cyclase**, and the formation of **cAMP**, which leads to a pharmacological response. These receptors are referred to as **metabotropic** (Figure 7.1).

G-proteins: heterotrimeric proteins (α, β and γ subunits), and at rest the α subunits bind GDP, but following coupling to an activated receptor a conformation change results in exchange of GDP for GTP and the α-GTP subunit dissociates. This leads to the α-GTP subunit interacting with coupled enzymes such as adenylyl cyclase and phospholipases (releasing membrane-derived second messengers) or ion channels. There are many subtypes and they can be stimulatory or inhibitory. They undergo a cycle such that activated α-GTP has intrinsic GTPase activity, and when α-GDP is formed the subunit can reassociate with the β and γ subunits (Figure 7.2).

Intracellular or nuclear receptors: located within the cell and are activated by lipophilic molecules such as steroids, which pass through the membrane and enter the cytoplasm. Once the receptor is activated the resulting complex influences DNA transcription, resulting in the production or suppression of mRNA and target proteins, and so their effects are delayed.

Receptors coupled to enzymic activity (catalytic receptors): activation of these receptors results in activation of enzymic activity. For example, an insulin receptor has intrinsic tyrosine kinase activity, such that activation leads to autophosphorylation of tyrosine residues on the receptor, which is coupled to the cellular responses.

Receptors linked to ion channels (ligand-gated ion channels): these are **ionotropic** receptors and activation leads to altered channel function. For example, at neuromuscular junctions (NMJs) acetylcholine activates N receptors and this leads to channel opening (Chapter 22). This is part of the receptor complex and results in ion (predominantly Na^+) influx and depolarisation of the skeletal muscle, which ultimately leads to contraction (Figure 7.3).

Responses linked to ionotropic receptors can be inhibitory. For example, in the central nervous system (CNS) the inhibitory neurotransmitter gamma-amino butyric acid (GABA) acts at the $GABA_A$ receptor and causes activation of its chloride channel. This results in the influx of Cl^- and hyperpolarisation, which reduces cell excitability. Benzodiazepines (e.g. diazepam) modulate the $GABA_A$ receptor and augment the actions of GABA.

Drug–receptor interactions

Agonists: cause receptor activation and a response, which may be either excitatory or inhibitory. A **full agonist** causes a maximum response (Figure 7.4).

Antagonist: binds to a receptor. While not causing a direct response, it prevents the receptor activation by an agonist.

Competitive antagonism: the antagonist binds at the same site as the agonist and so reduces the action of the agonist by competition. The competition may be overcome by increasing the concentration of the agonist (Figure 7.4).

Non-competitive antagonism: the antagonist binds at a site distinct from the agonist and prevents its action. For example, it might block the channel associated with the receptor or interfere with the transduc-

tion mechanism. The effects of the antagonist cannot be overcome by increasing the concentration of the agonist (Figure 7.4).

Irreversible antagonism: often due to the antagonist chemically modifying the receptor so that it prevents the action of an agonist; this cannot be reversed.

Partial agonist: causes a response but cannot elicit a full response even at its highest concentration.

Spare receptors: a full agonist can cause a maximum response without needing to occupy all receptors, and the unoccupied receptors are 'spare'. A partial agonist, even when it occupies all of its receptors, cannot elicit the maximum response and it does not have a receptor reserve of 'spare' receptors.

Inverse agonism: the drug binds to a receptor which itself has intrinsic activity, i.e. in the resting state the receptor is causing a basal response. When the drug binds it reduces the intrinsic activity and may cause a response that is opposite to that caused by an agonist.

Receptor desensitisation: repeated exposure of a receptor to an agonist may lead to a reduction in responses.

Description of drug actions

Pharmacological effects are described as concentration-dependent, with increasing concentrations causing a larger response until a maximum is achieved. The log concentration-response curve is usually sigmoidal (Figure 7.4).

EC_{50}: the agonist concentration that yields the half-maximal response, where the maximum is the maximal response caused by the specific agonist (Figure 7.4). It is a measure of **potency**.

Affinity: this is a measure of how well a drug binds to a receptor. The affinity constant is K_A ($molar^{-1}$), and $1/K_A$ is the dissociation constant, K_d, the concentration at which the drug occupies half of the receptor population. A high-affinity drug will have a low K_d.

Efficacy: how effective an agonist is at causing a response. A full agonist has high efficacy, an antagonist has zero efficacy and a partial agonist is intermediate.

Drugs can also act at other sites, which include the following.

Pumps and transporters: in the cell membrane, these systems are responsible for influx or efflux of ions, transmitters or substrates (e.g. glucose).

• Proton pump inhibitors suppress acid production from parietal cells and are used in peptic ulceration (Chapter 42).

• Inhibitors of neurotransmitter transporters are antidepressants, e.g. serotonin-selective reuptake inhibitors (SSRIs) (Chapter 57).

Ion channels: voltage-operated ion channels may be activated or inhibited by drugs, e.g. Calcium channel blockers (Chapter 32), local anaesthetics (Chapter 19).

Extracellular enzymes: usually specifically inhibited by drugs, either competitively or irreversibly, e.g. ACE inhibitors (Chapter 32).

Intracellular enzymes: usually specifically inhibited by drugs, either competitively or irreversibly, and alter enzymic activity associated with cellular processes such as synthesis or degradation, e.g. statins (Chapter 35).

DNA: anticancer drugs target rapidly dividing cells by interfering with purine/pyrimidine synthesis, chemically modifying or damaging DNA or the spindle fibres involved in mitosis (Chapter 65).

Bacterial cells and organelles: antibiotics target cellular processes such as protein synthesis (e.g. erythromycin) or bacterial structures such as the cell wall (e.g. penicillins).

General principles of cellular metabolism

Fergus Doherty

Figure 8.1 An overview of metabolism. Metabolism can be divided into energy-producing (largely in the form of ATP) catabolism and energy-consuming (largely as ATP) anabolism

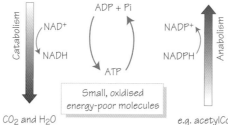

Larger, more reduced energy rich molecules, e.g. complex lipids, carbohydrates, proteins

Stage 1: breakdown of complex molecules to building blocks, e.g. polysaccharides to monosaccharides

Stage 2: conversion of building blocks to to acetate (as acetylCoA) – involves oxidation generating NADH and sometimes $FADH_2$

Stage 3: oxidation of acetate (acetylCoA) to CO_2 and H_2O (citric acid cycle)

Catabolism

NAD^+

NADH

ADP + Pi

ATP

$NADP^+$

NADPH

Anabolism

Anabolism involves the formation of building blocks, e.g. amino acids, fatty acids, in reactions often involving reduction with NADPH, and the incorporation of the building blocks into large molecules, e.g. proteins, complex lipids

CO_2 and H_2O (and NH_3 from amino acids)

Small, oxidised energy-poor molecules

e.g. acetylCoA, pyruvate, amino acids, fatty acids, monosaccharides

Note: the reducing power in NADH, formed from NAD^+ in catabolism, can be transferred to $NADP^+$ to give NADPH used in anabolic pathways. Some of the ATP generated in catabolism can be used to drive anabolic reactions

Figure 8.2 The 'energy currency' of the cell is ATP. Energy released during catabolism is used to drive the synthesis of ATP and this ATP can be hydrolysed to release energy to drive anabolic processes

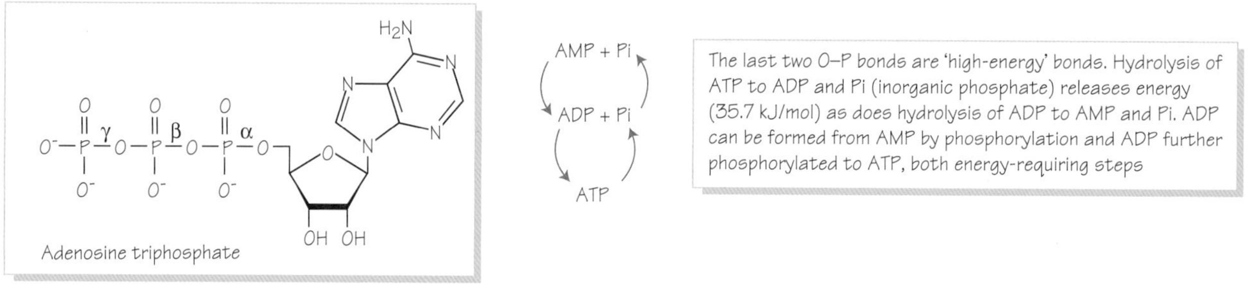

Adenosine triphosphate

AMP + Pi

ADP + Pi

ATP

The last two O–P bonds are 'high-energy' bonds. Hydrolysis of ATP to ADP and Pi (inorganic phosphate) releases energy (35.7 kJ/mol) as does hydrolysis of ADP to AMP and Pi. ADP can be formed from AMP by phosphorylation and ADP further phosphorylated to ATP, both energy-requiring steps

Figure 8.3 Enzymes involved in metabolism are often subject to regulation by covalent modification by the addition or removal of phosphate groups. The resulting change in enzyme activity can alter the rate of the metabolic pathway involved

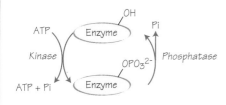

ATP

Kinase

ATP + Pi

Enzyme

OH

Pi

OPO_3^{2-}

Enzyme

Phosphatase

Enzymes that regulate metabolic pathways are often themselves regulated by addition (phosphorylation) or removal (dephosphorylation) of phosphate groups, by kinases and phosphatases respectively, on hydroxyl-containing amino acids (usually serine or threonine). ATP is the phosphate donor. The activity of the modified enzyme may increase or decrease. Phosphorylation/dephosphorylation in turn is often regulated by signalling pathways starting at the cell surface with hormone binding to a receptor. Signalling pathways may contain 'cascades' of different kinases, one phosphorylating many molecules of the next to amplify the original signal and produce a large metabolic effect

 Medical Sciences at a Glance, First Edition. Edited by Michael D Randall. © 2014 John Wiley & Sons, Ltd. Published 2014 by John Wiley & Sons, Ltd.

Metabolism can be described as the sum of the chemical reactions in an organism that produce and maintain its molecular structure, and the chemical reactions that make energy available for those processes. Metabolism can therefore be divided into anabolism and catabolism.

Anabolism

This is the production of complex molecules from more simple precursors, e.g. the synthesis of amino acids from simpler carbon skeletons and a source of amino groups, the synthesis of proteins from amino acids. These are energy-requiring processes where energy is usually consumed in the form of adenosine triphosphate (ATP). The end products are often more reduced than the simple precursors, and so reducing power, in the form of NADPH, is often required (Figure 8.1).

Catabolism

This is the destruction or disassembly of complex molecules, often ultimately leading to the release of chemical energy, which is usually stored in the form of ATP (Figure 8.1). Examples of catabolism include the breakdown of complex lipids (fats) to glycerol and fatty acids, and the oxidation of the resulting fatty acids in mitochondria (β-oxidation) to acetyl coenzyme A, which in turn can be further oxidised to carbon dioxide and water (TCA cycle). Both processes lead to the reduction of NAD$^+$ to NADH, which in turn can be used to drive the formation of ATP.

Energy requirements

It follows from the above that to maintain cells and, in addition, to support cell growth and division, energy is continually required. Note that many key molecules, especially proteins, once made do not last forever but rather are subject to turnover, that is continual synthesis and degradation back to amino acids. This turnover requires energy, therefore simply to maintain the normal complement of cellular proteins, outside of growth, requires energy input. The average daily energy requirement of a sedentary women is just under 2000 kcal/day, rising to 3080 kcal/day for a very active person. This energy is supplied by the oxidation of fuel molecules: carbohydrates, fats (lipids) and proteins, with carbohydrate being the major fuel for most humans. To sustain growth or support pregnancy, the calorific requirement will rise. If the calorific intake does not match the demands made on the organism then mechanisms will be invoked to try and match those demands by utilising stored fuels, such as fat reserves, and even by the breakdown of body proteins and oxidation of the resulting amino acids. It is recommended that human calorific intake should be 55% from carbohydrates, 30% from fats (lipids) and 15% from protein.

High-energy phosphates

Cellular oxidation releases some energy as heat but most is trapped in the form of a 'high-energy' molecule. These high-energy molecules include ATP (and also adenosine diphosphate, ADP) and creatine phosphate. ATP consists of an adenine base attached to a ribose sugar (adenosine) (Figure 8.2a). Three phosphate groups are attached sequentially to carbon atom 5 of the ribose (Figure 8.2b). To add a phosphate to adenosine monophosphate (AMP) to form ADP requires more energy than for most covalent bonds. This may be explained in a simple way as being necessary to overcome the resistance of AMP (already negatively charged due to the phosphate) to the addition of another negative charge. To add yet another phosphate requires even more energy because of the two phosphate groups on ADP. It follows that more energy is released when these bonds between the phosphates are broken. ATP, therefore, can serve as a short-term energy 'store' and is referred to as the 'energy currency' of the cell. The oxidation of fuels ultimately leads to phosphorylation of ADP to ATP and the ATP is used to drive energy-requiring processes as the hydrolysis of ATP to ADP is linked to an energy-requiring reaction. Another important high-energy phosphate is creatine phosphate, which is abundant in muscle. When ATP is used to support muscle contraction the resulting ADP is phosphorylated to ATP by transfer of the high-energy phosphate from creatine phosphate.

How is ATP generated? The oxidation reactions in cells, which are exergonic (release energy), are coupled to the reduction of a small molecule, most often nicotinamide adenine dinucleotide or NAD$^+$ to NADH, i.e. an electron is transferred from the molecule oxidised to NAD$^+$. Under aerobic conditions NADH is then re-oxidised by the electron transport chain in mitochondria, which pumps protons across the **inner mitochondrial membrane** (IMM). The subsequent flow of these protons back across the IMM drives the phsophorylation of ADP by inorganic phosphate to form ATP. The electrons are ultimately transferred to molecular oxygen to form water.

Enzymes and regulation (Chapter 9)

Metabolic reactions, like all biological reactions, are catalysed by enzymes. Organisms need to regulate these metabolic pathways to match the supply of energy (catabolism) with their requirements (anabolism). Regulation of these enzymes is therefore key to regulating the pathway. Enzyme activity responds to changes in substrate concentration, but enzymes may also be regulated by changes in the concentration of small molecules that may not be the substrate but, for example, the end product of a pathway. As the concentration of the end product increases this will inhibit the activity of an early enzyme in that pathway, thus preventing an unwanted build-up of end product and wastage of the starting material. This is an example of 'end product inhibition or 'negative feedback'. Enzymes may also be regulated by covalent modification, especially addition of a phosphate to the protein, known as phosphorylation. This modification may activate or inhibit the enzyme. **Phosphorylation** and **dephosphorylation** of specific enzymes, by **kinases** and **phosphatases**, is often in turn regulated by hormone signals and in this way hormones can regulate metabolic pathways (Figure 8.3).

9 Enzymes

Michael D Randall

Figure 9.1 Rate of reaction plot for enzymic reactions that obey Michaelis-Menten kinetics

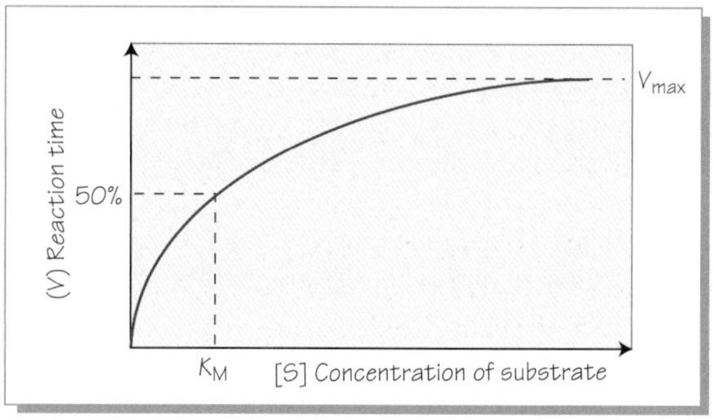

Figure 9.2 The double reciprocal or Lineweaver-Burke plot

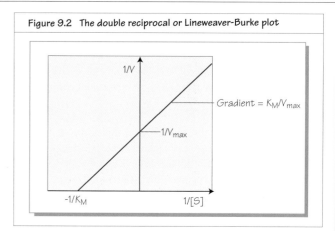

Figure 9.3 The characteristic effects of a competitive and a non-competitive inhibitor on enzymic activity as shown on the Lineweaver-Burke plot

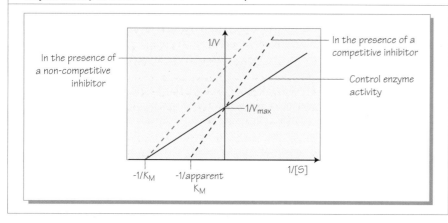

Medical Sciences at a Glance, First Edition. Edited by Michael D Randall. © 2014 John Wiley & Sons, Ltd. Published 2014 by John Wiley & Sons, Ltd.

Enzymes are biological catalysts that are involved in most biochemical reactions. As with catalysts in chemistry, they speed up chemical reactions and this is achieved by lowering the activation energy for a chemical reaction. Most enzymes are proteins, an important exception being rRNA, which has peptidyl transferase enzyme activity (Chapter 15).

Characteristics of enzymes

The proteinacious nature of enzymes means that they often show:

Activation: many enzymes are released as inactive precursors that can be activated, for example by hydrolysis, which then liberates the active enzyme. An example of this is the coagulation cascade in blood, in which the activation of a coagulation factor from its precursor involves cleavage.

pH dependence: changes in pH can affect the protein structure and function. For example, gastric enzymes such as **pepsins** are activated at acidic pH in the stomach but inactivated as they enter the small intestine at pH 5.3.

Temperature sensitivity: many enzymes show temperature dependence and undergo substantial increases in activity with small increases in temperature. Enzymic activity is usually optimal at the physiological temperature of 37°C. Increasing temperature can destroy the protein structure and lead to **denaturation**.

Enzyme kinetics
Michaelis-Menten kinetics

This is a relatively simple model that accounts for enzyme kinetics. It takes account of the substrate concentration in relation to the rate of reaction.

The Michaelis-Menten equation is summarised:

$$V = \frac{V_{max}[S]}{[S] + K_M},$$

where V = rate of reaction (number moles produced per unit time), V_{max} = maximum rate of reaction, [S] = concentration of substrate, K_M = Michaelis constant.

The K_M is defined as the concentration of substrate at which the rate of reaction (V) is half of the maximal reaction (V_{max}). The K_M value is typically in the range of 10^{-1}–10^{-6} M, where a low concentration indicates high affinity of the enzyme for the substrate. As it is the concentration at which half of the enzyme's active sites are occupied by substrate, it is affected by factors such as pH and temperature. The V_{max} occurs when all of the active sites are occupied and the enzyme is **saturated**, and is therefore dependent on the quantity of enzyme present.

Figure 9.1 summarises the plot reaction for an enzyme that obeys Michaelis-Menten kinetics.

Enzyme inhibition

Enzymes can be inhibited by **competitive** and **non-competitive inhibitors**. Competitive inhibitors literally compete with the substrate for the active site and so the inhibition can be overcome by increasing the concentration of the substrate. Generally, the competitive inhibitor is similar to the substrate but unreactive. An example of this are the statins, which inhibit the HMG CoA reductase enzyme in cholesterol synthesis.

A non-competitive inhibitor may bind at a site distinct from the active site and decreases enzymic activity. In contrast to competitive inhibitors, the effects of non-competitive inhibitors cannot be overcome by increasing the concentration of the substrate. Examples include heavy metals such as Pb^{2+} binding to enzymes and reducing their activity.

Irreversible inhibitors bind to the enzyme and this interaction is irreversible and the enzymic activity is blocked. An example of this is the interaction between penicillins and the transpeptidases responsible for cross-linking peptidoglycans in the bacterial cell wall.

Characteristically, a competitive inhibitor does not affect V_{max}, but there is an apparent decrease in K_M, whereas a non-competitive inhibitor decreases V_{max} and K_M remains unchanged. The effects of inhibitors can be analysed by the double reciprocal plot (1/V vs 1/[S]; the Lineweaver-Burke plot) (Figures 9.2 and 9.3).

Allosteric modulation

As enzymes are invariably proteins with quaternary structures, the binding of modulatory molecules can lead to conformational changes, which can result in increased or decreased enzymic activity. This allows physiological control of enzymic activity in relation to the body's needs. A key example of this is phosphorylation of pyruvate dehydrogenase, which reduces activity, whereas dephosphorylation increases activity.

Key enzymic activities

The suffix '-ase' usually indicates an enzyme, here are some key terms and enzymes.

ATPase: involved in ATP dephosphorylation to provide energy, e.g. to drive pumps (e.g. $3Na^+/2K^+$ ATPase) (Chapter 18).

Cofactors: these are non-protein components that are required for correct enzymic activity. Examples include ions such as Zn^{2+}, haem groups and coenzyme A. A prosthetic group is present when the cofactor is bound and a coenzyme is a more loosely associated.

Cyclases: these lead to formation of cyclic structures via cyclisation, e.g. adenylyl cyclase leads to the formation of cAMP as a second messenger from ATP (Chapter 7).

Isomerases: lead to isomerisation.

Kinases: phosphorylate targets, e.g. tyrosine kinases leads to phosphorylation of kinases in cell signalling (Chapter 7).

Ligases: connect molecules via covalent bonds.

Lipases: breakdown lipids, e.g. breakdown of lipids in digestion (Chapter 43).

Oxidases: lead to oxidation.

Phosphatases: dephosphorylate targets.

Proteases: break down proteins. Involved in protein digestion, and many coagulation factors when active are serine proteases, which cleave at serine residues.

Reductase: lead to reduction, e.g. dihydrofolate reductase involved in folate metabolism in purine synthesis (Chapter 65).

Synthase: a synthetic enzyme, e.g. nitric oxide synthase (Chapter 31).

Transferases: transfer a functional group, e.g. choline acetyltransferase in the synthesis of acetylcholine (Chapter 20).

10 Central metabolic pathways

Fergus Doherty

Figure 10.1   The formation of acetylCoA

AcetylCoA is formed by the β-oxidation of fatty acids and the oxidative decarboxylation of pyruvate, following transport across the inner mitochondrial membrane, by pyruvate dehydrogenase (PDH), a multi-enzyme complex in the mitochondrial matrix. PDH is regulated by phosphorylation (inactivates) and dephosphorylation (activates) by a kinase and phosphatase, which are in turn allosterically and hormonally regulated. The reverse reaction is catalysed by a separate enzyme in gluconeogenesis–pyruvate carboxylase

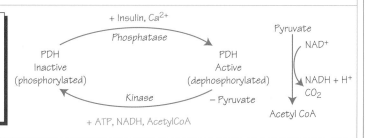

Figure 10.2   The TCA cycle

The TCA cycle takes place in mitochondria and starts with the condensation of the two carbon acetyl CoA with oxaloacetate to form citrate. Two carbon atoms are lost as CO_2 for each round of the cycle, which generates NADH and $FADH_2$, which yield ATP via oxidative phosphorylation, and a molecule of GTP, which can be used to phosphorylate ADP to ATP. The acetylCoA can come from the PDH reaction (above) or from the β-oxidation of fatty acids

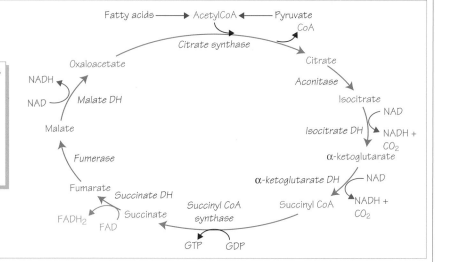

Figure 10.3   Oxidative phosphorylation

ATP is generated from reduced co-enzymes NADH and $FADH_2$ via the electron transport chain on the inner mitochondrial membrane and the activity of ATP synthase. The flow of electrons from along the chain drives the pumping of protons from the matrix to the intermembrane space to create an electrochemical gradient. The flow of these protons through the ATP synthase back into the matrix drives a conformational change in the synthase, which in turn leads to the phosphorylation of ADP to ATP. An ATP/ADP exchanger in the inner membrane allows ATP to cross out of the matrix in exchange for ADP

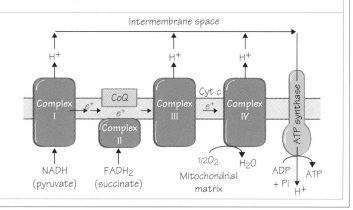

 Medical Sciences at a Glance, First Edition. Edited by Michael D Randall. © 2014 John Wiley & Sons, Ltd. Published 2014 by John Wiley & Sons, Ltd.

Catabolism of lipids, carbohydrates and the carbon skeletons of some amino acids converge on acetylCoA. **AcetylCoA** is a precursor for ketone bodies (acetoacetate and β-hydroxybutyrate) and for the biosynthesis of fatty acids (under anabolic conditions), and is also fed into the tricarboxylic acid cycle (**TCA cycle, citric acid cycle, Krebs cycle**), which generates substantial amounts of energy in the form of ATP and reduced co-factors (**NADH, FADH$_2$**) which in turn generate ATP via the electron transport chain.

The Link Reaction – pyruvate dehydrogenase

Pyruvate, generated by the **glycolytic pathway** or from **amino acid metabolism**, can be transported across the inner mitochondrial membrane into the matrix and oxidatively decarboxylated to acetyl-coenzyme A (acetylCoA) by the multi-enzyme complex **pyruvate dehydrogenase** (PDH). The product of the reaction, acetylCoA, can enter the TCA cycle. Pyruvate dehydrogenase is regulated by phosphorylation and dephosphorylation by a dedicated kinase and phosphatase. Phosphorylation by the kinase, which is allosterically activated by high levels of 'high-energy' molecules (ATP, acetylCoA, NADH, inactivates PDH (Figure 10.1). In this way, PDH responds to the energy needs of the cell, only producing acetylCoA when energy, generated from the TCA cycle, is required. In skeletal muscle, calcium ions, which increase during muscle contraction, also stimulate the PDH phosphatase, which in turn activates PDH by dephosphorylation. The phosphorylation status of PDH is also regulated in the liver by the hormones insulin and glucagon. During the fed state (high blood glucose) the high insulin:glucagon ratio activates PDH phosphatase and PDH is dephosphorylated and active, the resulting acetylCoA being used in the TCA cycle or for fatty acid synthesis. During fasting/starvation the high glucagon:insulin ratio favours PDH phosphorylation and inhibition, therefore sparing pyruvate for gluconeogenesis.

The TCA cycle

In many tissues, the major fate for acetylCoA will be oxidation via the TCA cycle to CO$_2$ and H$_2$O (Figure 10.2). Most of these reactions take place in the mitochondrial matrix and start with condensation of acetylCoA with oxaloacetate to form citrate (citrate can act as a source of acetylCoA for fatty acid synthesis), which is then isomerised to isocitrate. The oxidative decarboxylation of isocitrate to α-ketoglutarate generates CO$_2$ and NADH (+ H$^+$) and the α-ketoglutarate is oxidatively decarboxylated to succinylCoA and produces another molecule of NADH. SuccinylCoA is cleaved to succinate, yielding the high-energy phosphate molecule GTP (which subsequently generates ATP), and then oxidised to fumarate, yielding FADH$_2$. Fumarate is hydrated to form malate, which is oxidised to oxaloacetate, producing another NADH, and the oxaloacetate can accept another acetylCoA to repeat the cycle. In this way, oxaloacetate acts as a 'carrier' for acetate, which is completely oxidised to CO$_2$ and H$_2$O yielding 3 x NADH, 1 x FADH$_2$ and 1 x GTP (=ATP). Each NADH generates around 3 ATP and the FADH$_2$ 1 ATP via the electron transport chain, so there is a yield of 12 ATP for each acetate oxidised.

The electron transport chain (ETC) and oxidative phosphorylation

Reduced coenzymes, NADH and FADH$_2$, produced by the TCA cycle, the PDH reaction, oxidation of fatty acids and other reactions, can be oxidised in mitochondria via the electron transport (respiratory chain) to reduce oxygen to water and phosphorylate ADP to ATP (oxidative phosphorylation) (Figure 10.3). The **electron transport chain**, located in the convoluted inner mitochondrial membrane, which is impermeable to most ions, comprises **Complexes I-IV** of various proteins and coenzyme Q (ubiquinone). A hydride (H$^-$) from NADH and a proton (H$^+$) are transferred to Complex I (NADH dehydrogenase) to reduce the coenzyme FMN to FMNH$_2$. Hydrogens from the coenzyme FADH$_2$ (e.g. from the oxidation of succinate) are transferred to Complex II. The hydrogens from both Complex I and Complex II are transferred to coenzyme Q, which transfers electrons to Complex III (cytochrome bc$_1$). Complex III donates electrons to cytochrome c and from there they are transferred to Complex IV (cytochromes a + a$_3$). Cytochrome a$_3$ is then able to donate the electrons to O$_2$, which combines with H$^+$ in solution to form water. As oxygen is required as the final electron acceptor this is aerobic respiration and the ETC is also called the respiratory chain.

It is thought that the flow of electrons along the ETC drives the **pumping of protons** out of the mitochondrial matrix and into the inter membrane space to create a proton (charge and pH) gradient (the **chemiosmotic hypothesis**). The inner mitochondrial membrane is impermeable to protons except for Complex V (ATP synthase). Flow of protons down the concentration gradient through ATP synthase results in a conformation change (rotation) in the protein, which in turn provides the energy for phosphorylation of ADP to ATP by the synthase.

Oligomycin is a small molecule that blocks the proton channel in Complex V (ATP synthase), thus preventing the flow of protons into the matrix and the production of ATP. The build up of the proton gradient prevents any further electron flow along the ETC – electron transport and phosphorylation are coupled. These processes can be uncoupled by molecules that allow the protons to flow back across the inner mitochondrial membrane without passing through Complex V, such as 2,4-dinitrophenol, when the energy is dissipated as heat. Toxic doses of salicylate (aspirin) have the same effect. Uncoupling proteins (e.g. **UCP1** or thermogenin) are found in brown adipose tissue and therefore lead to heat generation (non-shivering thermogenesis), although humans have little brown adipose tissue.

11 Fat metabolism

Fergus Doherty

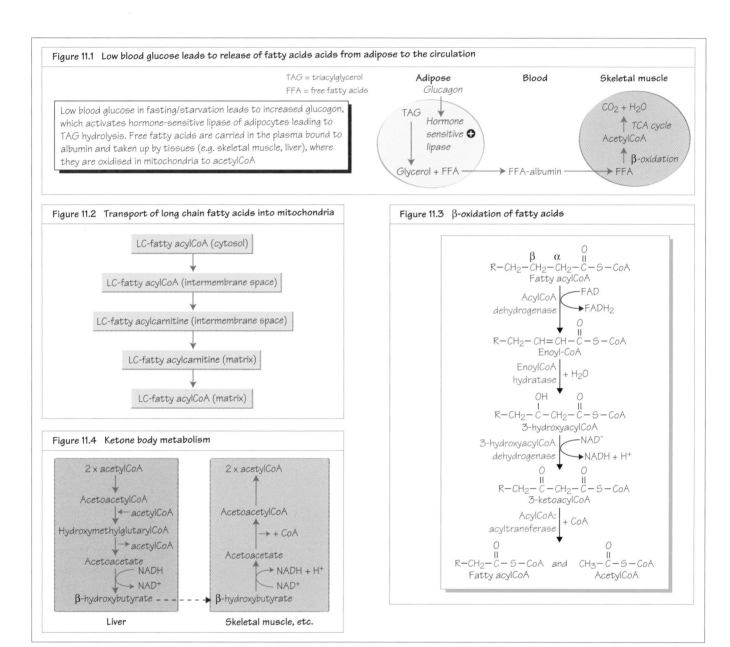

Figure 11.1 Low blood glucose leads to release of fatty acids acids from adipose to the circulation

TAG = triacylglycerol
FFA = free fatty acids

Low blood glucose in fasting/starvation leads to increased glucogon, which activates hormone-sensitive lipase of adipocytes leading to TAG hydrolysis. Free fatty acids are carried in the plasma bound to albumin and taken up by tissues (e.g. skeletal muscle, liver), where they are oxidised in mitochondria to acetylCoA

Adipose   Blood   Skeletal muscle

Glucagon

TAG
Hormone sensitive ⊕ lipase
Glycerol + FFA ⟶ FFA-albumin ⟶ FFA

$CO_2 + H_2O$
↑ TCA cycle
AcetylCoA
↑ β-oxidation

Figure 11.2 Transport of long chain fatty acids into mitochondria

LC-fatty acylCoA (cytosol)
↓
LC-fatty acylCoA (intermembrane space)
↓
LC-fatty acylcarnitine (intermembrane space)
↓
LC-fatty acylcarnitine (matrix)
↓
LC-fatty acylCoA (matrix)

Figure 11.3 β-oxidation of fatty acids

$$R-CH_2-CH_2-CH_2-\overset{\overset{O}{\|}}{C}-S-CoA$$
β α
Fatty acylCoA

AcylCoA dehydrogenase — FAD → FADH₂

$$R-CH_2-CH=CH-\overset{\overset{O}{\|}}{C}-S-CoA$$
Enoyl-CoA

EnoylCoA hydratase | + H_2O

$$R-CH_2-\overset{\overset{OH}{|}}{C}-CH_2-\overset{\overset{O}{\|}}{C}-S-CoA$$
3-hydroxyacylCoA

3-hydroxyacylCoA dehydrogenase — NAD⁻ → NADH + H⁺

$$R-CH_2-\overset{\overset{O}{\|}}{C}-CH_2-\overset{\overset{O}{\|}}{C}-S-CoA$$
3-ketoacylCoA

AcylCoA: acyltransferase | + CoA

$$R-CH_2-\overset{\overset{O}{\|}}{C}-S-CoA \quad \text{and} \quad CH_3-\overset{\overset{O}{\|}}{C}-S-CoA$$
Fatty acylCoA   AcetylCoA

Figure 11.4 Ketone body metabolism

2 x acetylCoA
↓
AcetoacetylCoA
↓ ← acetylCoA
HydroxymethylglutarylCoA
↓ → acetylCoA
Acetoacetate
⤵ NADH
⤶ NAD⁺
β-hydroxybutyrate ------→ β-hydroxybutyrate

2 x acetylCoA
↑
AcetoacetylCoA
↑ → + CoA
Acetoacetate
⤸ NADH + H⁺
⤷ NAD⁺
β-hydroxybutyrate

Liver   Skeletal muscle, etc.

 Medical Sciences at a Glance, First Edition. Edited by Michael D Randall. © 2014 John Wiley & Sons, Ltd. Published 2014 by John Wiley & Sons, Ltd.

Lipids (fats and oils) are a high-energy source yielding twice the energy per gram of protein and carbohydrate. Around 30% of calorific intake by humans is currently recommended, as an upper limit, to be in the form of lipid. Lipids are utilised as a fuel during fasting, starvation and stress, when fatty acids are mobilised from the storage lipid triacyglycerol, stored in adipose tissue, and are metabolised by tissues such as skeletal muscle and liver, but not by the brain or erythrocytes. Fatty acid oxidation yields energy and **acetylCoA (acetylCoA)**, which feeds into the **tricarboxylic acid (TCA) cycle** or in the liver is used to make **ketone bodies**.

Lipolysis

Low blood glucose concentrations trigger the release of glucagon by the pancreas, which in turn activates a hormone-sensitive lipase in adipose cells (adipocytes), which in turn hydrolyses triacyglycerol to free fatty acids and glycerol (Figure 11.1). **Glucagon** binding to its cell-surface receptor leads to an increase in intracellular cAMP, which activates **protein kinase A**, which phosphorylates and activates **hormone-sensitive lipase**. The resulting free fatty acids are released to the circulation, bound to the plasma protein albumin, from where they can be taken up by other tissues. Fatty acids freely pass the plasma membrane into the cytosol but cannot cross the blood–brain barrier. The glycerol, released from triacyglycerol breakdown, is transported to liver, phosphorylated to glycerol 3-phosphate and converted to **dihydroxyacetone phosphate** (DHAP). DHAP can be used in glycolysis or more likely converted to glucose via gluconeogenesis to provide glucose for glucose-dependent tissues.

Metabolism of fatty acids

Activation of fatty acids and transport into mitochondria

Long-chain (>12 C) fatty acids are activated in the cytosol by esterification to **coenzyme A (CoA)**, an ATP-consuming process, to form acylCoA esters (Figure 11.2). Oxidation of fatty acids occurs in the mitochondria, but the inner membrane is impermeable to acylCoA. Consequently the acyl group is transferred to carnitine and the acylcarnitine is transferred to the matrix using a shuttle system. Once in the matrix the long-chain acyl group is transferred to CoA and the carnitine exported to the cytosol via the shuttle. Short (2–4 C) and medium-chain (6–10 C) fatty acids pass directly into the mitochondrial matrix and form acylCoA there.

Oxidation of fatty acids

Fatty acids are oxidised in the mitochondria by **β-oxidation**, which cleaves two carbons off the fatty acid from the carboxyl end, as ace-

tylCoA, for each round of oxidation (Figure 11.3). First the fatty acyl CoA is oxidised by a family of **acylCoA dehydrogenases** to yield $FADH_2$ and an enoylCoA with a double bond between carbon atoms 2 and 3 (the β-carbon). This is then hydrated to form a hydroxyl group at position 3 and further oxidised to yield a carbonyl group at position 3 (a ketoacylCoA) and NADH (and H^+). The ketoacylCoA is cleaved between carbons 2 and 3 to yield acetylCoA and a fatty acylCoA shortened by two carbons. The shortened fatty acylCoA enters β-oxidation again until it is all converted to acetylCoA. The $FADH_2$ and NADH produced can be oxidised via the electron transport chain (ETC) to generate 2 and 3 ATP. Each acetylCoA generates 12 ATP via the TCA cycle and the electron transport chain, so large amounts of ATP are generated from the complete oxidation of fatty acids. Very-long-chain fatty acids are first subject to β-oxidation in peroxisomes until short enough to be oxidised in mitochondria. Various additional enzymatic steps are also available to allow the oxidation of unsaturated and odd-numbered fatty acids. **ω-oxidation** (from the methyl end) occurs in the endoplasmic reticulum, especially if there is a problem with β-oxidation, and leads to the excretion of dicarboxylic acids.

Ketone bodies

In the initial stages of starvation, fatty acids are mobilised from adipose and oxidised in liver and skeletal muscle (low insulin results in low glucose uptake by muscle), sparing glucose for glucose-dependent tissues. The brain and red blood cells cannot utilise fatty acids. From about three days of starvation the high levels of acetyl-CoA in the liver from fatty acid oxidation cannot all be consumed in the TCA cycle and are surplus to the liver's energy needs. The acetylCoA is diverted to the formation of the ketone bodies, acetoacetone and β-hydroxybutyrate (Figure 11.4), and individuals are said to be **ketotic**. β-hydroxybutyrate is formed from the reduction of acetoacetate resulting from the high levels of NADH generated by fatty acid oxidation. The ketone bodies are released to the circulation and utilised by the kidneys and then the brain, so that eventually 75% of the brain's energy needs are met by ketone bodies. The liver cannot utilise ketone bodies, which in other tissues are converted to acetylCoA which enters the TCA cycle. High levels of ketone bodies reduce skeletal muscle breakdown during starvation. When the ketone body concentration in the plasma reaches 7 mM the tissues are saturated and ketones appear in the urine (ketonuria). Very high levels of plasma ketones reduce blood pH, leading to a form of metabolic acidosis – **ketoacidosis** – which can be life threatening and can occur in uncontrolled diabetes.

12 Glucose metabolism

Fergus Doherty

Figure 12.1 Hormonal changes in response to glucose ingestion

Following a meal containing carbohydrate, glucagon levels fall and insulin levels rise, which promotes insulin uptake by tissues and therefore a drop in blood glucose. The fall in blood glucose eventually leads to a drop in insulin and a rise in glucagon, which triggers glucose release from the liver, therefore these hormone help to maintain glucose homeostasis

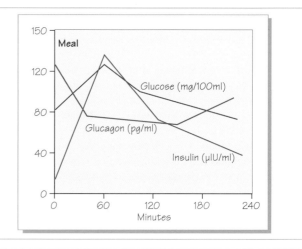

Figure 12.2 Glucose metabolism

Glycolysis and gluconeogenesis showing key enzymes (italics). Glycolysis is an energy-yielding pathway ending in pyruvate, found in all cells. In aerobic conditions pyruvate is oxidatively decarboxylated to acetate (as acetylCoA), which can then enter the TCA cycle. In anaerobic conditions pyruvate is reduced to lactate to regenerate NAD$^+$, tissues such as skeletal muscle release lactate, which can be utilised by the heart after conversion back to pyruvate and then to acetylCoA, or converted to pyruvate and then to glucose (gluconeogenesis) in the liver

Gluconeogenesis occurs in the liver when blood glucose is low and is the formation of glucose from amino acids via pyruvate, or glycerol (from triacylglycerol) via dihydroxyacetone phosphate. Much of gluconeogenesis is the reverse of glycolysis except for the steps shown in green. Removal of the phosphate from glucose by glucose-6-phosphatase allows the glucose to be released from the liver to the blood

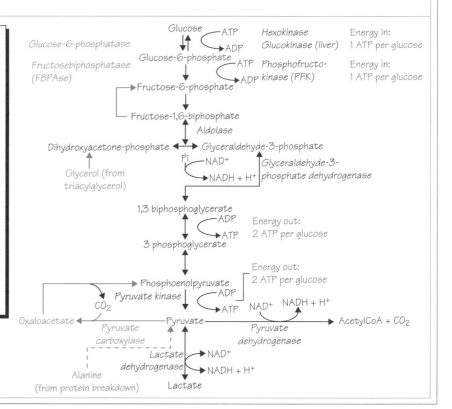

Medical Sciences at a Glance, First Edition. Edited by Michael D Randall. © 2014 John Wiley & Sons, Ltd. Published 2014 by John Wiley & Sons, Ltd.

Approximately 55% of the energy needs of the average human are met by the metabolism of carbohydrates, of which the major component is glucose. The glucose concentration in the blood is maintained at 4–8 mmol/L (glucose homeostasis) largely by the action of hormones such as **insulin** and **glucagon** (Figure 12.1 and Chapter 46). The majority of carbohydrates in the diet are polysaccharides, which are digested in the gastrointestinal tract to mono- and disaccharides by amylases and other enzymes.

Glucose uptake

Glucose is transported into the enterocytes of the gastrointestinal tract by an energy-requiring process against a concentration gradient and then passes down a concentration gradient into the plasma (Chapter 43). Uptake of glucose from the plasma into tissues is mediated by a family of **glucose transporters (GLUTs)**. GLUT4 in adipose and skeletal muscle is dependent on insulin for activity, while GLUT 1 and 3 (brain, erythrocytes) are not. GLUT2 in liver and kidney is insulin independent and can also transport glucose out to the plasma. On entry into the cell, glucose is phosphorylated by **hexokinase** (all tissues) or **glucokinase** (liver) to **glucose-6-phosphate**, which traps it in the cell. Glucokinase is only active at high glucose concentrations.

Glucose metabolism (Figure 12.2)

Glycolysis

All cells are capable of glycolysis. The first stage of glycolysis consumes ATP due to glucose phosphorylation, and then as **glucose-6-phosphate** is converted to fructose-6-phosphate and then phosphorylated by the regulatory enzyme of glycolysis, **phosphofructokinase-1** (PFK-1), to fructose-1,6-bisphosphate. PFK-1 is activated by low ATP concentrations and high ADP and AMP concentrations, as the purpose of glycolysis is to produce ATP. Fructose-1,6-bisphosphate is cleaved to two three-carbon glyceraldehyde-3-phosphate, which is subject to oxidation, generating two molecules of NADH in total, and phosphorylation (not requiring ATP) before 4 ATP is generated for every glucose molecule in energy-yielding steps, leading to the formation of the end product pyruvate. The net yield is 2 ATP for each molecule of glucose, but a further 6 ATP can be generated from the oxidation by the electron transport chain of the 2 NADH produced, and in aerobic conditions the pyruvate can be converted to acetylCoA, which enters the TCA cycle (Chapter 10) to generate more ATP. Under anaerobic conditions, e.g. in skeletal muscle or in erythrocytes (without mitochondria), NADH cannot be oxidised in this way, but instead pyruvate is reduced to lactate to regenerate NAD^+ to allow glycolysis to continue. Lactate from these tissues is released to the plasma and converted back to pyruvate in the heart, which respires aerobically, or the liver, where the pyruvate is used to synthesise glucose (**gluconeogenesis**), which is released back to the circulation (the **Cori cycle**).

Pentose phosphate pathway

In some tissues (adipose, liver), when glucose concentrations are high glucose-6-phosphate is fed into the pentose phosphate pathway. This pathway generates NADPH, a co-factor used in the biosynthesis of fatty acids which is important in both these tissues, and ribose-5-phosphate used in nucleotide biosynthesis.

Glycogen metabolism

Glucose comes not only from the diet but also from body stores of glycogen, a glucose polymer, in particular in the skeletal muscle and liver. When blood glucose levels are low, glucagon released from the pancreas causes the activation of **glycogen phosphorylase**. This breaks down glycogen to glucose-1-phosphate, which is converted to glucose-6-phosphate, which in turn can enter glycolysis. Low cellular concentrations of ATP and high AMP in muscle also activate this enzyme. While muscle utilises the glucose-6-phosphate, in liver much of this will be converted to glucose by glucose-6-phosphatase and the resulting glucose will be released to the circulation to maintain glucose homeostasis.

Gluconeogenesis

The liver is capable of producing glucose, not just from glycogen but also from other, non-carbohydrate, sources (gluconeogenesis). Alanine, produced in skeletal muscle from amino acids released following protein degradation during fasting/starvation (low blood glucose, low insulin, high glucagon), is taken up by the liver, deaminated (to form urea) and the resulting pyruvate can be converted back to glucose by gluconeogenesis and released to the plasma.

Glucose utilisation and homeostasis

Following ingestion of carbohydrate the plasma concentration rises to 7–8 mmol/L, triggering the release of insulin from the pancreas, which stimulates glucose uptake into muscle and adipose as well as glycogen synthesis in liver and muscle. The result is a lowering of blood glucose concentration. During fasting, blood glucose levels drop to about 4 mmol/L, triggering glucagon release and a fall in insulin. This stimulates glycogen breakdown, allowing the liver to release glucose to the blood, while gluconeogenesis in the liver increases and glycolysis decreases. In this way blood glucose levels are kept from falling too low, as the brain and erythrocytes are dependent on glucose as a fuel.

13 Amino acid metabolism

Jane Arnold

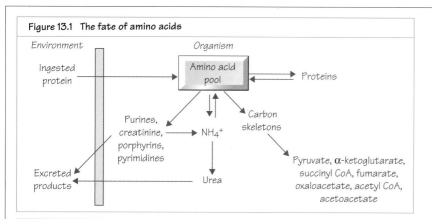

Figure 13.1 The fate of amino acids

Table 13.1 Glucogenic and ketogenic amino acids

Ketogenic	Both	Glucogenic	
Leu	Iso	Ala	Cys
Lys	Trp	Gly	Ser
	Phe	Asp	Asn
	Tyr	Met	
	Thr	Val	Glu
		Gln	His
		Pro	Arg

Figure 13.2 Transamination and deamination reactions

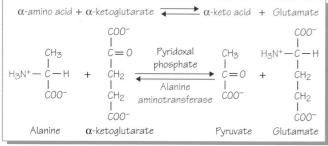

(a) Transamination reaction

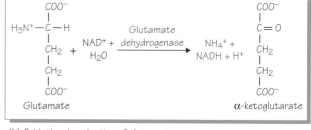

(b) Oxidative deamination of glutamate

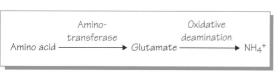

(c) Overall reaction of ammonium ion production

Figure 13.3 The urea cycle

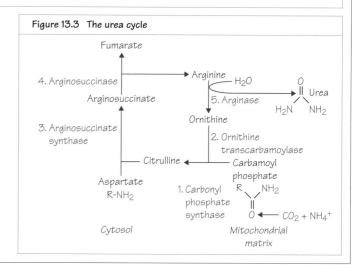

Amino acid synthesis

Of the 20 amino acids needed for protein synthesis, humans are only able to make 11. These are termed the **non-essential amino acids** and are made by either *de novo* pathways or by conversion from existing amino acids. These pathways involve, in the first instance, the addition of an amino group to a carbon skeleton via a **transaminase reaction**. The other nine amino acids are termed **essential amino acids** and have to be obtained from the diet. In a well-nourished adult approximately 50 g of dietary protein is required daily.

The amino acid pool and protein turnover

A major source of amino acids is from the hydrolysis of dietary protein as well as from the breakdown of cellular protein. These sources, in addition to synthesised amino acids, give rise to a pool of free amino acids within the body (Figure 13.1). Cellular protein is continuously undergoing synthesis and breakdown in a process known as **protein turnover**, which allows damaged or abnormal proteins to be removed from the body. This is a highly regulated process and approximately 400 g of cellular protein is degraded and re-synthesised each day. In a well-nourished adult the rate of protein synthesis is equal to the rate of protein degradation.

Formation of nitrogen-containing molecules

Amino acids are precursors to a number of important nitrogen-containing molecules. These include **porphyrins** (e.g. heme groups), **purines** and **pyrimidines** (e.g. nucleotides for DNA synthesis; Chapter 15), **neurotransmitters** (e.g. dopamine, noradrenaline) and **creatine** (found in muscle as the high-energy molecule creatine phosphate) (Figure 13.1).

Catabolism of amino acids

Unlike fatty acids and carbohydrate, amino acids cannot be stored in the body. Consequently any surplus amino acids have to be broken down. This involves the removal of the α-amino group to form an ammonium ion, which will in turn be converted to urea via the urea cycle. The remaining carbon skeletons are then further metabolised to form intermediates used in energy production. The main reactions are are as follows.

Removal of the α-amino group via transamination

The α-amino group of the amino acid is removed by an enzyme reaction known as **transamination** and is catalysed by an **aminotransferase** enzyme (also called a transaminase). Two of the most important aminotransferases are alanine aminotransferase (ALT) and aspartate aminotransferase (AST), which are highly expressed in the liver (Chapter 44). In this reaction the α-amino group of the amino acid is transferred to α-ketoglutarate to produce the corresponding α-keto acid and glutamate, e.g. alanine aminotransferase transfers the amino group of alanine to α-ketoglutarate to form glutamate and its corresponding α-keto acid, pyruvate (see Figure 13.2a). Similarly, aspartate aminotransferase catalyses the deamination of aspartate to form glutamate and its corresponding α-keto acid, oxaloacetate. All aminotransferases require pyridoxal phosphate (derived from vitamin B6) as a cofactor. These reactions are near equilibrium, so they can also be used to synthesise amino acids, e.g. alanine will be produced when levels of pyruvate and glutamate are high and alanine levels are low.

Formation of the ammonium ion via oxidative deamination

Following on from transamination, the enzyme glutamate dehydrogenase releases the amino group from glutamate to form the ammonium ion and α-ketoglutarate (Figures 13.2b and 13.2c). This enzyme can use either NAD^+ or $NADP^+$ as a coenzyme.

Formation of urea

A series of reactions known as the urea cycle takes place in the liver, where the highly toxic ammonium ion is converted into urea (Figure 13.3). The first two reactions of the urea cycle occur in the mitochondria to produce citrulline, which is then transported into the cytosol, where the remaining reactions occur. Urea is then transported in the blood to the kidneys, where it is excreted as urine. The two nitrogen atoms in urea come from one **ammonium ion** and one molecule of **aspartate.**

Metabolism of the remaining carbon skeletons

The carbon skeletons of amino acids are an important energy source and are used under certain metabolic conditions, e.g. short-term starvation, for energy production. Amino acids are defined as being glucogenic or ketogenic (Table 13.1). Glucogenic amino acids are those that will form pyruvate, or the TCA cycle intermediates α-ketoglutarate, oxaloacetate, succinyl CoA, or fumarate. They will primarily be used in gluconeogenesis to form glucose (in the liver) and are an important source of glucose in short-term starvation. Ketogenic amino acids form acetylCoA or the ketone body acetoacetate. Leucine and lysine are the only two amino acids that are purely ketogenic. The ability of amino acids to be converted into these metabolic intermediates means that amino acids, when in excess, have the ability to form **glucose, fatty acids** (from acetylCoA) and **ketone bodies**.

Aminoacidopathies

There are more than a hundred genetic defects in amino acid metabolism. One of the most clinically important is phenylketonuria. This is due to a defect in the enzyme phenylalanine hydroxylase.

14 Principles of molecular genetics

Stuart Brown

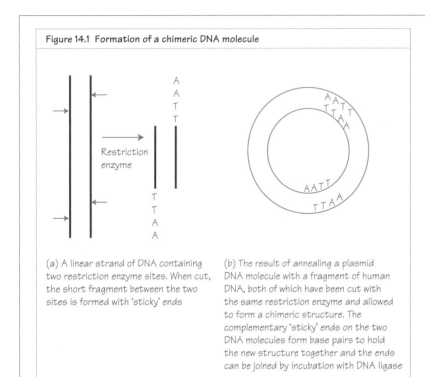

Figure 14.1 Formation of a chimeric DNA molecule

(a) A linear strand of DNA containing two restriction enzyme sites. When cut, the short fragment between the two sites is formed with 'sticky' ends

(b) The result of annealing a plasmid DNA molecule with a fragment of human DNA, both of which have been cut with the same restriction enzyme and allowed to form a chimeric structure. The complementary 'sticky' ends on the two DNA molecules form base pairs to hold the new structure together and the ends can be joined by incubation with DNA ligase

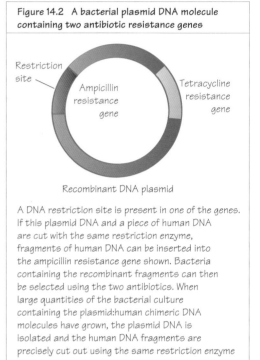

Figure 14.2 A bacterial plasmid DNA molecule containing two antibiotic resistance genes

Recombinant DNA plasmid

A DNA restriction site is present in one of the genes. If this plasmid DNA and a piece of human DNA are cut with the same restriction enzyme, fragments of human DNA can be inserted into the ampicillin resistance gene shown. Bacteria containing the recombinant fragments can then be selected using the two antibiotics. When large quantities of the bacterial culture containing the plasmid:human chimeric DNA molecules have grown, the plasmid DNA is isolated and the human DNA fragments are precisely cut out using the same restriction enzyme

Prior to the development of molecular genetic techniques our understanding of genetic disease and potential treatments was based on the analysis of pedigrees and studying abnormal proteins. The knowledge gained from understanding the structure of a gene and gene cloning techniques has revolutionised knowledge of the cause of genetic diseases and potential treatments, including gene therapy.

Gene cloning

The basis of gene cloning technology owes its origins to the realisation that two different practical techniques (the use of **restriction enzymes** and the use of **bacterial plasmids**) could be utilised to generate **chimeric DNA** molecules in large quantities. Restriction enzymes are **endonucleases** that recognise and cut DNA at specific sequences within the molecule (Figure 14.1a). They recognise short four- or six-base pair sequences and either cut at opposite ends of these sequences, generating overlapping ends known as **'sticky' ends** because they can reanneal using allowed base pair rules, or they cut both strands at the same site to generate 'blunt' ends.

Plasmids are small circular DNA molecules that can be present in a bacterial cell and replicate along with the bacterial genome (Figure 14.1b). They can code for proteins such as antibiotic-resistance proteins (Figure 14.2) and are responsible for creating many multi-drug-resistant bacteria.

 Medical Sciences at a Glance, First Edition. Edited by Michael D Randall. © 2014 John Wiley & Sons, Ltd. Published 2014 by John Wiley & Sons, Ltd.

The combination of these two technologies led to the production of **recombinant DNA molecules**. If a plasmid preparation is cut with a particular restriction enzyme, small lengths of DNA with identical sticky ends will form. Similarly, if a piece of human DNA is cut with the same restriction enzyme, short sequences of DNA will result with the same sticky ends. The two sets of DNA pieces can be incubated together and allowed to reanneal. The annealed DNA pieces can then be covalently joined *in vitro* using DNA ligase. The result will be a mixture of reformed plasmid molecules in addition to some plasmids into which human DNA sequences have been inserted. It is now possible to use selection techniques to select for only the chimeric human/plasmid molecules. These chimeric DNA molecules will be replicated by the host bacteria. The plasmid acts as the **vector**, to produce large quantities of the human molecules. The human DNA sequences can then be extracted using the same restriction enzyme that was used to cut the DNA initially.

Libraries

If a sample of total human DNA is treated with a restriction enzyme and the fragments are inserted into a vector, the **chimeric molecules** generated will contain the sum total of all the DNA sequences present in the human genome. The product of this process has been called a **human genomic library**. It can be prepared from the DNA of human tissue or human cell lines and will not be dependent on the source of DNA. Much of our understanding of the sequences in human genes has come from studies on human DNA libraries. However, these sequences cannot be used to generate human proteins in a bacterial protein synthesising system because bacterial cells cannot process the complex intron/exon structure of human genes.

If the total mRNA is isolated from a specific human tissue or cell line it can be **reverse transcribed** into **complementary DNA** *in vitro* using the RNA virus enzyme reverse transcriptase. The complementary DNA sequences can be ligated into a particular vector. The vector will then contain DNA copies of all the mRNA molecules present in that tissue. This is known as a **complementary DNA (or cDNA) library**. Unlike the genomic library, a cDNA library will be specific to the tissue used to isolate the mRNA because different tissues express different genes at different times. cDNA libraries can be used to produce large quantities of proteins.

Isolation of a specific DNA sequence

If cellular DNA is isolated from human tissue and treated with a restriction enzyme, thousands of fragments result. These can be separated on a polyacryamide gel. The different size fragments will migrate to different positions in the gel based on their molecular weights. A specific fragment can be identified using a specific 'probe' for that fragment. Probes are any molecule that can be used to detect a specific polynucleotide or polypeptide sequence. For example, a small piece of radioactively labelled DNA complementary to the sequence to be isolated can be used to detect the required DNA fragment. It can be incubated with the gel containing all the human fragments and it will specifically bind to the complementary sequence and can be detected using autoradiography. Once detected, the DNA fragment can be cut from the gel, ligated into a plasmid and grown in a suitable bacterial host to produce large quantities of the DNA sequence. Similar strategies are now used to detect RNA and peptide sequences on gels.

The use of a DNA probe to detect a DNA sequence on a gel is called a **Southern blot**. A **Northern blot** is used to detect RNA sequences

on a gel and the use of an antibody to probe a gel containing a mixture of polypeptides is called a **Western blot**.

DNA sequencing

It is possible to sequence DNA molecules to test whether the sequence isolated from a Southern blot or a DNA library is the correct one. **DNA polymerases** replicate DNA by adding new deoxyribonucleotides at the 3′ end of the growing DNA chain. If a dideoxynucleotide, i.e. one with no 2′ or 3′ hydroxyl group on the deoxyribose ring, is used as a substrate in a DNA synthesis reaction the incorporation of a dideoxynucleotide will terminate DNA synthesis, as there will be no 3′ hydroxyl group to accept a new deoxynucleotide. To sequence a DNA strand a mixture of deoxynucleotides and dideoxynucleotides is added to the reaction mixture. DNA synthesis will terminate at random when a dideoxynucleotide is inserted, producing many DNA strands of different length. Careful analysis of these fragments allows the sequence to be determined. Automation of this process has finally led to techniques able to sequence the complete three billion bases in the human genome.

Practical applications
Gene mapping

In order to attempt to correct genetic disease it is necessary to know the location of the defective gene. Prior to the development of modern recombinant DNA technology this used to be performed by extensive analysis of a set of hybrid cells. For example, when human and mouse cells are fused the resulting hybrid cell is viable and gradually loses human chromosomes. It was possible to map a human gene to a human chromosome using these cells. This technique was limited. The gene to be mapped not only had to produce a protein that could be detected in the cells but also be different from the mouse counterpart. With modern technology it is now possible to use molecular probes for specific genes to locate the gene on a specific human chromosome using Southern blot analyses without any knowledge of the gene product. In addition, the automation of DNA sequencing has finally led to the sequencing of the complete human genome.

Protein synthesis

Using a cDNA library it is now possible to generate human proteins in large quantities for research purposes or for treatment of human diseases. This has been especially important in the production of proteins that are only present in very small quantities in cells and hence are very difficult to purify by conventional techniques. It is now possible to produce proteins for treatment of disease, such as insulin, human growth hormone and interferon, or for diagnostic purposes, such as HIV detection, in large quantities.

Prenatal diagnosis of disease

It is now possible to use Southern blotting techniques to analyse a chorionic villus sample or amniotic fluid for the presence of an abnormal gene in a fetus. Sickle cell anaemia and cystic fibrosis are just two diseases that can be detected using this new technology.

The ultimate goal of the new technology is to be able to replace a missing gene in order to correct a genetic disease. It is now possible to clone a gene such as adenosine deaminase or the cystic fibrosis transmembrane conductance regulator gene and, using a suitable vector such as a viral vector or a liposome, introduce the synthetic gene back into the patient's cells. Although still in its infancy this technology is showing great promise.

Stuart Brown

Figure 15.1 DNA and chromatin structures

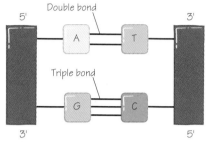

(a) A diagram of a DNA double helix showing the base pairs that form perpendicular to the direction of the helix. Adenine pairs with thymine: forms two hydrogen bonds, while guanine pairs with cytosine: forms three hydrogen bonds. The two phosphodiester backbone strands consist of alternating deoxyribose and phosphate molecules and are shown running antiparallel, i.e. one strand runs 5' to 3' and the other runs 3' to 5'

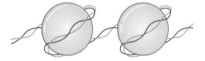

(b) In mammalian cells DNA does not exist without being combined with proteins. Two copies of histone proteins H2a, H2b, H3 and H4 form spherical structures around which DNA can wrap. In this way the strand of DNA is more condensed. Histone H1 attaches to the DNA linker region between the histone octamers to protect the DNA from degradation. This 'beads-on-a-string'-type structure then coils in several further modification steps until a chromosome is formed

Figure 15.2   A DNA replication fork

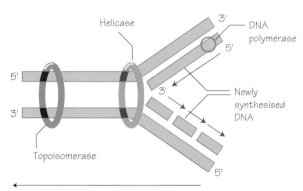

The double-stranded DNA unwinds to expose the two separate DNA strands. DNA polymerases then copy the template strands to form two new daughter DNA strands. DNA polymerases can only travel in the 5' to 3' direction and thus a complex series of events has to occur to copy both template strands. The 3' to 5' template strand can be copied continuously by a DNA polymerase travelling in the 5' to 3' direction. The other template strand has to be unwound to allow a DNA polymerase to attach and synthesise short DNA sequences in the opposite direction to the direction of replication. These short sequences, known as Okazaki fragments, are then joined together by a DNA ligase to form the new DNA molecule

Deoxyribonucleic acid (DNA)

DNA is the hereditary material in prokaryotic and eukaryotic cells. It consists of four nitrogenous bases, **adenine (A), guanine (G), cytosine (C)** and **thymine (T)**, attached to deoxyribose (a pentose sugar) molecules (Figure 15.1a). The deoxyribose molecules are linked by covalent ester bonds to phosphate molecules to produce a long thin polymer. The monomeric units of this polymer are known as **nucleotides**. A single nucleotide consists of a base bound to a deoxyribose molecule with a phosphate attached. Since the polymer is made up of nucleotides, DNA is called a polynucleotide. In prokaryotes such as *Escherichia coli*, there is a single DNA polynucleotide chain consisting of 4×10^6 bases. This DNA is known as the genome. In humans, there is a separate DNA molecule in each of the 46 chromosomes. The total number of bases in the human genome is 3×10^9.

DNA polymers can be described in terms of the position of the chemical bonds joining the sugar and the phosphate. The five carbon atoms in deoxyribose are numbered 1′ to 5′ (the primes are added to differentiate the carbon atoms in the sugar from those in the base). In a DNA polymer, phosphate molecules are attached at the 5′ and 3′ carbons of a deoxyribose. Thus at the ends of the polymer there will be a deoxyribose with either a free 3′ hydroxyl group or a free 5′ phosphate group. The ends are known as the 5′ or 3′ ends and the polymer can be described as having a direction, i.e. 5′ to 3′ or 3′ to 5′.

DNA sequence

Each nucleotide in the DNA helix can be described by the letter representing the specific base it contains. By convention the base sequence is written in the 5′ to 3′ direction. Thus the sequence AATTGCC would represent a base sequence with an adenine base at the 5′ end and a cytosine base at the 3′ end.

The DNA double helix

DNA strands in human cells are wound around each other to form a **double helix** with the deoxyribose–phosphate hydrophilic backbone on the outside and the bases on the inside. The strands run in an antiparallel direction, i.e. one strand runs 5′ to 3′ and the other 3′ to 5′. Thus the DNA helix is asymmetric. The bases are attached at the 1′ position on the sugar. The bases on opposite strands of the helix form hydrogen bonds with each other and the numerous hydrogen bonds formed in the base pairs contribute to the force stabilising the helix structure. The hydrogen-bonded base pairs are known as base pairs and can only form in certain specific combinations: A pairs with T via two hydrogen bonds and G with C via three hydrogen bonds. The base pairs are perpendicular to the direction of the helix. The base pairs are hydrophobic and stack on top of each other. This '**hydrophobic stacking force**' provides another main source of force holding the DNA helix together.

In the most common form of DNA, known as the B form, the helix is a right-handed double helix with 10 bases per turn, i.e. the angle of rotation between base pairs is 36°. Although the B form of DNA is the most common form found, DNA can form an A form right-handed helix in which the base pairs are tilted with respect to the helix direction or even a Z form left-handed helix. The Z form is thought to exist in cells but its role is still not totally understood.

DNA organisation in human cells

Double-stranded DNA does not exist alone in human cells. Two molecules of histone proteins H2A, H2B, H3 and H4 form a cylindrical structure around which the DNA strand is wrapped (Figure 15.1b). Two turns of DNA (147 base pairs) are wrapped around each octamer and the DNA linking these structures is protected by binding a histone H1 molecule. This fundamental form of DNA wrapped around the histones is known as the 'beads-on-a-string' structure. It represents the most uncondensed form of DNA in a cell. Higher-order structures in which the DNA is gradually more and more condensed form by the coiling of the 'beads-on-a-string' structure into a coil and then a coiled coil and ultimately into the highly condensed form known as the chromosome. Only the most condensed form of DNA and histone is called a chromosome. The other forms are called chromatin. **Chromatin** can exist in a cell in two forms: heterochromatin, which is highly condensed; and euchromatin, which is less condensed and is the form that would be present during transcription. This condensation process is the means by which the vast amount of DNA, approximately 2m in total length, can be contained in the nucleus of a human cell, with a diameter of only approximately 10 μm.

DNA replication

Watson and Crick deduced the structure of DNA in 1953. They postulated that the helix structure would enable the molecule to be replicated by unwinding the helix and producing new copies using the separate strands of the parent helix as a template. This is indeed the case. Each strand of the DNA molecule contains the genetic information and thus can act as a template for the synthesis of two new daughter DNA strands each containing the same genetic information as the parental strand (Figure 15.2).

DNA polymerases are the enzymes responsible for replication. There are several different DNA polymerases found in bacterial and human cells. *E. coli* contains five different DNA polymerases known as **pol I, II, III, IV** and **V**. Although all possess similar properties, pol III is the main replication enzyme. The others have roles in DNA repair. In humans, there are 15 DNA polymerases. DNA pol α, δ and ε are involved in nuclear DNA replication, and pol γ is responsible for replication of mitochondrial DNA. Several others are involved in DNA repair and not too well understood.

Despite the fact that several forms of DNA polymerase exist they have similar properties:
- they require all four deoxyribonucleotide triphosphates as substrates;
- they require a divalent cation, e.g. magnesium ions;
- they cannot initiate DNA synthesis without a primer;
- they cannot join two DNA molecules together;
- most of them have endonuclease activity.

Several of these properties are to ensure the great accuracy required to copy such large sequences of nucleotides faithfully, without making errors. The accuracy of human DNA replication is estimated at one error for every 10^{10} bases copied. This is essential to avoid the introduction of mutations that could lead to genetic disease.

Due to the restrictions on the properties of DNA polymerases, several other proteins and enzymes are required to completely replicate a DNA molecule:
- **RNA primase** to generate the RNA primer
- **DNA ligase** to join single DNA strands together
- **helicases** and **topoisomerases** to wind or unwind the helix when required
- *single-stranded binding proteins* to protect the unwound single stranded DNA strands.

In humans, the process is complicated further by the fact that the DNA is in the form of chromatin. The chromatin must be unwound before replication starts and rewound after replication.

Ribonucleic acid (RNA)

RNA has a very similar structure to DNA, except that:
- it is usually single stranded;
- it contains ribose sugars instead of deoxyribose;
- it contains uracil as a base instead of thymine.

There are three different major types of RNA in a cell:
- **messenger RNA (mRNA)**
- **ribosomal RNA (rRNA)**
- **transfer RNA (tRNA)**.

All three forms are coded for by genes in DNA and are required for protein synthesis.
- mRNA is the RNA copy of a gene that is used to code for proteins.
- rRNA, together with several proteins, forms the small and large subunits of the ribosome, which is used in protein synthesis.
- tRNA is responsible for delivering the correct amino acid to the ribosome for protein synthesis to occur.

Stuart Brown

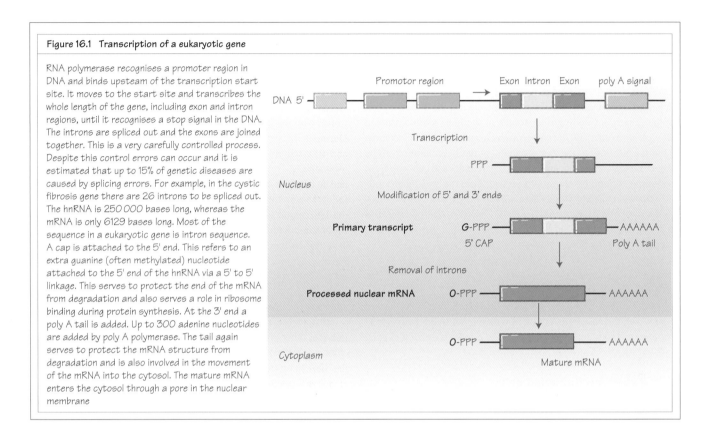

Figure 16.1   Transcription of a eukaryotic gene

RNA polymerase recognises a promoter region in DNA and binds upsteam of the transcription start site. It moves to the start site and transcribes the whole length of the gene, including exon and intron regions, until it recognises a stop signal in the DNA. The introns are spliced out and the exons are joined together. This is a very carefully controlled process. Despite this control errors can occur and it is estimated that up to 15% of genetic diseases are caused by splicing errors. For example, in the cystic fibrosis gene there are 26 introns to be spliced out. The hnRNA is 250 000 bases long, whereas the mRNA is only 6129 bases long. Most of the sequence in a eukaryotic gene is intron sequence. A cap is attached to the 5' end. This refers to an extra guanine (often methylated) nucleotide attached to the 5' end of the hnRNA via a 5' to 5' linkage. This serves to protect the end of the mRNA from degradation and also serves a role in ribosome binding during protein synthesis. At the 3' end a poly A tail is added. Up to 300 adenine nucleotides are added by poly A polymerase. The tail again serves to protect the mRNA structure from degradation and is also involved in the movement of the mRNA into the cytosol. The mature mRNA enters the cytosol through a pore in the nuclear membrane

Gene sequences occupy only about 2% of the human genome. Following the successful genome project that enabled the sequence of bases in the human genome (3 billion) to be elucidated, it is now thought that there are only approximately 20–25 000 genes in the human genome. The term **genotype** is used to describe the genes present in a genome. However, in different cells and tissues not all the same genes will be expressed. The term **phenotype** is used to describe which genes are expressed in different cells or tissues. **Gene expression** refers to the processes in which the information in a gene in DNA is used to produce the corresponding protein in a cell. It involves the **transcription** of the DNA sequence into RNA and then the **translation** of RNA into proteins. Gene expression is very carefully regulated in order to control not only how much of a protein is made but also when particular proteins are synthesised, e.g. during development or differentiation of cell types. Although cells can control transcription and translation, the major control of gene expression is at the level of transcription.

Transcription (Figure 16.1)

Cells contain three different types of RNA molecules: **mRNA, rRNA** and **tRNA** (Chapter 15). All three types of RNA are transcribed from genes present in DNA. Only mRNA, however, is used as a template for new protein synthesis. rRNA and tRNA are used in the translation process. In eukaryotic cells, transcription is carried out by three different **DNA-dependent RNA polymerases**:
- **pol I** transcribes rRNA genes and is located in the nucleolus;
- **pol II** transcribes mRNA genes;
- **pol III** transcribes tRNA genes and other small RNA molecules.

Pol II and III are found in the nucleus. RNA polymerase enzymes are multisubunit structures containing approximately 16 subunits and are more complex than the single RNA polymerase enzyme found in bacteria.

To understand the series of events that produce an mRNA molecule from a gene it is necessary to understand the eukaryotic gene structure. Eukaryotic genes are made up of **exons**, regions of DNA that will code for the mature mRNA, and **introns**, regions of DNA that will be transcribed into RNA but later removed during post-**transcriptional processing**. RNA polymerase II will transcribe the full length of the gene using the template strand as a template so that the mRNA sequence is the same as that in the DNA-coding strand. Only one DNA strand is copied. This initial product is called heterogeneous nuclear RNA (**hnRNA**). Three important post-transcriptional processing events occur while the hnRNA is still in the nucleus (see Figure 16.1).

Following completion of these events the product is mRNA. It now moves out of the nucleus, through the nuclear pores, and is located in the cytosol where translation occurs.

Control of transcription

As mentioned above, transcription is very well regulated, specifically transcription initiation. This regulation is exerted through a combination of special DNA sequences and proteins known as transcription factors, which recognise and bind to the control elements in DNA. One major DNA control element is the **promoter** situated at the 5′ end of the gene. Eukaryotic promoters have several features in common. The promoter sequence will allow the polymerase to bind and start transcription at the correct base. A specific conserved sequence was identified approximately 25–35 bases upstream of the transcription start site. This sequence is rich in A and T bases and is known as the **TATA box**. There are other special DNA sequences up to 200 bases upstream of the transcription start site that also help regulate the level of gene transcription, and even others that can be many hundreds or thousands of bases upstream of the gene. The latter are known as **enhancers or silencers** because they can increase or decrease the frequency of transcription.

The DNA-controlling elements at the 5′ end of the gene bind other proteins known as transcription factors. The initiation of transcription can be controlled by many of these proteins forming a multisubunit transcription complex at the promoter site. These will form in some cell types but not others, or at different times during development, and hence control transcription. Transcription factors have several distinctive protein motifs that enable them to bind to DNA and to other proteins in the complex. These motifs include zinc fingers, helix loop helix motifs and leucine zippers.

A recent development has been the discovery of **alternative splicing**. During the removal of introns from a hnRNA the exons may be spliced in different ways in different tissues. This increases the diversity of proteins that can be made from the relatively small number of genes present in the human genome. An example of this phenomenon is **tropomyosin**. This is used in different contractile systems in different cells and the specific form required is produced by alternative splicing of the single hnRNA rather than having different tropomyosin genes in the different cell types.

Translation

The final stage in gene expression is translation. Translation is the term used for the process of translating mRNA into protein. In a eukaryotic cell, this can occur in the cytosol when synthesising soluble proteins destined for use in that cell, or at the endoplasmic reticulum membrane when synthesising proteins destined for secretion from the cell or ones that will be membrane bound. Note the information instructing the protein to its final destination was originally in the DNA.

Translation requires the use of all three RNA species: the mRNA is used as the template for protein synthesis; rRNA, together with many proteins, forms the complex ribosomes that carry out the synthesis reactions; and the tRNA is responsible for selecting the correct amino acid and placing it at the ribosome for incorporation into the growing peptide.

Like DNA replication and transcription, translation occurs in three stages: initiation, elongation and termination. Each stage is well controlled by protein factors and each requires GTP as an energy source. During initiation a ribosome assembles at the start site on the mRNA and tRNA brings the first amino acid, usually methionine, to the growing complex. A second amino acid is attached to the ribosome and a **peptidyl transferase enzyme** activity, unusually present in the rRNA molecule, forms the first peptide linkage. This completes the initiation reactions. The ribosome begins to translocate along the mRNA in the 5′ to 3′ direction as tRNA molecules bring more amino acids to join the growing chain. These are the elongation reactions. Finally, the ribosome reaches a stop or termination signal in the mRNA and the complex stops and releases the complete peptide. Several **post-translational modifications** can occur to produce the mature protein: the peptide may be gylcosylated, phosphorylated or acetylated; it may be present in the form of a proprotein or preproprotein that is cleaved to produce the smaller mature proteins as in the case of insulin; or it may carry a signal peptide that will direct it to the site or organelle in the cell where it will function. Finally, the signal peptide may direct it to the endoplasmic reticulum and it may be used as a membrane protein or even be secreted from the cell.

The genetic code

An mRNA molecule is translated into a peptide using the genetic code. This is a triplet code in which three bases in RNA, i.e. originally in DNA and called a codon, code for a specific amino acid. The four bases in DNA can code for 64 different codons. Three of these are called termination or nonsense codons (UAG, UGA and UAA) and do not code for amino acids. One is the initiation codon (AUG) and codes for methione. Other important features of the genetic code are:
• it is degenerate: up to six different codons may code for the same amino acid;
• it is not ambiguous: a particular codon always codes for a particular amino acid;
• apart from the start and stop signals there is no other punctuation.
Thus when a ribosome starts synthesising a peptide at the first AUG codon in the mRNA it sets the reading frame: the next three bases will be the second codon and so on. Point mutations that add or delete one or two bases in a gene will alter the reading frame of a gene and alter the peptide sequence synthesised. This type of mutation is called a frameshift mutation. If three bases are deleted, the reading frame may not be altered but the peptide will be missing one amino acid; this is one of the common mutations responsible for cystic fibrosis.

The fact that the code is degenerate is an advantage to the cell. Some point mutations in DNA may result in an altered codon in the mRNA, but this new codon may also code for the same amino acid as the non-mutated codon: thus a normal protein is synthesised. This type of mutation is called a silent mutation.

17 Medical genetics

Stuart Brown

Figure 17.1 Examples of human chromosome structures

Short or
p arm
Centromere
Long or
q arm
2
1
1
2
a
b
c
d
e
f
g
h
i
a
b
h
g
f
e
d
c
i

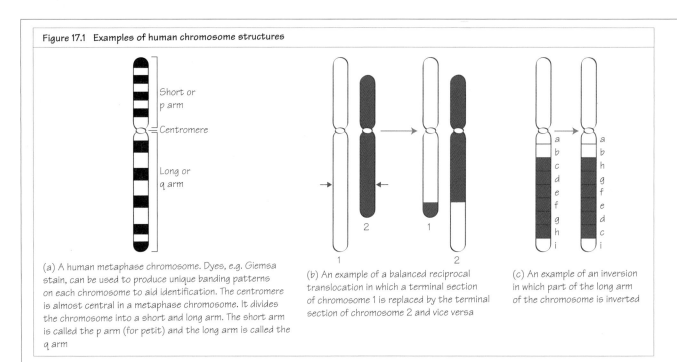

(a) A human metaphase chromosome. Dyes, e.g. Giemsa stain, can be used to produce unique banding patterns on each chromosome to aid identification. The centromere is almost central in a metaphase chromosome. It divides the chromosome into a short and long arm. The short arm is called the p arm (for petit) and the long arm is called the q arm

(b) An example of a balanced reciprocal translocation in which a terminal section of chromosome 1 is replaced by the terminal section of chromosome 2 and vice versa

(c) An example of an inversion in which part of the long arm of the chromosome is inverted

Figure 17.2 Common features associated with Down's syndrome

- Characteristic facial features
- Mental retardation
- Immune system abnormalities
- Increased risk of certain cancers, e.g. leukaemia
- Alzheimer-like dementia
- Infertility
- Cardiac, respiratory and gastrointestinal tract problems
- Possible epilepsy

Figure 17.3 A mechanism for tripet repeat sequence expansion

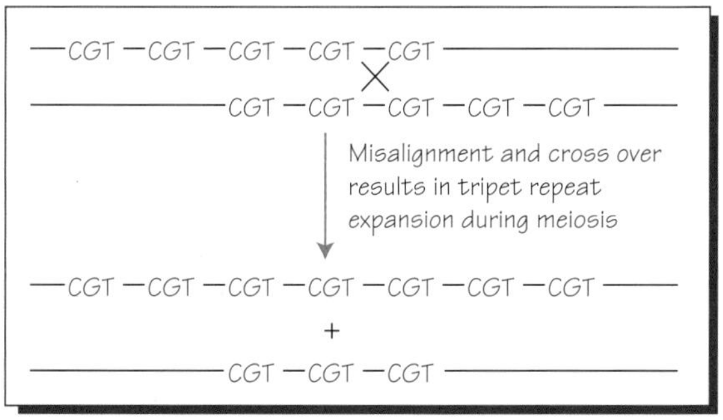

—CGT —CGT —CGT —CGT —CGT
CGT —CGT —CGT —CGT —CGT
Misalignment and cross over results in tripet repeat expansion during meiosis
—CGT —CGT —CGT —CGT —CGT —CGT —CGT
+
CGT —CGT —CGT

Figure 17.4 Possible effects of a point mutation

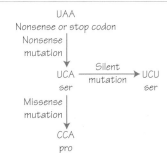

UAA
Nonsense or stop codon
Nonsense
mutation
UCA
ser
Silent
mutation
UCU
ser
Missense
mutation
CCA
pro

Point mutation may result in an altered phenotype, e.g. if the mutation alters the particular amino acid in a protein or if protein synthesis is prematurely terminated. However, since the genetic code is degenerate, i.e. up to 6 codons may code for a particular amino acid, the mutation may be silent. In the example shown both UCA and UCU code for serine

Genetic disease is a common cause of illness and even death. Approximately 3% of babies are affected by a genetic disease. Genetic diseases can be considered to be caused by chromosomal defects or single or multiple gene defects. One per cent of children admitted to hospitals suffer from chromosomal defects, 5–10% from single gene defects and 35–45% from multi-gene defects. Chromosomal defects are relatively common, with 15% of all conceptions affected, and if severe they usually result in miscarriage.

Chromosome structure

Human cells are **diploid**, i.e. there are two copies of each chromosome. They are the result of an 8000-fold condensation of chromatin during mitosis. The human genome consists of 23 pairs of chromosomes: 22 pairs of autosomes and a pair of sex chromosomes, XX for a female and XY for a male. The chromosome content of a cell is known as the **karyotype**. Each cell in an individual contains the same genome, known as the genotype. The expression of certain genes in different tissues refers to the phenotype.

Cytogenetic analysis shows that humans contain metaphase chromosomes (Figure 17.1).

Sources of genetic variation

• During reproduction the fertilisation of an ovum of one individual by the sperm of another.
• Human genes are inherited according to Mendelian laws. Offspring inherit one chromosome from each parent.
• During meiosis crossing-over of DNA between two chromatids occurs.

Mutations

A mutation is any permanent heritable change in DNA sequence. A mutagen is an agent that increases the mutation rate. There are two major types of mutation.

Chromosomal defects

During cell division the following changes in chromosome structure or content can occur.
• Gain of a whole set of chromosomes to form a tetraploid.
• Changes in the number of copies of a single chromosome arising from non-disjunction during meiosis, a failure to separate chromosomes correctly; the resulting cells are aneuploid, e.g. the gain of a chromosome results in a triploid cell. Triploidy is deleterious to the cell. Down syndrome results from the presence of three copies of chromosome 21. Fewer than 30% of Down fetuses survive to birth (Figure 17.2). For trisomy 18 (Edward's syndrome) and trisomy 13 (Patau syndrome) fewer than 10% survive to birth. Sex chromosomes are an exception to this. Aneuploidy is usually much less severe if a cell contains 47XXX, 47XXY, or 47XYY. This is as a result of the inactivation of all but one X chromosome in a somatic cell during the early stages of embryogenesis (known as the Lyon hypothesis) or the small number of genes on the Y chromosome.
Changes in chromosome structure can occur (Figure 17.1).
• Triplet repeat sequences occur in normal chromosomes. For example, the normal myotonin gene contains between five and 35 copies of a CTG sequence. The number of these repeats can increase during meiosis (Figure 17.3). In patients suffering from myotonic dystrophy, the number of these repeat sequences increases to greater

than 50 and may be over 1000. A similar situation occurs in a number of other diseases, including Huntington's disease. It is possible to estimate in which generation a future offspring will inherit sufficient triplet repeats to be affected by the disease. This phenomenon is known as anticipation.

Point mutations

A **point mutation** is the alteration of a single base in DNA. Point mutations can be caused by the following
• Spontaneous changes in DNA structure:
  – a defective DNA polymerase may introduce errors during replication;
  – a nucleotide may be in the incorrect tautomeric (isomeric) form such that it pairs with the wrong base.
• Chemicals can alter the H-bonding capacity of DNA bases.
• Physical agents such as X-rays or UV light can interact with DNA to cause breaks or cross-links.
Point mutations can have various effects on cells (Figure 17.4).
• They may have no effect. Following completion of the Human Genome Project in 2003 the 4 billion bases that make up the human genome have been sequenced and the number of genes present is estimated to be between 20 000 and 25 000. Thus genes occupy less than 10% of the genome. Mutations in the majority of DNA will not affect cell behaviour.
• In addition, the mutation may be **silent**.
• The mutation may be a **missense mutation**. This may have a range of effects on the host. For example, sickle cell anaemia is caused by a single base change resulting in a glutamate residue being replaced by valine at position 6 in the beta chain of haemoglobin. This substitution of a non-polar amino acid for a polar amino acid causes the red cells to 'sickle'. Sickle cell anaemia was the first haemoglobinopathy to be discovered and although more than 4000 are now known, it is still the most serious.
• The mutation may be a **nonsense mutation**. If the mutation results in the formation of a nonsense codon, no amino acid is inserted into the protein and the synthesis is prematurely terminated.

Treatment of genetic disease

The treatment of genetic disease has usually concentrated on the manipulation of the environment rather than genetic manipulation. The emphasis has been on prevention rather than cure. It is possible to avoid genetic disease by screening and prenatal diagnosis. It is also possible to reduce the effects of a genetic disease on an individual by altering the diet, e.g. for phenylketonuria or familial hypercholesterolemia. It is possible to replace certain materials or even organs in an individual, e.g blood transfusions in haemophilia patients or even liver transplants for patients with familial hypercholesterolemia. Cancer can be considered a genetic disease and great emphasis has been placed on avoiding the mutagens present in sunlight or cigarette smoke.

More recently considerable effort has been placed on **gene therapy**, the introduction of genetic material into a patient to replace the absent or damaged gene. Numerous trials have been undertaken and although progress has been slow, it is possible to treat diseases such as cystic fibrosis by introducing copies of the normal gene into the lungs of affected individuals. Viral and liposome vectors have been developed to deliver the new gene sequences and long-term success in the near future is possible.

Michael D Randall

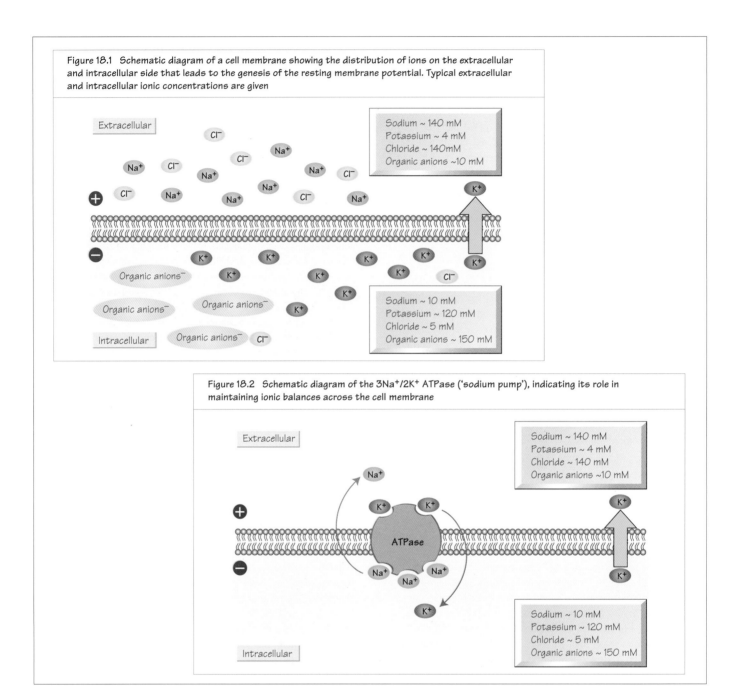

Figure 18.1 Schematic diagram of a cell membrane showing the distribution of ions on the extracellular and intracellular side that leads to the genesis of the resting membrane potential. Typical extracellular and intracellular ionic concentrations are given

Extracellular

Sodium ~ 140 mM
Potassium ~ 4 mM
Chloride ~ 140mM
Organic anions ~10 mM

Sodium ~ 10 mM
Potassium ~ 120 mM
Chloride ~ 5 mM
Organic anions ~ 150 mM

Intracellular

Figure 18.2 Schematic diagram of the $3Na^+/2K^+$ ATPase ('sodium pump'), indicating its role in maintaining ionic balances across the cell membrane

Extracellular

Sodium ~ 140 mM
Potassium ~ 4 mM
Chloride ~ 140 mM
Organic anions ~10 mM

ATPase

Sodium ~ 10 mM
Potassium ~ 120 mM
Chloride ~ 5 mM
Organic anions ~ 150 mM

Intracellular

Physiological processes (e.g. nervous conduction, the release of transmitters and hormones, muscle contractility) depend on cell excitability. Therefore, excitability and excitation of cells is tightly regulated.

Resting membrane potential (V_m)

Each cell in the body has an **electrical potential difference** which is determined by the distribution of ions across the cell membrane (Chapter 2). The potential difference across the membrane is the **membrane potential**. In the resting state the inside of the cell is negative on the intracellular side with respect to the outside, and this is the **resting membrane potential** (Figure 18.1). A typical value for a neurone is **−70 mV**, for skeletal muscle it is **−90 mV**. The resting membrane potential is determined by ionic balances across the cell membrane. The movement of ions is determined by both their electrical gradients and chemical gradients as driving forces; this is the **electrochemical potential gradient**. The ionic balance is governed by relative **membrane permeability**. For example, if we consider K^+ and organic anions, both have high intracellular concentrations and the chemical gradient favours their movement out of the cell. However, the membrane is more permeable to K^+ compared with the organic anions, and so the net efflux is K^+ unaccompanied by the anions. This results in the cell becoming more negative with respect to the outside. The balance of electrical and chemical work for K^+ is summarised by the **Nernst equation**:

$$E = \frac{RT}{F} \log_e \frac{[K]_o}{[K]_i}$$

where: E = membrane potential; $[K]_o$ = extracellular potassium; R = gas constant; $[K]_i$ = intracellular potassium; T = Absolute temperature; F = Faraday's constant.

At physiological temperatures the equation can be simplified to:

$$E = 61.5 \log_{10} \frac{[K]_o}{[K]_i}$$

When the electrical and chemical gradients are in balance there is no net flux of ions and E is the **Nernst potential** for the ion in question (e.g. for K^+ it is approximately −90 mV; for Na^+ it is approximately +65 mV).

As the membrane potential is governed by a number of ions, the equation can be modified to include each ion (the **Goldman field equation**), but the contribution of each is determined by **membrane permeability**:

$$E = \frac{RT}{F} \log_e \frac{P_k[K]_o + P_{Na}[Na]_o + P_{Cl}[Cl]_i}{P_K[K]_i + P_{Na}[Na]_i + P_{Cl}[Cl]_o}$$

where P_{ion} takes account of the ion's permeability.

In the resting state, the cell membrane is substantially more permeable to K^+, such that the membrane is typically 70- to 100-fold more permeable to K^+ compared with Na^+. The consequence of this is that the resting membrane potential of cells lies close to the equilibrium potential for K^+ (approx. −90 mV). Hence the major determinant of membrane potential is the extracellular K^+ concentration. By contrast, as the membrane is relatively impermeable to Na^+ in the resting state then changes in extracellular Na^+ concentration have little impact on the resting membrane potential.

The sodium pump (3Na⁺/2K⁺ ATPase)

This is a membrane transporter that uses ATP to pump $3Na^+$ ions out of the cell in exchange for $2K^+$ ions into the cell (Figure 18.2). While the sodium pump is **electrogenic**, its primary role is to maintain or replenish ionic balances, with Na^+ concentrations being high extracellularly/low intracellularly and K^+ concentrations being low extracellularly/high intracellularly. Hence the role of the pump is to maintain concentration gradients. The pump is in opposition to the electrical gradient for K^+ and since the membrane is relatively permeable to K^+ these ions pass out of the cell through K^+ channels to approach the Nernst potential for K^+. This leads to the setting up of the resting membrane potential. Only a small proportion of K^+ ions pass out to establish the resting membrane potential, with little impact on the concentration gradient.

While the membrane potential is small, the narrow width of the cell membrane (~10 nm) means that the electrical gradient is large (7 million volts per metre). This means that proteins within the cell are under an appreciable electrical force, and so changes in membrane potential lead to conformational changes in these proteins, which have significant regional charges. These conformational changes underpin activities such as the opening of voltage-operated ion channels.

Maintenance of the resting membrane potential is crucial to excitability. When a cell starts to depolarise (e.g. the propagation of an action potential, in response to activation of receptors, stimulation of mechanoreceptors) the change in potential may take the cell to threshold potential (Chapter 19). At this point the changes in the electrical field lead to conformation changes in **voltage-operated** (or gated) **ion channels** (VOCs). For example, at threshold in a neurone this leads to activation of voltage-operated Na^+ channels and the initiation of the action potential. Other examples of excitation may lead to the release of neurotransmitters and hormones. In pancreatic beta-cells, increases in ATP levels lead to closure of K^+ channels and this initiates depolarisation, which opens voltage-operated Ca^{2+} channels and the influx of Ca^{2+} leads to insulin secretion. This couples insulin secretion to states of raised ATP and glucose.

Hypokalaemia

A small reduction in extracellular K^+ below its normal range (3.5–5.3 mM) leads to the resting membrane potential becoming more negative with respect to the outside (**hyperpolarisation**). As a consequence the cell becomes less excitable, as it is more difficult for the cell to reach threshold potential and generate an action potential. A common cause of hypokalaemia is the use of diuretics (drugs that act on the kidney to promote fluid loss and are used in chronic heart failure and hypertension; Chapter 32). Diuretics reduce circulating volume, which activates the renin-angiotensin-aldosterone system (RAAS) (Chapters 32 and 38). The increased levels of aldosterone act on the distal convoluted tubules in the kidney to promote Na^+ reabsorption with the loss of K^+ from the body (Chapter 38).

Correction of hypokalaemia can be achieved by the use of K^+ supplements, K^+ rich foods (e.g. bananas) or K-sparing diuretics (e.g. spironolactone) that interfere with the actions of aldosteorone.

Hyperkalaemia

Increases in extracellular K^+ levels lead to cells becoming less negative with respect to the outside (**depolarisation**) and this results in cell excitation. For this reason, KCl should never be given by rapid intravenous injection as widespread cellular depolarisation is likely to prove fatal, often through abnormalities in cardiac rhythm. Hyperkalaemia is often associated with renal disease or the use of ACE inhibitors (Chapter 32), which block the RAAS and reduce K^+ loss (Chapter 38).

19 Nervous conduction

Michael D Randall

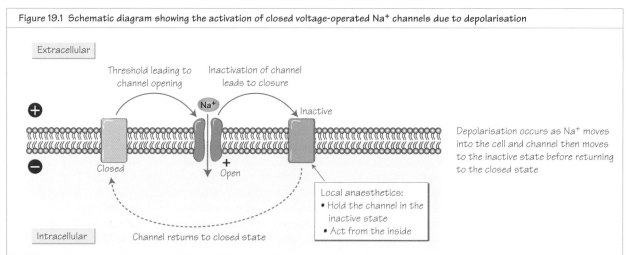

Figure 19.1 Schematic diagram showing the activation of closed voltage-operated Na⁺ channels due to depolarisation

Extracellular

Threshold leading to channel opening

Inactivation of channel leads to closure

Na^+

Inactive

Closed

Open
+

Depolarisation occurs as Na^+ moves into the cell and channel then moves to the inactive state before returning to the closed state

Local anaesthetics:
- Hold the channel in the inactive state
- Act from the inside

Intracellular

Channel returns to closed state

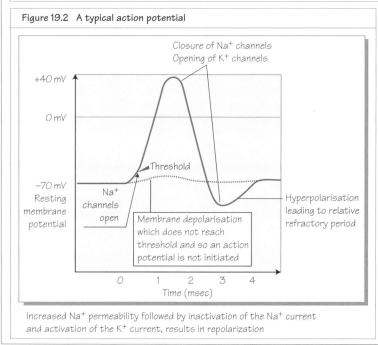

Figure 19.2 A typical action potential

Closure of Na^+ channels
Opening of K^+ channels

+40 mV

0 mV

Threshold

−70 mV
Resting membrane potential

Na^+ channels open

Membrane depolarisation which does not reach threshold and so an action potential is not initiated

Hyperpolarisation leading to relative refractory period

Time (msec)

Increased Na^+ permeability followed by inactivation of the Na^+ current and activation of the K^+ current, results in repolarization

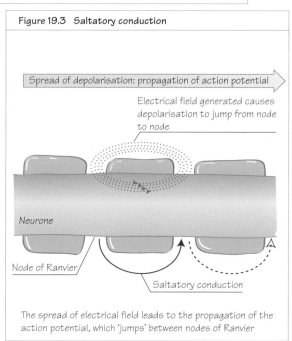

Figure 19.3 Saltatory conduction

Spread of depolarisation: propagation of action potential

Electrical field generated causes depolarisation to jump from node to node

Neurone

Node of Ranvier

Saltatory conduction

The spread of electrical field leads to the propagation of the action potential, which 'jumps' between nodes of Ranvier

Extracellular [K⁺] essentially determines resting **membrane potential** $(\mathbf{V_m})$ and ensures that excitation occurs at an appropriate time (Chapter 18). Excitation forms the basis of nervous conduction and also ensures the coupling of physiological responses (e.g. muscle contraction). Na⁺ ions play a central role in the initiation and propagation of excitation (Figure 19.1).

Neurones typically have a $\mathbf{V_m = -70\,mV}$, and following excitation (e.g. activation of receptors, the spread of nervous impulses) there is local **depolarisation** (i.e. the intracellular potential difference becomes less negative) and the membrane reaches **threshold**. At threshold, **voltage-operated Na⁺ channels** ('fast' sodium channels) undergo a conformation change and the channel opens. The increase in Na⁺ permeability causes an influx of Na⁺ ions down their **electrochemical gradient** and, as determined by the **Nernst equation**, the movement of ions attempts to take the membrane towards the equilibrium potential for Na⁺ (+65 mV).

Ion channels

Excitability is governed by ion channels. These are proteins that span the membrane and are permeable to specific ions. Their activity may be sensitive to voltage (voltage-operated) and their opening and closure are determined by the electrical environment. Other channel types are receptor-operated, in which events such as mechanical changes (e.g. stretch in **muscle spindle fibres**) cause the channel to open, leading to depolarisation (the **receptor generator potential**), which may lead to the initiation of action potentials.

The action potential

From **threshold** (approx. −50 mV) both the chemical and electrical gradients favour Na⁺ influx (Figure 19.2). As the membrane depolarises to a potential of 0 mV, the electrical gradient dissipates and is no longer apparent at 0 mV. At this point it is the chemical gradient that continues to drive Na⁺ influx such that the membrane potential becomes positive. As the membrane depolarises from 0 mV the electrical gradient starts to oppose force generated by the chemical gradient. The interplay of the chemical and electrical driving forces mean that there is depolarisation until (an **overshoot**) a peak membrane potential of approx. +40 mV is reached.

As the Na⁺ channels open this leads to the next step, which is channel closure. At the same time, the depolarisation due to the Na⁺ channels, leads to the activation of voltage-sensitive K⁺ channels. The closure of Na⁺ and activation of K⁺ channels limits the depolarisation. More importantly, the opening of K⁺ channels leads to K⁺ efflux and this leads to the membrane to repolarise, i.e. initiates the return of the membrane potential to the resting membrane potential and may overshoot to a **hyperpolarised** (more negative) and less excitable state.

Refractory period

The action potential is followed by a period (a few milliseconds) in which the cell cannot be excited. It has two components.

• **Absolute refractory period**: during which the cell cannot be excited, even at high stimuli. This is because the Na⁺ channel has three kinetic states: **Close – Open – Inactivated**. Once the channel has opened it enters the inactive state before returning to the closed state. While in the inactive state the channel is closed and it cannot be activated. The period of time the channel is in the inactive state is the absolute refractory period.

• **Relative refractory period**: once the Na⁺ channel returns to the closed state, the hyperpolarisation due to the K⁺ efflux results in reduced excitability, with the Na⁺ channels further from threshold and less likely to open. However, with increased stimulus (e.g. greater activation of mechanoreceptors and summation of receptor generator potentials) an action potential can be initiated, hence this refractory period is 'relative'.

The refractory period means that there is a maximum frequency of nervous impulses (~300 per second) and so nervous information is **frequency encoded** (the number of impulses correlates with the size of the stimulus).

Nervous conduction

The action potential is responsible for the transmission of electrical information. For this to occur, the action potential must spread or be propagated along the neurone. This is achieved by local depolarisation causing an adjacent region of the membrane to reach threshold, which causes the voltage operated Na⁺ channels to open, leading to depolarisation and the genesis of an action potential along the nerve.

Saltatory conduction

To achieve rapid nervous conduction consistent with a fast-reacting nervous system, large nerves have a sheet of myelin to insulate the nerve (Figure 19.3). At intervals of 1–2 mm the myelin is absent and these areas are the **nodes of Ranvier**. This means that the wave of depolarisation 'jumps' from node to node and this leads to rapid conduction of electrical activity, referred to as 'saltatory conduction'.

Speed of conduction

Larger diameter neurones are myelinated and have high conduction velocities. For example, Aα motor neurones have a diameter of 12–20 μm and conduction velocity of 70–120 m/s, whereas smaller nerves are unmyelinated and condition rates are slower, e.g. C pain fibres are unmyelinated with a diameter of ~1 μm and conduction velocities of 0.5–2.3 m/s.

Local anaesthetics

These are drugs (e.g. lidocaine) that block the transmission of pain by inhibiting action potential propagation. Local anaesthetics block action potential conduction in sensory nerves. They block voltage-operated Na⁺ channels by binding to the channel in the 'Inactive' state. The channel is then held in the inactive state, and this prevents further activation and the propagation of action potentials. Many local anaesthetics show **use-dependence**, which means that as the frequency of action potentials increase, the level of blockade increases.

For local anaesthetics to act they must penetrate the cell membrane to act on the channel from the inside and this only occurs when the drug is in the uncharged form. Local anaesthetics are often weak bases and so show pH-dependence. As they are weak bases they are protonated (charged) at lower pHs and only at higher pH does the uncharged form predominate and it is in this form that the drug can penetrate the cell membrane and act on the channel from the intracellular side.

Cardiac action potentials (Chapter 30)

The classic neuronal action potential is not the only form of an action potential. Cardiac activity also involves the propagation of electrical activity. In the ventricles, the Na⁺-channel-led depolarisation also activates voltage-operated Ca²⁺ channels, resulting in Ca²⁺ influx and cardiac contraction. The opening of the Ca²⁺ channels is prolonged, resulting in a plateau of the action potential.

20 Synaptic transmission

Michael D Randall

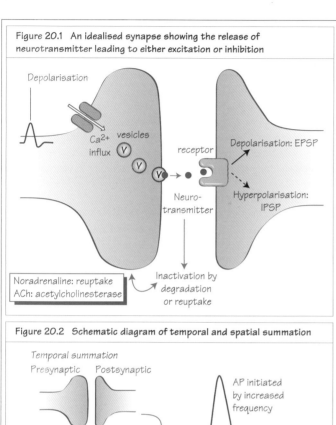

Figure 20.1 An idealised synapse showing the release of neurotransmitter leading to either excitation or inhibition

Depolarisation

Ca²⁺ influx

vesicles

receptor

Neuro-transmitter

Depolarisation: EPSP

Hyperpolarisation: IPSP

Noradrenaline: reuptake
ACh: acetylcholinesterase

Inactivation by degradation or reuptake

Figure 20.2 Schematic diagram of temporal and spatial summation

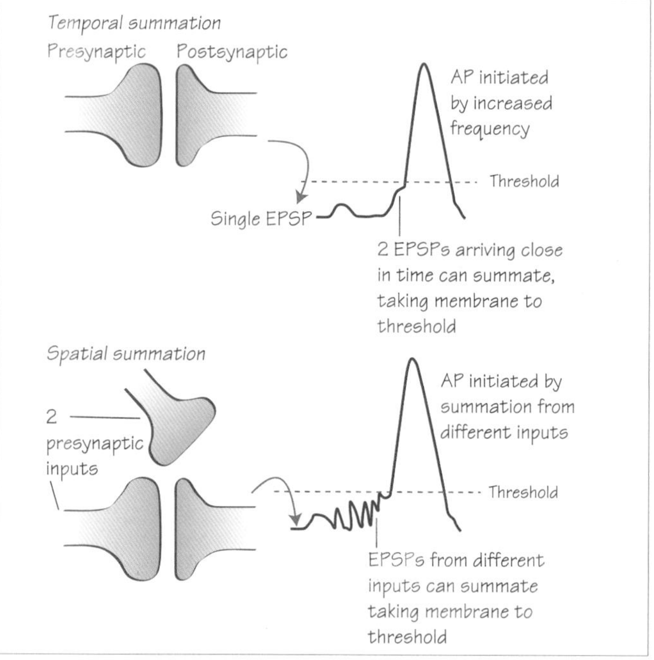

Temporal summation
Presynaptic   Postsynaptic

AP initiated by increased frequency

Single EPSP

Threshold

2 EPSPs arriving close in time can summate, taking membrane to threshold

Spatial summation

2 presynaptic inputs

AP initiated by summation from different inputs

Threshold

EPSPs from different inputs can summate taking membrane to threshold

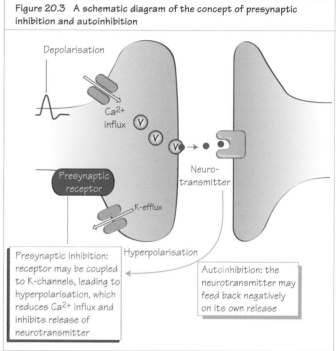

Figure 20.3 A schematic diagram of the concept of presynaptic inhibition and autoinhibition

Depolarisation

Ca²⁺ influx

Presynaptic receptor

K-efflux

Neuro-transmitter

Hyperpolarisation

Presynaptic inhibition: receptor may be coupled to K-channels, leading to hyperpolarisation, which reduces Ca²⁺ influx and inhibits release of neurotransmitter

Autoinhibition: the neurotransmitter may feed back negatively on its own release

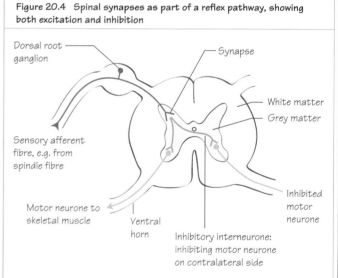

Figure 20.4 Spinal synapses as part of a reflex pathway, showing both excitation and inhibition

Dorsal root ganglion

Synapse

White matter

Grey matter

Sensory afferent fibre, e.g. from spindle fibre

Motor neurone to skeletal muscle

Ventral horn

Inhibitory interneurone: inhibiting motor neurone on contralateral side

Inhibited motor neurone

Nervous activity involves the spread of electrical charge via the generation and propagation of action potentials. Communication between neurones is predominantly via chemical transmission at synapses, in which an impulse in one fibre leads to the release of neurotransmitter, which acts on an adjacent neurone. In the autonomic nervous system a **presynaptic fibre** may synapse with a single **postsynaptic fibre**, which then releases neurotransmitters to control the target tissue. Synaptic transmission ensures that nervous conduction is **orthodromic**, i.e. unidirectional. In the central nervous system (CNS) a neurone may make up to 10 000 synapses with other neurones, reflecting the complexity and integration of connections with the CNS.

General principles

The arrival of the action potential at the presynaptic terminal leads to depolarisation, which activates voltage-sensitive Ca^{2+} channels resulting in Ca^{2+} influx. The rise in intracellular Ca^{2+} then leads to **exocytosis** of neurotransmitter vesicles and the release of neurotransmitter into the **synaptic cleft**. The neurotransmitter then binds to receptors on the postsynaptic terminal, leading to activation or inhibition of the neurone. The activation often involves depolarisation, leading to an **EPSP (excitatory postsynaptic potential)**, and inhibition often leads to hyperpolarisation with an **IPSP (inhibitory postsynaptic potential)**. The neurotransmitter is then degraded or taken up by transport mechanisms (Figure 20.1).

Temporal and spatial summation of impulses

The post-synaptic events, whether excitatory or inhibitory, may be additive. For example, if two excitatory impulses are close in time (i.e. temporally close) then the EPSPs in the post-synaptic cell may combine, leading to greater depolarisation and so increasing the probability of the cell reaching threshold and initiating an action potential. This leads to an enhancement of excitation, termed **temporal summation** (Figure 20.2).

For a post-synaptic neurone that has multiple presynaptic inputs, then the EPSPs (or IPSPs) derived from different connections can summate (or act in opposition) and so determine whether the cell reaches threshold and sets up an action potential. This is termed **spatial summation** (Figure 20.2).

The consequence of these properties of summation mean that information may be reinforced by high-frequency stimulation and that there is integration information from the different inputs.

Presynaptic inhibition

Synaptic transmission may be modulated by **presynaptic inhibition** (Figure 20.3). Under these circumstances a neurotransmitter (e.g. endogenous opioids such as the enkaphalins) or drug (e.g. opioids such as morphine) acts on presynaptic receptors, leading to hyperpolarisation, and this opposes the release of neurotransmitters. An example of this is when opioids act at μ-opioid receptors, leading to an inhibition of adenylyl cyclase, leading to a reduction in cAMP and the activation of a K-conductance. This results in hyperpolarisation, which stabilises the cell membrane and opposes synaptic transmission. This can explain the ability of opioids to inhibit pain transmission via sensory nerves and to cause constipation via inhibition of parasympathetic nerves responsible for lower gastrointestinal motility. There may also be **autoinhibition**. For example, at noradrenergic synapses the released noradrenaline may stimulate the target post-synaptic adrenoceptors but also act on presynaptic α_2-adrenoceptors, which reduce further transmitter release. This leads to negative feedback.

Cholinergic transmission

Acetylcholine (ACh) is involved at all autonomic ganglia and activates nicotinic receptors to activate postsynaptic fibres. It is also released by postganglionic parasympathetic fibres to activate muscarinic receptors on the target organ/tissue. ACh is also the neurotransmitter at neuromuscular junctions to stimulate nicotinic receptors on skeletal muscle. Once released, ACh is metabolised by **acetylcholinesterase (AChE)**, leading to inactivation and the reuptake of choline into the presynaptic terminal.

Noradrenergic transmission

Noradrenaline is the neurotransmitter that is released by sympathetic nerves and acts on the target tissues/organs. It activates alpha (α_1 and α_2)-adrenoceptors and beta (β_1 and β_2)-adrenoceptors. The activity of noradrenaline is terminated by **neuronal and non-neuronal uptake** via specific transporters. Following reuptake noradrenaline is metabolised by **monoamine oxidases**.

The neuronal reuptake of noradrenaline is a site of drug action and is inhibited by tricyclic antidepressants (e.g. amitripyline), which increase the levels of noradrenaline in the synaptic cleft. Some older antidepressants also act via inhibition of the monoamine oxidases.

Ionotropic neurotransmission

Ionotropic transmission is when the postsynaptic receptor is coupled to ion channels (ligand-gated), leading to a rapid depolarisation (excitation) or hyperpolarisation (inhibition). It occurs when a rapid 'on-off' response is required.

Metabotropic neurotransmission

Metabotropic transmission is when the postsynaptic receptor activation leads to a biochemical response in the target tissue, e.g. β-adrenoceptors activating adenylyl cyclase, leading to an increase in cAMP. In the heart, β_1-adrenoceptors increase cAMP, leading to an increase force and rate of contraction; in the airways, β_2-adrenoceptors increase intracellular cAMP, leading to relaxation of bronchial smooth muscle.

Inhibitory neurotransmission

Inhibition of nerve activity in the nervous system is key to nervous control. In the spinal cord, glycine, and in the brain, GABA, are examples of inhibitory transmissions. Both cause cellular hyperpolarisation by setting up IPSPs through inotropic receptors. In the spine, this dampens reflexes by having inhibitory modulation. In the brain, GABA is a key inhibitory transmitter that acts at $GABA_A$ receptors, in which the receptor complex is associated with a chloride channel, which in opening allows chloride influx and hyperpolarisation. The **benzodiazepines** (e.g. diazepam) enhance the actions of GABA at the $GABA_A$ receptors, leading to enhanced inhibition, resulting in sedation and anticonvulsive effects.

Spinal reflexes (Figure 20.4)

Synaptic transmission underpins spinal reflexes. The simple monosynaptic pathway involves sensory information (e.g. from spindle fibres, pain receptors) arriving at the dorsal root and activating a motorneurone via an excitatory synapse. This can lead to a simple reflex arc, e.g. the patella tendon reflex. The communication is more complex in that the sensory nerve can activate an inhibitory interneurone, which then inhibits for example a motor neurone on the contralateral side, resulting in inhibition of an opposing muscle.

21 Autonomic nervous system

Michael D Randall

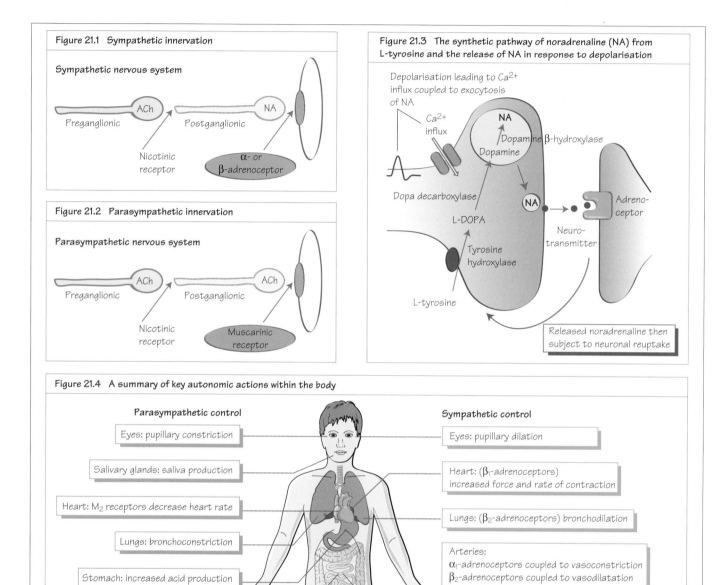

Figure 21.1 Sympathetic innervation

Sympathetic nervous system

Preganglionic — ACh — Postganglionic — NA

Nicotinic receptor

α- or β-adrenoceptor

Figure 21.2 Parasympathetic innervation

Parasympathetic nervous system

Preganglionic — ACh — Postganglionic — ACh

Nicotinic receptor

Muscarinic receptor

Figure 21.3 The synthetic pathway of noradrenaline (NA) from L-tyrosine and the release of NA in response to depolarisation

Depolarisation leading to Ca²⁺ influx coupled to exocytosis of NA

Ca²⁺ influx

NA

Dopamine β-hydroxylase

Dopamine

Dopa decarboxylase

L-DOPA

Tyrosine hydroxylase

L-tyrosine

NA

Neuro-transmitter

Adreno-ceptor

Released noradrenaline then subject to neuronal reuptake

Figure 21.4 A summary of key autonomic actions within the body

Parasympathetic control

- Eyes: pupillary constriction
- Salivary glands: saliva production
- Heart: M_2 receptors decrease heart rate
- Lungs: bronchoconstriction
- Stomach: increased acid production
- Gastrointestinal tract: increased motility
- Bladder: (M_3 receptors) contraction and micturition

Sympathetic control

- Eyes: pupillary dilation
- Heart: (β_1-adrenoceptors) increased force and rate of contraction
- Lungs: (β_2-adrenoceptors) bronchodilation
- Arteries: α_1-adrenoceptors coupled to vasoconstriction β_2-adrenoceptors coupled to vasodilatation
- Gastrointestinal tract: (β-adrenoceptors) decreased motility
- Bladder: (β-adrenoceptors) relaxation and storage of urine (α-adrenoceptors) contraction of neck and urethra

The autonomic nervous system regulates involuntary actions such as breathing, the regulation of cardiac contractions, blood pressure control, gastrointestinal secretions and motility, control of pupil diameter, sweating, bladder control and sexual function.

The autonomic nervous system is divided into the **sympathetic** and **parasympathetic** systems (Figures 21.1 and 21.2). Both systems involve preganglionic and postganglionic fibres. In both cases, **acetylcholine** (ACh) is the neurotransmitter at the ganglionic synapse, where it stimulates ligand-gated **nicotinic receptors**, leading to the activation of the postganglionic fibres. These in turn lead to the activation of target receptors on the innervated tissue.

 Medical Sciences at a Glance, First Edition. Edited by Michael D Randall. © 2014 John Wiley & Sons, Ltd. Published 2014 by John Wiley & Sons, Ltd.

Parasympathetic control

In the parasympathetic nervous system, the ganglion is generally located close to, or in, the innervated organ and generally leads to more localised control. The postganglionic neurotransmitter is Ach, which acts at muscarinic receptors.

Muscarinic receptors are G-protein-coupled receptors (GPCRs) in which the subtypes M_1, M_3 and M_5 are coupled via $G_{q/11}$ to Ca^{2+} mobilisation; and M_2 and M_4 are G_i-linked to inhibition of formation of the second messenger cAMP (Chapter 7).

Sympathetic control

Anatomically this tends to provide more 'global' control, with the autonomic ganglia or synapses being located more centrally and closer to the spinal cord. The postganglionic neurotransmitter is noradrenaline (Figure 21.3), which acts at α- or β-adrenoceptors, depending on the tissue. An exception are the sweat glands, which are functionally sympathetic but have ACh as the neurotransmitter, which stimulates muscarinic (M) receptors.

An extension of the sympathetic nervous system is the adrenal medulla, which is essentially a sympathetic postganglionic fibre where ACh acts at nicotinic receptors to stimulate the release of adrenaline (and some noradrenaline) into the circulation. Adrenaline then exerts sympathetic actions (e.g. increase in heart rate and bronchodilation). This forms part of the 'fright, flight or fight' response.

Adrenoceptors

α_1-adrenoceptors are coupled via G-proteins ($G_{q/11}$) to activation of phospholipase C, which liberates inositol trisphophate (IP_3) and diacyl glycerol (DAG), leading to increases in intracellular Ca^{2+}.

α_2-adrenoceptors are negatively coupled via G_i to adenylyl cyclase, leading to reductions in cAMP.

β_1- and β_2-adrenoceptors are also GPCRs in which G_s is coupled to the activation of adenylyl cyclase and elevations in cAMP.

Autonomic regulation (Figure 21.4)

Cardiac control (Chapter 30)

Sympathetic: noradrenaline acts at β_1-adrenoceptors to increase the force (inotropy) and rate of cardiac contractions, (positive chronotropy).

Parasympathetic: ACh acts at M_2 receptors to reduce the heart rate (negative chronotropy).

Pharmacology: β-adrenoceptor antagonists (beta-blockers) are used to block cardiac β_1-adrenoceptors in the treatment of angina (e.g. atenolol) and heart failure (e.g. bisoprolol) (Chapter 35).

Vascular control (Chapter 31)

Sympathetic: noradrenaline acts at α_1- and α_2-adrenoceptors on vascular smooth muscle on arteries to cause vasoconstriction, and β_2-adrenoceptors (in skeletal muscle) to cause vasodilatation.
• α_1-adrenoceptor antagonists (e.g. prazosin) are used as antihypertensives but their use is limited by widespread side effects through interference of sympathetic control.
• Adrenaline is used to increase cardiac output and cause bronchodilation in anaphylactic shock.
• Sympathomimetic agents: these agents mimic the sympathetic nervous system and are widely used as decongestants. These actions can be direct (due to receptor agonism, e.g. phenylephrine) or indirect (by displacing and releasing noradrenaline, e.g. pseudoephedrine). They cause local vasoconstriction, reducing blood flow and mucus.

Central control of the cardiovascular system

In the cardiovascular control centres of the central nervous system noradrenaline activates α_2-adrenoceptors to decrease sympathetic outflow and increase vagal output.

Respiratory control (Chapter 26)

Sympathetic: circulating adrenaline acts at β_2-adrenoceptors to cause bronchodilation.

Parasympathetic: ACh acts at M_3 receptors to cause bronchoconstriction and increase mucus secretion.
• β_2-adrenoceptor agonists (e.g. salbutamol) are bronchodilators and are used as 'relievers' in asthma. Longer-acting β_2-agonists (e.g. salmeterol) are used for longer-term control as 'preventers' in asthma and chronic obstructive pulmonary disease (COPD).
• Muscarinic receptor antagonists (e.g. ipratropium) block parasympathetic bronchoconstriction and are used as bronchodilators in COPD.
• Beta-blockers (even β_1-selective) are contraindicated in asthma as they can block bronchial β_2-adrenoceptors, causing severe bronchospasm.

Gastrointestinal control (Chapters 42 and 43)

Salivary glands: parasympathetic control via ACh acting at M_3 receptors stimulates the production of saliva and increases blood flow. Sympathetic stimulation leads to the production of viscous saliva.

Gastric acid secretion: ACh acts at M_1 and M_3 receptors on parietal cells to stimulate gastric acid production.

Gastrointestinal motility: Muscarinic receptors are coupled to increased motility. Muscarinic receptor antagonists reduce motility and lead to constipation. They are sometimes used as antispasmodic agents.

Bladder control (Chapter 40)

Parasympathetic: ACh acts at M_3 receptors, which are coupled to contraction of the detrusor muscle, and at M receptors at the trigone and sphincter muscles leading to relaxation. These actions lead to bladder voiding.

Sympathetic: noradrenaline acts at β_2- and β_3-adrenoceptors to relax the detrusor muscle and at α_1-adrenoceptors at the trigone and sphincter muscles, leading to contraction.

Pharmacology: muscarinic receptor antagonists (e.g. oxybutynin) are used to relax the bladder and reduce the symptoms of overactive bladder. α_1-adrenoceptor antagonists (e.g. tamsulosin) are used to relax prostatic smooth muscle and so reduce prostatic obstruction.

Visual system

Sympathetic: α-adrenoceptors are coupled to pupilary dilation.

Parasympathetic: M_3 receptors are coupled to pupilary constriction.

Pharmacology: muscarinic receptor antagonists (e.g. tropicamide) are used as eye drops to dilate the pupils in ophthalmic examinations. Muscarinic agonists (e.g. pilocarpine) are used to constrict the pupils (miosis), which reduces pressure in closed-angle glaucoma.

Co-transmission

In addition to the 'classical' mediators of autonomic transmission, other mediators may also act in concert to form co-transmission. These are termed 'NANC' transmitters, as they are non-adrenergic and non-cholinergic. Important examples of co-transmitters include the purine ATP and neuropeptide Y (sympathetic), and vasoactive intestinal polypeptide and nitric oxide (parasympathetic), and these may be released in addition to the classical transmitter. Their release may enhance the actions of the 'classical' transmitter or be released differentially under certain circumstances (e.g. at different frequencies of stimulation).

22 Neuromuscular transmission

Michael D Randall

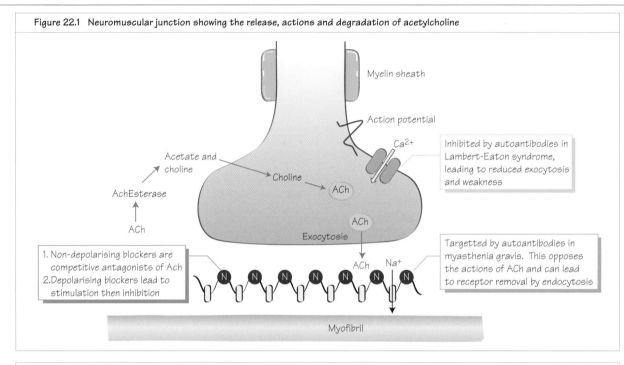

Figure 22.1 Neuromuscular junction showing the release, actions and degradation of acetylcholine

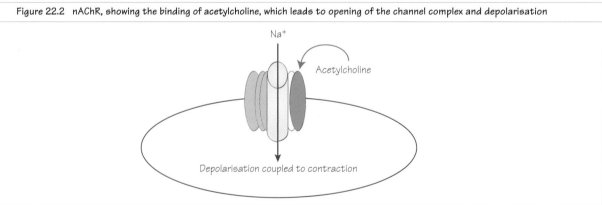

Figure 22.2 nAChR, showing the binding of acetylcholine, which leads to opening of the channel complex and depolarisation

Medical Sciences at a Glance, First Edition. Edited by Michael D Randall. © 2014 John Wiley & Sons, Ltd. Published 2014 by John Wiley & Sons, Ltd.

Neuromuscular junction (NMJ)

The neuromuscular junction (NMJ) is a specialised synapse between motor neurones and skeletal muscle, which enables nervous control of skeletal muscle contraction. At the NMJ, the neurone and skeletal membrane are brought into close contact by folding and the outside of the neurone is held in place by a **Schwann cell**. Anatomically, a collection of neuromuscular junctions form a **motor end plate**.

At the NMJ action potentials in the motor neurone cause depolarisation of the presynaptic terminal (**bouton**), which leads to the opening of voltage-operated (gated) Ca^{2+} channels and the influx of Ca^{2+} ions. The influx of Ca^{2+} ions then stimulates the **exocytosis** of synaptic vesicles containing the neurotransmitter **acetylcholine (ACh)** (Figure 22.1).

When released, ACh diffuses across the synaptic cleft (typically 50 nm) and stimulates postsynaptic **ionotropic nicotinic receptors**. The **nicotinic acetylcholine receptor** (nAChR) is an ion-channel complex of five transmembraneous subunits (α_2, β, δ, γ) and opens on activation by ACh. The open ion-channel complex is permeable to both Na^+ (influx) and K^+ (efflux), and following activation there is transient cellular depolarisation, which leads to a **miniature end plate potential (mEPP)** of typically 0.4 mV. The vesicles of ACh are of a relatively consistent size and so the transmission is quantal, with packages of excitation leading to steps in excitation. The mEPPs generated at the NMJ summate to form **excitatory post-synaptic potentials** (EPPs) and once threshold is reached lead to actions potential via voltage-operated Na^+ channels (sensitive to tetrodotoxin), which are propagated across the skeletal muscle by spreading depolarisation. The depolarisation of the skeletal muscle is coupled (via the T-tubular system) to Ca^{2+} release from the intracellular sarcoplasmic reticulum stores and the increase in intracellular Ca^{2+} leads to contraction of the skeletal muscle (Figures 22.1 and 22.2).

The actions of ACh (and therefore the signal for contraction) are terminated by **acetylcholinesterase (AChE)**, which breaks down ACh into acetate and choline. The choline is then recycled by reuptake by the presynaptic terminal. The reuptake mechanism can be blocked by hemicholinium.

Neuromuscular blockers

Neuromuscular transmission is targeted therapeutically by neuromuscular blockers, which are used in surgery to prevent muscle contraction, e.g. to prevent abdominal muscle contractions during abdominal surgery. Neuromuscular blockers are divided into two main classes.

Non-depolarising blockers (e.g. tubocurarine, pancuronium)

These drugs were developed from the neurotoxin curare, which was used in South American poisoned arrows.

These are competitive receptor antagonists of ACh at the nAChR. The onset of blockade leads to paralysis, as they block the actions of ACh. The blockade is dose-dependent and may be overcome by inhib-itors of AChE, which lead to increased levels of ACh to compete with the blocker.

Depolarising blockers (e.g. suxamethonium)

These are actually agonists at the nAChR and the onset of action is initially accompanied by stimulation, which leads to muscle twitches. However, the activation of the nAChR leads to prolonged depolarisation of the skeletal muscle and inactivation of the voltage-operated Na^+ channels that propagate the action potentials. It is the inactivation of these Na^+ channels that leads to failure of neuromuscular control and paralysis. In contrast to non-depolarising blockade, the inhibition by depolarising agents cannot be reversed by inhibition of AChE.

Toxins and the neuromuscular transmission

The exocytosis of vesicles can be blocked by **botulinum toxin**, which prevents fusion of the vesicles with the cell membrane, and this inhibition of release leads to paralysis.

The nAChR is sensitive to blockade by **α-bungarotoxin**. This is a snake-derived venon that binds irreversibly to the nAChR and is used extensively on neurophysiology to investigate the regulation of NMJs.

Inhibitors of acetylcholinesterase (AChE)

These prevent the breakdown of ACh and are used therapeutically in myasthenia gravis (MG). Inhibition also occurs with organophosphorus insecticides and nerve toxins, which lead to perpetual activation of neuromuscular transmission. Hence they are used in insecticides and nerve gases to disrupt neuromuscular control, leading to death.

AChE inhibitors are also used therapeutically to enhance the actions of ACh in the brain to improve cognitive function in Alzheimer's disease (Chapter 57).

Pathophysiology
Myasthenia gravis

This is a rare disease that affects neuromuscular transmission. It is associated with muscle weakness and an inability for prolonged muscle contraction due to impaired neuromuscular transmission. MG is caused by autoantibodies which bind to and block the nAChRs, so preventing the actions of ACh and muscle contraction. In some cases, the antibodies lead to endocytosis of the receptors and their removal from the membrane. To overcome the impaired actions of ACh inhibitors of AChE (e.g. neostigmine) are used to prevent the breakdown of ACh and so enhance its actions.

Lambert-Eaton myasthenic syndrome

This is characterised by the production of antibodies against the presynaptic Ca^{2+} channels involved in stimulating exocytosis of ACh vesicles. In this condition there is reduced ACh release, leading to weakness. However, the inhibitory effects of the antibodies can be overcome by increased Ca^{2+} influx and so the weakness can improve on exercise.

23 Structure of the respiratory system

Siobhan Loughna and Deborah Merrick

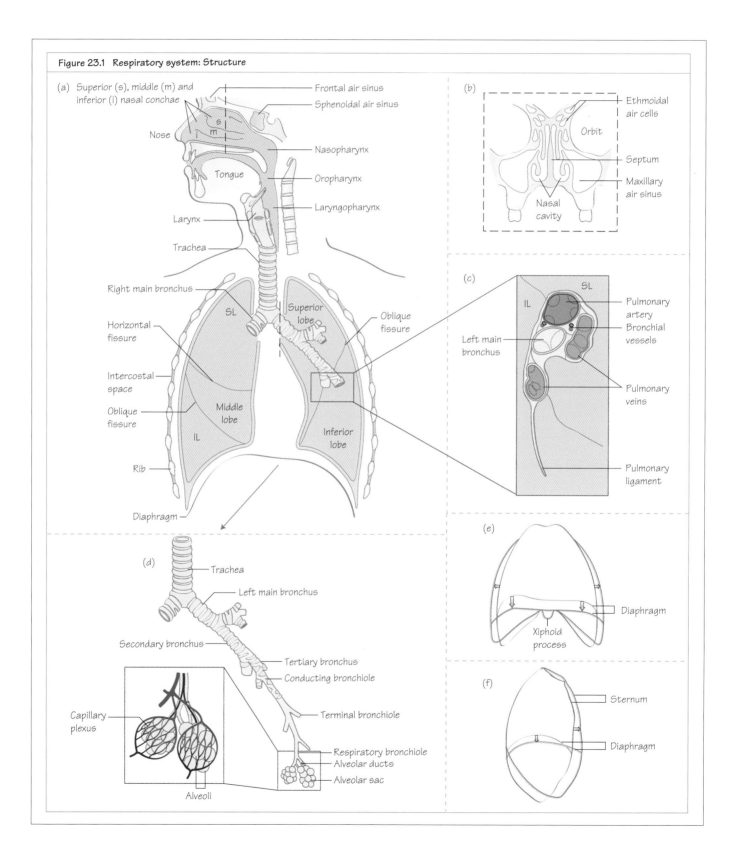

Figure 23.1 Respiratory system: Structure

The respiratory tract extends from the lips and nostrils to the alveoli of the lungs (Figure 23.1). It comprises a network of conducting and respiratory airways allowing air to pass into (inspiration) and out of (expiration) the lungs for gas exchange. The respiratory tract can be divided into upper and lower respiratory tracts for descriptive purposes.

Upper respiratory tract
Nasal cavities
These extend from the nostrils anteriorly to the posterior nasal apertures (choanae) posteriorly, and are divided into right and left halves by the nasal septum. Except for the vestibule of the nose, mucosa lines the nasal cavity. Air passing over the mucosa is warmed, filtered and moistened in preparation for efficient gas exchange, before passing further into the respiratory tract. The mucosa lining the majority of the respiratory tract is composed of **pseudostratified ciliated columnar epithelium** (respiratory epithelium). In certain areas within the nasal cavity the mucosa is modified for the specialised function of olfaction (olfactory epithelium). The nasal conchae, which increase the surface area, further divide each nasal cavity into four spaces: spheno-ethmoidal recess, superior nasal meatus, middle nasal meatus and inferior nasal meatus (Figure 23.1). The **paranasal sinuses** are air-filled cavities found within the frontal, maxilla, sphenoid and ethmoid bones (Figures 23.1 and 23.2). They communicate with the nasal cavities via small apertures.

Oral cavity
This extends from the lips anteriorly to the oropharynx posteriorly. It is divided into the oral vestibule and oral cavity proper. The oral vestibule is the slit-like space between the lips cheeks, teeth and gingivae. The oral cavity proper is the space posterior and medial to upper and lower dental arches; it contains the teeth and tongue.

Pharynx and larynx
This is the superior expansion of the alimentary system and is involved in the conduction of air to the larynx, trachea and lungs. It is a fibromuscular passage divided into three regions (Figure 23.1): **nasopharynx** (posterior to the nasal cavity), **oropharynx** (posterior to the oral cavity) and the **laryngopharynx** (posterior to the larynx). The **larynx** connects the oropharynx to the trachea. It has various important functions, including routing air into the lower respiratory tract, maintaining a patent respiratory tract and voice production.

Lower respiratory tract
Trachea and bronchial tree
The trachea is a fibrocartilaginous tube that extends from the larynx inferiorly and is characterised by C-shaped rings of hyaline cartilage contained within its walls. At vertebral level T4/5, the trachea bifurcates into two primary bronchi, with one passing to each lung. Within the lung, each bronchi divides repeatedly to form the bronchial tree (Figure 23.4). Each main bronchus divides into secondary bronchi (three on the right, two on the left – one to each lobe), which in turn divide into tertiary bronchi. The branching continues through terminal and respiratory bronchioles to alveolar ducts, alveolar sacs and the basic unit of gas exchange, the alveolus. The bronchioles are lined by ciliated simple columnar epithelium, transitioning to simple cuboidal epithelium in smaller peripheral branches. The alveoli are composed of type I pneumocytes (lining cells) and type II pneumocytes (surfactant producing cells).

Lungs
The lungs are divided by horizontal and oblique fissures into lobes, three on the right and two on the left (Figure 23.1). The root of the lung is formed by structures that enter and leave the lung (Figure 23.3). These include the main bronchus, a pulmonary artery supplying blood to the lung and two pulmonary veins draining blood from the lung. The bronchial vessels supply structures at the root of the lung, supporting tissues of the lung and viscera pleura. Innervation of the lungs is via the pulmonary plexuses containing parasympathetic and sympathetic fibres. **Parasympathetic innervation** (vagus nerves) causes bronchoconstriction, vasodilatation (pulmonary vessels) and secretomotor. **Sympathetic innervation** is limited to mainly **circulating adrenaline**, which causes bronchodilation and inhibits secretions.

Pleura: a serous pleural sac that is composed of two membranes.
• Visceral pleura: covers the lungs and is adherent to its surface.
• Parietal pleura: lines the pulmonary cavities and is divided according to the region it lines: cervical, costal, diaphragmatic, mediastinal (Figure 23.1; right lung).
The mediastinal parietal pleura is continuous with the visceral pleura at the root of the lung. Serous pleural fluid is contained between the pleura membranes, allowing the two layers to glide over each other smoothly during respiration.

Thoracic wall
This is composed of bones, cartilages, muscles, vessels, nerves, fascia and skin. It provides protection for the thoracic organs and plays a role in respiration.

Thoracic cage: consists of 12 ribs and costal cartilages, 12 thoracic vertebrae and associated intervertebral discs, and the sternum. The ribs are described as true (1–7), false (8–10), or floating (11 and 12).

Intercostal muscles: comprise three muscle layers (external, internal and innermost) located within the intercostal spaces, between the ribs. These muscles receive innervation from the intercostal nerves (T1–T11) which run within the intercostal spaces. The intercostal muscles act as accessory muscles of respiration.

Diaphragm
The main muscle of respiration which forms the convex floor of the thoracic cavity. The diaphragm receives all motor innervation and some of its sensory innervation from the phrenic nerves (C3, 4, 5). The periphery of the diaphragm receives sensory innervation from the intercostal (T5–T11) and subcostal (T12) nerves.

Movements of the thoracic wall and diaphragm: change intrathoracic diameters and volumes during respiration, resulting in changes in intrathoracic pressure (Figures 23.5 and 23.6). During inspiration the vertical dimension of the central part of the thoracic cavity increases as the diaphragm descends. As the diaphragm relaxes, during expiration, the vertical dimension returns to a neutral position. The transverse dimension of the thoracic cavity also increases slightly during inspiration due to the intercostal muscles raising the lateral aspect of the ribs. The intercostal muscles also alter the anteroposterior dimension of the thorax by elevating the anterior ends of the ribs and sternum.

Lymphatic drainage of thoracic wall and respiratory tract
Lymph returns to the venous system via either the right lymphatic duct (draining right side of the thorax, head and neck and the right upper limb) or the thoracic duct (rest of body). Both lymphatic ducts drain into the junction of the subclavian and internal jugular veins (right and left venous angles respectively).

24 Respiratory physiology

Steven Burr

Figure 24.1 Factors affecting the distributions of inhaled gases

(a) As chest expands airways widen, resistance to airflow decreases and inflation is easier, limits exhalation not inhalation

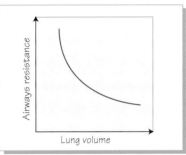

(b) As chest expands mechanical limits restrict volume, elastic forces increase and deflation is easier, limits inhalation not exhalation

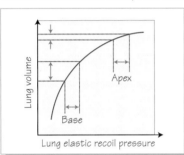

Same change in pressure yields a greater change in volume at bases than apical. Hence resting breathing is normally diaphragmatic

Figure 24.2 Alveolar gas exchange

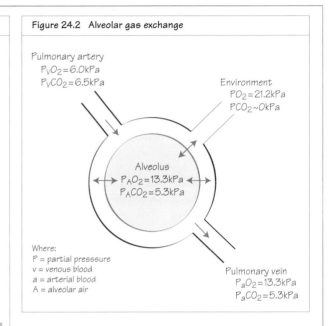

Pulmonary artery
$P_VO_2 = 6.0 kPa$
$P_VCO_2 = 6.5 kPa$

Environment
$PO_2 = 21.2 kPa$
$PCO_2 \sim 0 kPa$

Alveolus
$P_AO_2 = 13.3 kPa$
$P_ACO_2 = 5.3 kPa$

Where:
P = partial pressure
v = venous blood
a = arterial blood
A = alveolar air

Pulmonary vein
$P_aO_2 = 13.3 kPa$
$P_aCO_2 = 5.3 kPa$

Figure 24.3 Correlations between ventilation and perfusion

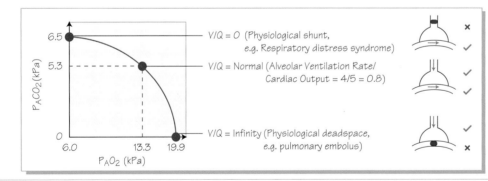

V/Q = 0 (Physiological shunt, e.g. Respiratory distress syndrome)

V/Q = Normal (Alveolar Ventilation Rate/ Cardiac Output = 4/5 = 0.8)

V/Q = Infinity (Physiological deadspace, e.g. pulmonary embolus)

The respiratory system serves to ensure that all tissues receive the O_2 they need and can dispose of the CO_2 they produce. Lungs exchange gases with atmosphere via the nasal cavity, which filters, warms and humidifies the air in preparation for efficient gas exchange. Blood carries gases to and from tissues, and has the intrinsic capacity to pick up O_2 and lose CO_2 if exposed to the right gaseous environment, and the lungs expose the blood to this type of environment.

Breathing

At rest we breathe at a respiratory rate of, on average, 12 breathes per minute, each with a volume of 0.5 L (with strenuous exercise this can rise to 120 L/min). The active inhalation phase lasts 2 s and the passive exhalation phase lasts 3 s. This normal respiration rate, depth and rhythm is called **eupnoea**. Breathing is therefore **tidal**, the last air to be inhaled is the first air to be exhaled. One-third of the air inhaled remains in the conducting airways at the end of inhalation and cannot take part in gas exchange. This relative proportion of **'dead space'** decreases with deeper breaths as the conducting airways contribute the same absolute volume. Thus deeper breaths are more efficient in moving air in and out of alveoli for gas exchange, but require more muscular effort. Two other critical internal factors that affect the distribution of inhaled gas and hence the efficiency of breathing, are airway resistance and lung compliance (Figure 24.1).

Airway resistance and conductance

Airway resistance is the opposition to airflow in the respiratory tree. Conductance (the reciprocal of resistance) is the change in flow for a unitary change in pressure, and usually limits exhalation. Airway resistance and conduction depend on friction and cross-sectional area. The major source of non-elastic resistance to air flow is friction in the respiratory passageways. **Resistance** in the respiratory tree is determined mostly by the diameters of the conducting tubules (i.e. trachea, bronchi, bronchioles, etc.). Gas flow stops at the terminal bronchioles, where airways have small diameters, but this is not a problem, as here diffusion is the main force driving gas movements. Therefore, the greatest resistance to gas flow occurs in the medium-sized bronchi and bronchioles. Although individual cross-sectional areas decrease with deeper penetration into the respiratory tree, total cross-sectional area increases. This means that there has to be very extensive damage to the small airways for ventilation to be affected.

Factors increasing airways resistance include: decreasing total lung volume; and increasing bronchomotor tone, age, mucus secretion and disease. Posture (through the effect of gravity) also affects airway resistance, as the height relative to heart affects blood vessel diameter and pressure on airways, while the abdominal contents either push up or pull down on the diaphragm altering lung volume by up to 1 L. Smooth muscle in the walls of the bronchioles has sensitive neural parasympathetic reflexes in response to inhaled irritants to prevent their deeper penetration (overreaction leads to asthma and can contribute to anaphylaxis).

Lung compliance and elastance

Compliance (the reciprocal of elastance, which is the ability to return to original shape after stretching) is the change in volume for a unitary change in pressure, and usually limits inhalation. As lung volume increases with expansion, then elasticity increases and compliance decreases (i.e. the more the lung inflates the harder it is to expand it further). Thus stiff lungs (e.g. with fibrosis) have low compliance and high elastic recoil (i.e. they are difficult to stretch and tend to return to resting position).

Surfactant decreases surface tension to maximise the compliance of lungs for inhalation. As surfactant becomes spread thinner during inflation it is less effective. So as alveoli become larger their surface tension decreases less, making it easier for small alveoli to expand and be recruited than it is for large alveoli.

It can be shown that for the same change in pressure, there is a greater change in lung volume at the lung base than at the apex (Figure 24.1b), because there is a greater range of mechanical movement at the diaphragm. Thus the lung acts as a more compliant structure at the lung base and it is easier to ventilate the lung base than the lung apex. We breathe from our lung bases at rest because of this reason.

With increasing age, tissue compliance increases (the lung is more compliant to air flow in, but does not collapse fully to push air out as elasticity has decreased), airways collapse more and thoracic compliance decreases (musculoskeletal elements become weaker and stiffer). The balance between lung tissue and thoracic compliance leads to peak ventilatory function in the third decade of life.

Diffusion and gas exchange

The lungs are a system for getting blood to one side and gas to the other side of alveolar membranes, so that gas exchange can occur between air and blood across the alveolar membrane (Figure 24.2). We inhale 21% O_2 and 0.03–0.04% CO_2, while exhaling 14% O_2 and 5% CO_2. Diffusion depends on large gradients for O_2 (19.9 kPa $P_AO_2 > 6.0$ kPa P_VO_2) and CO_2 (~0 kPa $P_ACO_2 < 6.5$ kPa P_VCO_2). Thus O_2 will diffuse into blood and CO_2 out of blood to achieve a P_aO_2 of 13.3 kPa and P_aCO_2 of 5.3 kPa. Diffusion also depends on a large combined alveolar surface area (70 m^2) and low diffusion resistance. Diffusion resistance depends on barrier thinness (0.5 μm, equal to one-tenth the width of an erythrocyte) and gas permeability (requiring low molecular weight and high solubility). O_2 exchange is complete within half a second of a blood cell arriving in a capillary. Erythrocytes spend about 1 s in a capillary, and so gas diffusion does not normally limit respiratory function.

Ventilation-perfusion coupling

To maximise the efficiency of gas exchange at the blood–gas interface, the amount of gas reaching the alveoli (ventilation) must be coupled to the flow of blood in pulmonary capillaries (perfusion). This is **ventilation-perfusion matching (V/Q)**, and it depends on local autoregulation of blood flow by altering vasomotor tone in response to P_AO_2 levels, and by altering bronchomotor tone in response to P_ACO_2 levels. Low O_2 causes vasoconstriction, while high O_2 causes vasodilatation. This is the opposite of what happens in the systemic circulation (e.g. low O_2 in a cerebral capillary would cause vasodilatation). High CO_2 dilates bronchioles, while low CO_2 constricts bronchioles. Thus gas is redirected to areas of the lung with adequate perfusion, while blood is similarly shunted to areas of the lung with adequate ventilation (Figure 24.3).

25 Gas transport

Steven Burr

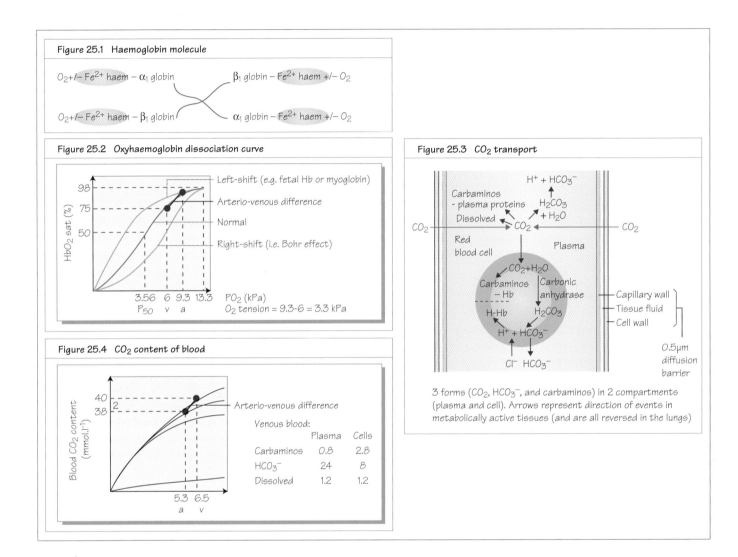

Figure 25.1 Haemoglobin molecule

$O_2 +/-$ Fe^{2+} haem – α_1 globin β_1 globin – Fe^{2+} haem $+/-$ O_2

$O_2 +/-$ Fe^{2+} haem – β_1 globin α_1 globin – Fe^{2+} haem $+/-$ O_2

Figure 25.2 Oxyhaemoglobin dissociation curve

HbO_2 sat (%)

98
75
50

Left-shift (e.g. fetal Hb or myoglobin)
Arterio-venous difference
Normal
Right-shift (i.e. Bohr effect)

3.56 6 9.3 13.3 PO_2 (kPa)
P_{50} v   a O_2 tension = 9.3-6 = 3.3 kPa

Figure 25.4 CO_2 content of blood

Blood CO_2 content (mmol.l^{-1})

40
38   2

Arterio-venous difference

Venous blood:

	Plasma	Cells
Carbaminos	0.8	2.8
HCO_3^-	24	8
Dissolved	1.2	1.2

5.3 6.5
a   v

Figure 25.3 CO_2 transport

$H^+ + HCO_3^-$
Carbaminos - plasma proteins
H_2CO_3
Dissolved $+ H_2O$
CO_2 — CO_2 — CO_2
Red blood cell   Plasma
$CO_2 + H_2O$
Carbaminos – Hb   Carbonic anhydrase
H-Hb H_2CO_3
$H^+ + HCO_3^-$
Cl^- HCO_3^-

Capillary wall
Tissue fluid
Cell wall

0.5µm diffusion barrier

3 forms (CO_2, HCO_3^-, and carbaminos) in 2 compartments (plasma and cell). Arrows represent direction of events in metabolically active tissues (and are all reversed in the lungs)

Medical Sciences at a Glance, First Edition. Edited by Michael D Randall. © 2014 John Wiley & Sons, Ltd. Published 2014 by John Wiley & Sons, Ltd.

Every minute at rest the human body consumes about 200 mL of oxygen (O_2) and produces about 200 mL of carbon dioxide (CO_2).

Oxygen

Forms of oxygen carriage and haemoglobin binding

O_2 is poorly soluble and so only 1.5% is transported dissolved in plasma. The remaining 98.5% is bound to **haemoglobin** (Hb) inside erythrocytes. Each erythrocyte contains 250–640 million Hb molecules (and there are 4.5–5.1 million erythrocytes per 1 mm^3 of blood). Hb is a protein composed of four polypeptide chain subunits. Each subunit is bound to an iron-containing porphyrin haem group. Because **ferrous** (Fe^{2+}) ions serve as O_2 binding sites, each Hb can rapidly and reversibly bind four O_2 molecules (Figure 25.1). A Hb molecule bound with O_2 is called **oxyhaemoglobin** (HbO_2), whereas a Hb molecule that has released its O_2 is called **deoxyhaemoglobin**. As O_2 binds it changes the optical absorption spectrum of the Hb and hence the colour of blood from cyan to red. Thus with an increase in the relative proportion of deoxyhaemoglobin to oxyhaemoglobin, a bluish discolouration of the skin and mucous membranes can be observed, which is referred to as **cyanosis**.

When the first O_2 molecule binds the first iron molecule, the Hb changes shape, and the affinity for the other three O_2 molecules progressively increases. Similarly, when the first O_2 is unloaded, the affinity for O_2 is decreased and it becomes progressively easier for the other three O_2 molecules to dissociate from the Hb. Hb is fully saturated when all four haem groups are bound to O_2. If fewer than all four haem groups are bound, the Hb is said to be partially saturated. Binding of the second is easier than the first, binding of the third is easier than the second, and binding of the fourth is easier than the third. The fourth O_2 molecule to bind has 300 times the affinity of the first. Thus, the affinity of Hb for O_2 changes depending on how much O_2 is bound to the Hb. The more saturated Hb is, then the easier it is to bind more O_2, and the harder it is to unbind O_2 from that Hb. So, binding gets more efficient as each O_2 binds, and release gets easier as each O_2 is released.

Oxyhaemoglobin dissociation curve

The association between O_2 and Hb is represented by a sigmoid-shaped (S-shaped) curve (Figure 25.2), because changes in affinity of Hb depend on O_2 saturation. The curve has a steep slope between 1 and 6 kPa PO_2 and a plateau between 9.3 and 13.3 kPa PO_2. The upper linear portion of the curve reflects where both O_2 loading in the lungs (from venous to arterial) and unloading in the tissues (from arterial to venous) occurs. Hb saturation (%; 'O_2 sats') depends on PO_2, not normally on Hb content. Near 100% Hb saturation implies healthy gas exchange, but could still occur with anaemia (reduced Hb content). O_2 content depends on both PO_2 and Hb content. So, low Hb content can cause tissue hypoxia, even if both PO_2 and Hb saturation are normal.

O_2 tension refers to the PO_2 difference between two sites, determining the direction and flow of O_2. Changes in O_2 tension do not correspond to equal changes in Hb saturation. As blood moves from arteries through tissues to veins there is a large decrease in PO_2 (13.3 to 6 kPa), associated with a much smaller decrease in Hb saturation (98% to 75%). PO_2 falls by more than 50%, whereas O_2 sats fall by less than 25%. This occurs because it is hardest to unload the first O_2 molecule and thus initially PO_2 falls without much decrease in O_2 sats. Hb is almost completely saturated at any PO_2 above 9.3 kPa, enabling normal O_2 delivery to tissues. When PO_2 decreases to below 9.3 kPa, Hb more readily gives up O_2. So, when blood arrives at tissues with low PO_2 it readily unloads O_2. A significant amount of O_2 is still available in venous blood and can be unloaded from blood to tissues if required (e.g. during vigorous exercise). Since Hb in arterial blood is 98% saturated, heavy breathing during exercise increases PO_2 above the normal 13.3 kPa, but causes almost no change in % saturation. Thus more Hb or increased cardiac output is needed to increase the transport of O_2.

Bohr effect

The Bohr effect is the decrease in affinity of Hb for O_2 (i.e. a 'right shift' in the dissociation curve; Figure 25.2). This occurs due to increased PCO_2 [H^+] or temperature in metabolically active tissues (or 2,3-diphosphoglycerate, which increases slowly in response to chronic hypoxia) when there is a need to unload O_2.

Carbon dioxide

There is almost three times as much CO_2 in *arterial* blood than there is O_2 (450–500 mL CO_2/L vs 200 mL O_2/L). CO_2 diffuses quicker across the lungs than O_2, and so exhalation of CO_2 is not limited by gas exchange. CO_2 is retained because it is not just a waste product of metabolism, it is critical for controlling the acidity of the body (see Chapter 27) and consequently for the control of ventilation (see Chapter 26). If O_2 consumption increases, then the removal rate of CO_2 from venous blood in the lungs needs to increase (e.g. via increasing ventilation or cardiac output) to keep arterial CO_2 constant.

Transformation and forms of carbon dioxide carriage

Dissolved CO_2 reacts with water in erythrocytes more efficiently than in plasma due to the presence of carbonic anhydrase. Within erythrocytes H^+ binds to Hb, so more CO_2 reacts and more bicarbonate is formed. Bicarbonate diffuses out of the erythrocyte in exchange for inward movement of chloride (known as the chloride shift), reaching equilibrium at 24 mmol/L of HCO_3^- in plasma. The third form of transport (after dissolved and as bicarbonate) is bound to protein (either Hb in erythrocytes or albumin in plasma) as carbamino compounds (Figure 25.3).

Carbon dioxide dissociation curve

Blood does not become saturated with CO_2 over the physiological range (Figure 25.4), unlike the oxyhaemoglobin dissociation curve, which does become saturated. Seventy per cent of CO_2 is transported as bicarbonate. There are more of all three forms (dissolved CO_2, HCO_3^- and carbaminos, in both plasma and erythrocytes) in venous blood, because PCO_2 is higher. However, the arteriovenous difference in CO_2 carriage needed for gas exchange is small. From P_aCO_2 of 5.3 kPa to P_vCO_2 of 6.5 kPa corresponds to a difference in blood CO_2 content of only 2 mmol/L.

Haldane effect

The Haldane effect is the increase in affinity of Hb for CO_2. This occurs due to the deoxygenation of Hb. CO_2 binds to the globin part of Hb, unlike O_2, which binds to the haem part of Hb. In metabolically active tissues, O_2 is unloaded, increasing affinity for CO_2, so CO_2 is loaded. In the lungs, O_2 is loaded, decreasing affinity for CO_2, so CO_2 is unloaded.

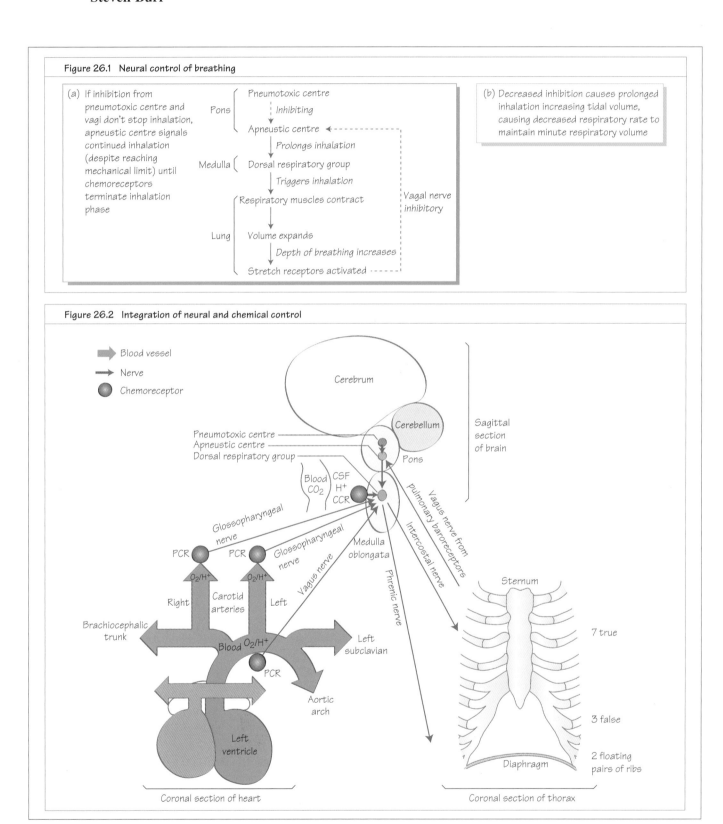

Figure 26.1 Neural control of breathing

(a) If inhibition from pneumotoxic centre and vagi don't stop inhalation, apneustic centre signals continued inhalation (despite reaching mechanical limit) until chemoreceptors terminate inhalation phase

Pons
Pneumotoxic centre
Inhibiting
Apneustic centre
Prolongs inhalation

Medulla
Dorsal respiratory group
Triggers inhalation
Respiratory muscles contract

Lung
Volume expands
Depth of breathing increases
Stretch receptors activated

Vagal nerve inhibitory

(b) Decreased inhibition causes prolonged inhalation increasing tidal volume, causing decreased respiratory rate to maintain minute respiratory volume

Figure 26.2 Integration of neural and chemical control

Blood vessel
Nerve
Chemoreceptor

Cerebrum
Cerebellum
Sagittal section of brain
Pneumotoxic centre
Apneustic centre
Dorsal respiratory group
Pons
Blood CO_2
CSF H^+ CCR
Glossopharyngeal nerve
Vagus nerve from pulmonary baroreceptors
Intercostal nerve
PCR
PCR
Glossopharyngeal nerve
Medulla oblongata
O_2/H^+
O_2/H^+
Vagus nerve
Phrenic nerve
Right
Carotid arteries
Left
Brachiocephalic trunk
Blood O_2/H^+
Left subclavian
PCR
Aortic arch
Left ventricle
Sternum
7 true
3 false
2 floating pairs of ribs
Diaphragm
Coronal section of heart
Coronal section of thorax

Neural generation of ventilatory pattern

We breathe automatically, and yet we can make instantaneous adjustments just by thinking about it. **Respiratory centres** in the **brainstem** maintain an optimum minute respiratory volume to meet the needs of metabolism, by controlling the relative contributions of both respiratory rate and tidal volume. The basic ventilatory rate and rhythm is produced by the **dorsal respiratory group** in the **medulla oblongata** by triggering the start of each inhalation (Figure 26.1). The duration of inhalation is prolonged by input from the **apneustic centre** in the **pons**, which itself receives inhibitory signals from both the **pneumotaxic centre** in the pons and vagal feedback from **lung baroreceptors** (which increases in response to progressive stretching). The lung baroreceptor (Hering-Breuer) reflex protects lungs from overinflation and is also implicated in fibrosis (where overstretching of unfibrosed areas prematurely curtails inhalation, decreasing tidal volume and increasing respiratory rate).

Chemical regulation of ventilatory pattern

The amount of O_2 consumed and CO_2 produced by the body varies depending on metabolic demand, and detection of chemical changes drives ventilation to match requirements. There are two types of chemoreceptor, which synapse with the respiratory centres in the brainstem to increase ventilation (Figure 26.2). **Central chemoreceptors** (CCRs) found on the ventrolateral surface of the medulla oblongata respond to increases in $[H^+]$ (and indirectly PCO_2) in cerebrospinal fluid (CSF). **Peripheral chemoreceptors** (PCRs) found within the aortic arch and carotid arteries respond when O_2 falls below $8\,kPa$ in arterial blood (functioning despite severe hypoxia, because of their extremely high blood supply in proportion to their size). PCRs respond quickly to large changes (as they are in main arteries), but CCRs dominate under normal conditions to determine fine control (being more sensitive, as CSF has less protein to buffer pH compared with blood). Thus rising CO_2 normally drives ventilation. While CCRs adapt on gradual exposure to sustained **hypocapnia** or **hypercapnia**, PCRs do not adapt, and produce a respiratory drive as long as P_aO_2 remains low (e.g. providing a fixed threshold for breath-holding). CCRs and PCRs work together synergistically, but their relative importance can change depending on the conditions.

If respiratory centres cannot respond quickly enough to changing P_aCO_2 and P_aO_2 (e.g. following stroke, head injuries, brain tumours, or when sleeping at high altitudes), then Cheyne-Stokes respiration occurs (a cycle of breaths becoming shallower and less frequent, followed by an overcompensatory hyperventilation).

Acclimatisation to altitude and hypocapnia

Ascent above $2500\,m$ leads to type I respiratory failure (hypoxia without hypercapnia). With increasing altitude, gravity is less, gases expand and the air becomes less dense. The volume fraction of O_2 remains the same, but because the total pressure decreases the P_AO_2 also decreases.

With sudden exposure, acute hypoxia is detected by peripheral chemoreceptors, which try to increase breathing, but as ventilation increases, P_aCO_2 falls and CSF becomes alkaline. Breathing more leads to death from alkalosis, but failing to breathe more leads to death from hypoxia. Peripheral receptors detect hypoxia but are overridden by central receptors detecting hypocapnia, and the hypoxic drive to increase ventilation is suppressed.

With gradual exposure, mountaineers can climb to $8850\,m$ without O_2, due to acclimatisation. Mild hypoxia stimulates ventilation enough to raise CSF pH slightly. Choroid plexus cells respond by exporting HCO_3^- from CSF to blood. CSF pH is corrected (even though P_aCO_2 remains low), hypoxic drive is expressed and ventilation can increase further. Over a period of hours, breathing becomes controlled around a new lower P_aCO_2. Over a period of days, the alkalinity of the blood is corrected as the exported bicarbonate is excreted by kidneys.

Hypoxic drive dependence with hypercapnia

Pulmonary pathology can lead to type II respiratory failure (**hypoxia with hypercapnia**). With mild hypercapnia, $[HCO_3^-]$ is matched to PCO_2 in CSF, but not in blood (which has a larger volume and is renal dependent). Choroid plexus cells respond by importing HCO_3^- from blood to CSF. Chronically, CSF pH is corrected and ventilation is normal (and inadequate), even though P_aCO_2 remains high (i.e. CO_2 trapping). Thus a gradually increasing P_aCO_2 is associated with inadequate drive for ventilation, which in turn becomes progressively more dependent on the hypoxic drive from PCRs. This is problematic when associated with the need to offset hypoxia by breathing supplemental O_2. Correcting low P_aO_2 removes the drive to breathe and results in a need for artificial ventilation. Hence O_2 therapy is administered at the lowest tolerable level and monitored closely.

Steven Burr

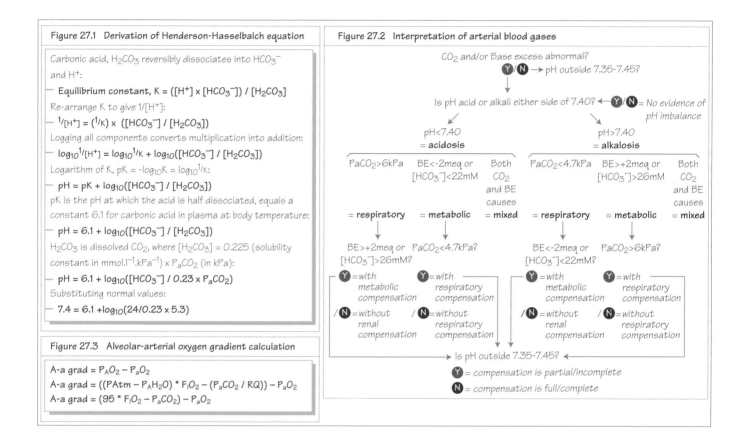

Figure 27.1 Derivation of Henderson-Hasselbalch equation

Figure 27.2 Interpretation of arterial blood gases

Figure 27.3 Alveolar-arterial oxygen gradient calculation

pH

The potential of hydrogen (pH) is a measure of the hydrogen ion concentration ($[H^+]$) in solution. It is conventionally expressed as $pH = \log_{10} 1/_{[H^+]} = -\log_{10} [H^+]$. The greatest range in $[H^+]$ is found in the gastrointestinal tract, where there are secretions in response to digestive requirements. There, gastric secretions can be as low as 1.1 and pancreatic secretions as high as 8.8. However, if blood becomes too acid or too alkaline there are serious consequences. If plasma pH falls below 6.8, enzymes are lethally denatured. If plasma pH rises above 7.6, free calcium concentration falls enough to produce fatal tetany. Therefore $[H^+]$ is kept within narrow bounds in blood. Mean normal extracellular $[H^+]$ is 40 nmol/L, equivalent to a pH of 7.4. The normal extracellular range is 35.5–44.7 nmol/L, which is equivalent to a pH range of 7.45–7.35 (as higher $[H^+]$ is more acidic and has a lower pH). Extracellular pH is kept close to 7.4, to maintain a gradient for $[H^+]$ removal from metabolically active tissues where the intracellular pH is normally 6.8–7.2.

Henderson-Hasselbalch equation

The dominant reaction governing extracellular $[H^+]$ and hence pH is: $CO_2 + H_2O = H_2CO_3 = HCO_3^- + H^+$ (Figure 27.1).

At a normal $PaCO_2$ of 5.3 kPa water in plasma dissolves 1.2 mmol/L. Dissolved CO_2 reacts with water forming H^+ and HCO_3. The reaction is reversible, with the amount reacting depending on [reactants] and [products]. If the amount of one constituent decreases, then the reaction is driven to produce more of that constituent in order to restore the equilibrium. At physiological equilibrium $[HCO_3] = 24$ mmol/L. and $[H^+] = 40$ nmol/L, so there is one million-fold less H^+ than HCO_3^- in blood. Thus changing how much CO_2 dissolves has a proportionally greater effect on H^+. Dissolved CO_2 depends directly on PCO_2. If PCO_2 rises, $[H^+]$ will rise; if PCO_2 falls, $[H^+]$ will fall. Thus, slow shallow breaths lead to less CO_2 exhaled, more CO_2 retained in blood, more free H^+ and consequently lower pH. Conversely, rapid deep breaths lead to more CO_2 exhaled, less CO_2 retained in blood, less free H^+ and consequently higher pH. Consequently, plasma pH depends primarily on the P_aCO_2 maintained by the lungs, and $[HCO_3^-]$, which is maintained by the kidneys. It is the relative not absolute values of these contributors that determine pH. A change in P_aCO_2 can be buffered by an equivalent relative change in $[HCO_3^-]$, and vice versa. The equation (Figure 27.1) enables calculation of the $[HCO_3^-]$ required to buffer an increase in P_aCO_2 and maintain a pH of 7.4. The required increase in $[HCO_3^-] = 10^{7.4-6.1+(\log 0.23 + \log PaCO2)}$ − existing $[HCO_3^-]$. For example, if P_aCO_2 increased from 5.3 kPa to 8 kPa, then $[HCO_3^-]$ has to increase by 12 (from 24 to 36) mmol/L to maintain pH at 7.4. In severe cases, the required increase is multiplied by the circulating volume (typically 5 L for an adult) and half this amount of sodium bicarbonate is administered either orally or intravenously before reassessing arterial blood gas status.

Acidosis, alkalosis and compensation

Acidosis and alkalosis refer to the process of becoming more acidic or alkali respectively. **Acidaemic** and **alkalemic** refer to the state of being more acid or alkali, while acidaemia and alkalemia specifically refer to the state of the blood. Changes in ventilation that cause acid-base imbalance are termed respiratory; all other non-ventilatory causes of acid-base imbalance are termed metabolic. Changes that act to restore normal acid-base balance are termed compensation. Causes of both imbalance and compensation can be respiratory, metabolic, or mixed/combined respiratory and metabolic (Figure 27.2). However, the lungs can adjust body pH much more rapidly than the kidneys. Altering ventilation can begin within seconds/minutes to compensate for acid-base imbalance, whereas altering kidney output takes hours/days to bring about effective renal compensation. Hence acute acid-base imbalances are likely to undergo complete respiratory compensation before renal compensation can take effect.

Respiratory alkali

Hyperventilation causes P_aCO_2 to fall (hypocapnia), for example to correct low P_aO_2 (hypoxia) on ascent to high altitude. So plasma pH rises = respiratory alkalosis. This can be compensated for (returning pH towards normal) by hypoventilation (if the cause of hyperventilation has ended), or by the kidneys increasing $[HCO_3^-]$ excretion.

Respiratory acid

Hypoventilation causes P_aCO_2 to rise (hypercapnia), for example when ventilation is impaired by disease. Plasma pH falls = respiratory acidosis. This can be compensated for by hyperventilation (if the cause of hypoventilation has ended), or by the kidneys increasing $[H^+]$ excretion.

Metabolic acid

If the tissues produce acid, for example with ketoacidosis (due to poorly controlled diabetes mellitus), this reacts with HCO_3^-. The fall in $[HCO_3^-]$ leads to a fall in pH = metabolic acidosis. This can be compensated for by increased ventilation to lower P_aCO_2, or by the kidneys increasing $[H^+]$ excretion.

Metabolic alkali

If plasma $[HCO_3^-]$ rises, for example vomiting causes loss of acid from the body (and hence a relative increase in plasma $[HCO_3^-]$), plasma pH rises = metabolic alkalosis. This can be compensated for by decreasing ventilation to raise P_aCO_2, or by the kidneys increasing $[HCO_3^-]$ excretion. Metabolic alkalosis can only be compensated for to a degree by hypoventilation because of the associated decrease in P_aO_2 leading to hypoxia.

Compensation

While renal metabolic compensation can occur at the same time as a non-renal metabolic cause of acid-base imbalance, respiratory compensation cannot occur at the same time as a respiratory cause of imbalance (i.e. hypoventilation and hyperventilation cannot occur together in time, although if the cause has stopped then compensation can follow).

Compensation may not occur, be partial, or complete. If neither P_aCO_2 nor $[HCO_3^-]$ have moved to compensate when one or the other would have been expected to change, then an apparently normal value can indicate an abnormality. Partial compensation occurs where there is evidence of P_aCO_2 or $[HCO_3^-]$ having moved to compensate, but the pH is not within the normal range. Complete compensation has occurred when the pH is within the normal range. Note that when deciding whether a case is either metabolic alkalosis with respiratory compensation or respiratory acidosis with metabolic compensation, assume that overcompensation does not occur (it would be inefficient for the body to expend resources in continuing to compensate beyond the midpoint pH of 7.40) unless there is evidence from the patient history to the contrary (e.g. imposing excessive or insufficient mechanical ventilation).

Arterial blood gases and alveolar-arterial gradient

Arterial blood gases are crucial for the management of all acute respiratory disorders and many chronic ones. Provided the patient has been at steady state for the preceding 20 minutes (i.e. breathing the same gas composition at the same rhythm), then a 0.5 mL blood sample is taken from their radial artery and analysed. Normal ranges are: pH = 7.40 (7.35–7.45); P_aO_2 = 10.6–13.3 kPa; P_aCO_2 = 4.7–6 kPa; and base excess (BE) = +2 to −2 meq/L (where BE is a derived value relative to a normal $[HCO_3^-]$ of 24 mmol/L). These values are a crucial indictor of prognosis as nobody dies with normal blood gases. Interpretation depends on identification of values that are clearly abnormal (severely so if O_2 is less than 8 kPa and/or CO_2 more than 7 kPa), and is supported by knowledge of the patient's history and whether there is any pre-existing disease (e.g. diabetes mellitus may contribute a metabolic acidosis).

Calculate the alveolar-arterial oxygen gradient (A-a grad, sometimes referred to as oxygen difference or A-a DO_2) to determine whether there is impaired gas transfer (indicating lung damage, as a large difference means poor gas exchange and a problem with the efficiency of ventilation-perfusion matching). A normal A-a grad (Figure 27.3) depends on atmospheric pressure (PAtm at sea level = 101.325 kPa), alveolar humidity (P_AH_2O is kept constant with normal respiratory tract physiology and hydration = 6.28 kPa), fractional concentration of oxygen in inspired gas (F_IO_2 for room air = 0.21093, but can differ if a patient is receiving supplemental oxygen) and aerobic metabolism (respiratory quotient = 1). The calculated A-a grad value is then classified as normal if it is less than a threshold determined by age (upper limits of normal A-a grad are: 2.5 kPa at 20 years; 3.2 kPa at 40 years; 3.7 kPa at 60 years; and 4.0 kPa at 80 years). For every 10% increase in F_IO_2, these normal A-a gradient thresholds increase by 0.66–0.93 kPa (a normal A-a gradient when breathing 100% oxygen = 8–9.3 kPa).

28 Respiratory pathophysiology

Steven Burr

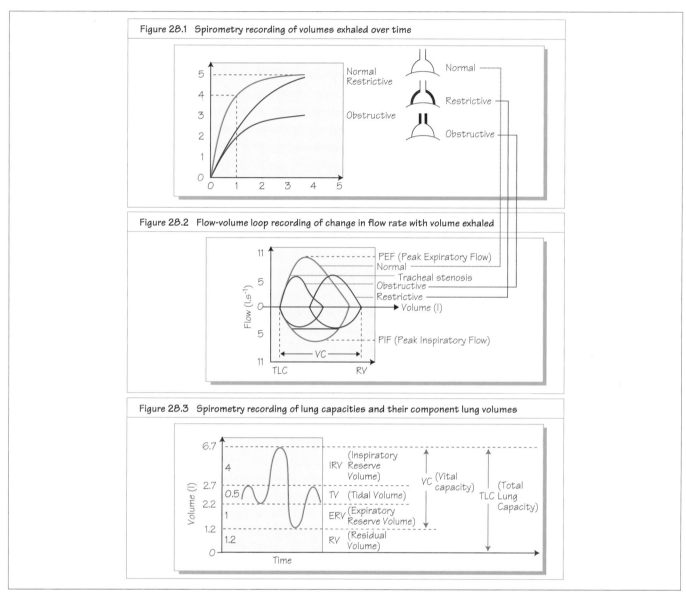

Figure 28.1 Spirometry recording of volumes exhaled over time

Figure 28.2 Flow-volume loop recording of change in flow rate with volume exhaled

Figure 28.3 Spirometry recording of lung capacities and their component lung volumes

The effect of disease on respiratory function is best demonstrated by changes in the measurements of air flow, lung volumes and gas transfer. Diagnosis, management and monitoring of respiratory problems rely on non-invasive measurements of the movement of air breathed in and out of the lungs, and the diffusion of gas between inspired air and the blood. Ventilation is assessed by both expiratory flow rate and lung volume measurements. Normal values will vary with gender, age, height, weight and ethnicity. Thus measured values are usually expressed as a percentage of average normal predicted values. Abnormal flow rates reflect changes in airway resistance indicating obstructive pathology; whereas abnormal lung volumes reflect changes in compliance indicating restrictive pathology.

Obstructive respiratory deficits

Increased airway resistance obstructs air flow and thus impairs exhalation. If airways are narrowed it is still possible to fill the lungs to capacity, but resistance will increase on exhalation, so air will come out more slowly. Possible pathological causes include **chronic obstructive pulmonary disease** (COPD), irreversible increases in airway resistance involving a combination of chronic bronchitis (recurrent inflammation with mucus secretion) and emphysema (permanent destructive enlargement of alveoli)), and **asthma** (reversible increases in airway resistance involving a combination of bronchoconstriction and inflammation).

Restrictive respiratory deficits

Decreased compliance restricts lung expansion and thus impairs inhalation. If lungs are difficult to fill to capacity because they are stiff, have weak muscles, or there is a problem with the chest wall, they will be less full before exhalation. Lung volume will be reduced, but air will come out at a normal rate. Possible physiological causes include obesity, pregnancy, or restrictive clothing. Possible pathological causes are parenchymal (e.g. pulmonary fibrosis, pulmonary oedema), chest wall (e.g. kyphoscoliosis, pneumothorax), or neuromuscular (e.g. myasthenia gravis). Mixed respiratory deficits are also possible (e.g. tumours or cystic fibrosis) or with a combination of obstructive and restrictive conditions (e.g. if both obese and asthmatic).

Spirometry

Spirometry records the volumes breathed in and out over time. Peak expiratory flow rate (PEFR) depends on the patient inhaling as deeply as possible and then exhaling as quickly as possible. Forced expiratory volume in the first second (FEV_1) and forced vital capacity (FVC) are measured by the same manoeuvre as PEFR, but the patient continues to try to breathe out until no more air can be exhaled (Figure 28.1). The FEV_1 is expressed as a percentage of FVC. PEFR is the simplest technique to perform, but it is less reliable for assessing conditions where airways are not affected uniformly. With variable airway damage, a very brief momentary high PEFR may still be achieved, whereas measuring over a whole second with FEV_1 would be a more reliable. With obstruction, FEV_1 will be less than 70% of predicted, but FVC will be more than 70% of normal. With restriction, FVC will be less than 70% of predicted, but FEV_1 will be more than 70% of FVC. A flow-volume loop is measured by the same manoeuvre as FEV_1 and FVC, but once no more air can be breathed out then the patient inhales as rapidly as possible until they can breathe no more air in (Figure 28.2). A flow-volume loop has the advantage of assessing inhalation as well as exhalation, along with producing shapes characteristic of certain conditions (Figure 28.2).

Lung volumes

The residual volume (and in turn total lung capacity and functional residual capacity) cannot be breathed out nor measured directly (Figure 28.3). Such unknown lung volumes can be measured indirectly by helium dilution. At a known point in the respiratory cycle (e.g. with only the residual volume remaining within the lungs) the patient starts breathing from (and to) a known volume (V1), which contains a known concentration of helium (C1). When the air between the unknown volume in the lungs and known volume containing helium have completely mixed, then the concentration of helium is re-measured (C2). Because helium is not normally present in air and is insoluble in blood, the helium will have redistributed equally only between the two volumes. The resulting dilution of the helium will be proportional to the increase in total volume. It is then possible to calculate the unknown volume that was in the lungs when the patient started breathing from V1. Thus the unknown lung volume = (C1/C2 − 1) × V1.

Effects of restrictive disease on lung volumes

A common effect of lung disease involving any kind of space-occupying lesion is that FRC, TLC and RV all decrease together. In contrast, weakness affecting both inspiratory and expiratory muscles causes FRC to remain unchanged. The lungs cannot be expanded fully, so the IRV and in turn TLC are decreased. Similarly, the lungs cannot be compressed fully, so the RV is increased by an amount equal to that by which the ERV is decreased (causing no overall change in FRC). The proportion of total lung capacity not involved in ventilation is often expressed as RV/TLC.

Effects of obstructive disease on lung volumes

The changes in lung volumes with COPD depend on the severity and relative contributions of chronic bronchitis and emphysema. FRC, TLC and RV all decrease slightly due to the reduction in airway volume associated with bronchoconstriction and mucus secretion caused by the chronic bronchitis. This has greatest effect on RV, because a larger proportion of RV is airways than for other lung volumes. However, if the emphysema is severe enough to collapse airways and trap air then RV will increase. In contrast, an upper tracheal stenosis or other localised obstruction (e.g. a tumour or foreign body obstruction) would not affect FRC, TLC, or RV.

Gas transfer

The efficiency of respiration can be limited by the diffusion of oxygen from alveolar air to pulmonary capillary blood. Gas transfer is measured using carbon monoxide (CO) as a surrogate for oxygen. The rate of transfer across the alveolar membrane can be calculated by fully exhaling then rapidly and maximally inhaling a single breath containing 0.3% CO, and holding that breath for 10 seconds before exhaling rapidly and maximally, and measuring the CO remaining in the exhaled air. Because P_VCO is negligible, and Hb is not saturated (because % CO is low), the rate of CO uptake, or permeability, is constant. A permeability factor (kCO) can be calculated from the decrease in alveolar fraction of CO over the time of the test (where: $kCO = \log_e (F_ACO_0 / F_ACO_t) / t$).

Alveolar volume (V_A; not alveolar ventilation rate)
V_A in litres = TLC − total dead space volume.
Normally = 4–5 L.

Total lung carbon monoxide transfer (T_LCO)
T_LCO in L/ min.$kPa^{-1} = (kCO \times V_A) / (PAtm − PH_2O)$.
Assume PAtm = 101.325 kPa, PH_2O = 6.28 kPa, and 1 mole of gas occupies 22.4 litres.
T_LCO in mmol.$min^{-1}.kPa^{-1}$ = (T_LCO in l.$min^{-1}.kPa^{-1}$ / 22.4) × 1000.
Normally T_LCO = 6–10 mmol/min.kPa^{-1}.

Factors that would decrease ventilation-perfusion matching and hence decrease T_LCO include: decreased alveolar surface area (e.g. caused by emphysema); thickened alveolar-capillary membrane (e.g. diffusion distance increase caused by pulmonary oedema); decreased pulmonary capillary blood flow (e.g. pulmonary embolus/ischaemia; cf. exercise increases T_LCO because pulmonary capillary blood flow increases); and decreased Hb (e.g. anaemia). With anaemia, a correction factor can be applied to adjust T_LCO, in order to assess gas exchange independently of Hb.

Coefficient of carbon monoxide transfer (KCO; not kCO)
$KCO = T_LCO / V_A$,
i.e. Efficiency per lung unit = gas exchange capacity/number of contributing units. Normally KCO = 1.25–1.75 mmol/min.kPa^{-1}/L.

Effects of restrictive disease on gas transfer

With incomplete lung expansion V_A is very low by definition, and this is normally associated with an increased KCO and hence only a slightly decreased T_LCO. The increased KCO is due to smaller alveoli having an increased surface area to volume ratio, thus increasing diffusing capacity. NB A low V_A with an apparently normal KCO would actually reflect impaired transfer.

Effects of obstructive disease on gas transfer

With COPD, V_A is effectively reduced slightly because there is increased mucus lining airspaces and trapping of air, leading to its exclusion from ventilation. There are larger airspaces and reduced alveolar surface area (emphysema), and increased diffusion distance due to mucus (from bronchitis); so KCO decreases and because $T_LCO = V_A \times KCO$, T_LCO is very low. With asthma the pulmonary microcirculation is maintained and cardiac output increases, so KCO increases and T_LCO decreases slightly.

Siobhan Loughna and Deborah Merrick

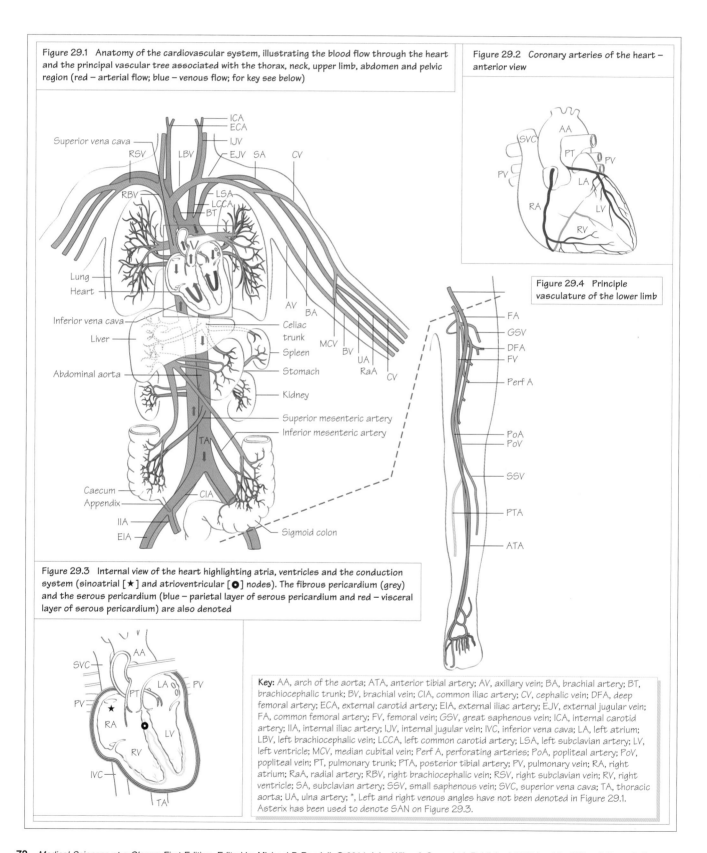

Figure 29.1 Anatomy of the cardiovascular system, illustrating the blood flow through the heart and the principal vascular tree associated with the thorax, neck, upper limb, abdomen and pelvic region (red – arterial flow; blue – venous flow; for key see below)

Figure 29.2 Coronary arteries of the heart – anterior view

Figure 29.4 Principle vasculature of the lower limb

Figure 29.3 Internal view of the heart highlighting atria, ventricles and the conduction system (sinoatrial [★] and atrioventricular [⊙] nodes). The fibrous pericardium (grey) and the serous pericardium (blue – parietal layer of serous pericardium and red – visceral layer of serous pericardium) are also denoted

Key: AA, arch of the aorta; ATA, anterior tibial artery; AV, axillary vein; BA, brachial artery; BT, brachiocephalic trunk; BV, brachial vein; CIA, common iliac artery; CV, cephalic vein; DFA, deep femoral artery; ECA, external carotid artery; EIA, external iliac artery; EJV, external jugular vein; FA, common femoral artery; FV, femoral vein; GSV, great saphenous vein; ICA, internal carotid artery; IIA, internal iliac artery; IJV, internal jugular vein; IVC, inferior vena cava; LA, left atrium; LBV, left brachiocephalic vein; LCCA, left common carotid artery; LSA, left subclavian artery; LV, left ventricle; MCV, median cubital vein; Perf A, perforating arteries; PoA, popliteal artery; PoV, popliteal vein; PT, pulmonary trunk; PTA, posterior tibial artery; PV, pulmonary vein; RA, right atrium; RaA, radial artery; RBV, right brachiocephalic vein; RSV, right subclavian vein; RV, right ventricle; SA, subclavian artery; SSV, small saphenous vein; SVC, superior vena cava; TA, thoracic aorta; UA, ulna artery; *, Left and right venous angles have not been denoted in Figure 29.1. Asterix has been used to denote SAN on Figure 29.3.

The cardiovascular system comprises the heart and an extensive network of vessels, called the vascular tree (Figures 29.1, 29.2 and 29.3). The heart is a four-chambered pump that ensures an adequate supply of oxygenated blood is provided to all tissues of the body. The right side of the heart receives deoxygenated blood destined for the lungs (via the pulmonary circulation). The left side receives oxygenated blood from the lungs, which is pumped at high pressure to the rest of the body (**systemic circulation**).

The heart and pericardium

The heart: is a muscular organ located in the middle **mediastinum** (Figure 29.1). The muscular layer of the heart is the **myocardium**, and an epithelial layer called the **endocardium** is the internal lining. The myocardium is composed of bundles of cardiac muscle, some of which have specialised functions in initiating and coordinating the contraction of the heart musculature (sinoatrial [SA] and atrioventricular [AV] nodes, Figure 29.3). The heart has three surfaces (sternocostal, diaphragmatic and the base) with the apex of the heart located approximately 9 cm to the left of the midline at the fifth intercostal space. The heart is divided into four chambers by septa: left and right atria and left and right ventricles (Figure 29.3). The right side of the heart pumps blood into the pulmonary circuit and the left side into the systemic circuit (denoted by blue and red arrows respectively in Figure 29.1). The heart cycle commences with ventricular expansion and filling (**diastole**), and ends with ventricular shortening and emptying (**systole**). Deoxygenated blood from the body enters the right atrium via the **inferior and superior vena cavae** (**IVC and SVC**); this blood enters the right ventricle via the tricuspid valve. Ventricular contraction leads to the blood going to the lungs via the pulmonary trunk through the pulmonary valve. Upon oxygenation, blood then returns to the heart via the pulmonary veins to enter the left atrium; the blood enters the left ventricle via the mitral valve. Ventricular contraction pumps the oxygenated blood into the aorta, through the aortic valve, from where it is distributed around the body via the vascular tree. **Coronary arteries** provide the blood supply to the heart. The main coronary arteries are the right and left coronary arteries, which arise from the aorta just superior to the aortic valve (Figure 29.2). Deoxygenated blood is returned to the heart via the coronary veins, with most blood entering the right atrium of the heart via the coronary sinus. The heart receives sympathetic and parasympathetic innervation via the cardiac plexuses.

The pericardium: is divided into fibrous (outer) and serous (inner) parts to form a sac that encloses the heart (Figure 29.3). The fibrous portion of the pericardium is strong and relatively nondistensible, preventing excessive movement of the heart. It attaches to the diaphragm inferiorly, and superiorly blends into adventitia of great vessels. The fibrous pericardium is lined internally by the parietal layer of serous pericardium, whereas the visceral layer of serous pericardium covers the surface of the heart. There is a potential space between the two serous layers and a lubricant produced by these layers prevents friction of the heart.

The vascular tree

Arteries and veins: carry blood from and to the heart respectively. Their walls contain three layers: **tunica intima** (inner endothelial lining), **tunica media** (middle smooth muscle layer) and **tunica adventitia** (outer connective tissue layer). Arteries have a more prominent tunica media and can be classed as elastic, muscular, or arterioles. **Capillaries** arise from terminal arterioles; blood contained within them moves into venules and then into progressively larger veins as they approach the heart. Veins carry blood at lower pressure and often contain valves to prevent retrograde blood flow.

Blood supply of the thorax: the **aorta** is the main arterial trunk, which takes oxygenated blood from the heart and passes it to numerous branches to be distributed around the body. Its main divisions are the ascending aorta, arch of the aorta, thoracic (descending) aorta and abdominal aorta (Figure 29.1). The arch of the aorta has three main branches: the brachiocephalic (divides into the right subclavian and right common carotid), the left common carotid and the left subclavian arteries. With regard to the venous system, the subclavian vein comes from the upper limb and the jugular vein from the neck; both enter the brachiocephalic vein (right and left), which in turn enter the SVC (Figure 29.1). The **azygos system** drains much of the thorax, also entering the SVC. The IVC enters the thorax from the abdomen via an opening in the diaphragm and immediately enters the right atrium of the heart (Figure 29.3).

Blood supply of the head and neck: within the neck, the common **carotid arteries** branches to form the internal and external carotid arteries (left and right; Figure 29.1). These arteries and their branches supply the head and neck region. Venous blood is returned from the brain, superficial head and neck via the internal **jugular veins**. These veins (left and right) terminate by joining the corresponding subclavian vein to form the brachiocephalic vein (Figure 29.1). External jugular veins receive blood from the exterior of the cranium and deep parts of the face, to enter the subclavian vein.

Blood supply of the upper limbs: the subclavian arteries continue as the axillary arteries in the upper limbs, which in turn continue as the brachial arteries. The blood supply to the limb is predominately via the **brachial** and **axillary** arteries and their branches, such as the ulnar and radial arteries (Figure 29.1). The main veins (on the right and left) are the basilic and cephalic veins, which both empty into the axillary veins followed by the subclavian veins and finally brachiocephalic veins, which unite to form the SVC to return deoxygenated blood to the right atrium of the heart.

Blood supply of the abdomen, pelvis and perineum: the majority of the abdominal viscera are supplied by three anterior branches of the abdominal aorta: **celiac trunk, superior and inferior mesenteric arteries** (Figure 29.1). The liver receives blood from the hepatic artery (branch of celiac trunk) and the hepatic portal vein. The latter carries poorly oxygenated blood rich in nutrients from the gastrointestinal viscera (**portal circulation**). The abdominal aorta bifurcates into left and right common iliac arteries (Figure 29.1). These further divide into internal and external iliac arteries; branches of the former supply the majority of the pelvic viscera (exceptions include testes and ovaries) and perineum. Venous blood from the abdomen, pelvis and perineum returns to the heart via the IVC and the azygos system.

Blood supply of the lower limbs: the external iliac artery continues in each lower limb as the common **femoral artery**, providing the main blood supply (Figure 29.4). The common femoral artery divides into the superficial and deep femoral arteries. The superficial femoral artery continues as the **popliteal artery** as it passes posterior to the knee. The popliteal artery divides into the anterior and posterior **tibial arteries**, with the posterior branch giving rise to the fibular (peroneal) artery. The veins of the lower limbs are divided into a deep and superficial group. The deep group consists of the popliteal vein, which continues as the femoral vein in the thigh (Figure 29.4). The superficial group consist of the small saphenous vein (enters into the popliteal vein) and the great saphenous vein (enters the femoral vein).

30 Cardiac physiology

Michael D Randall

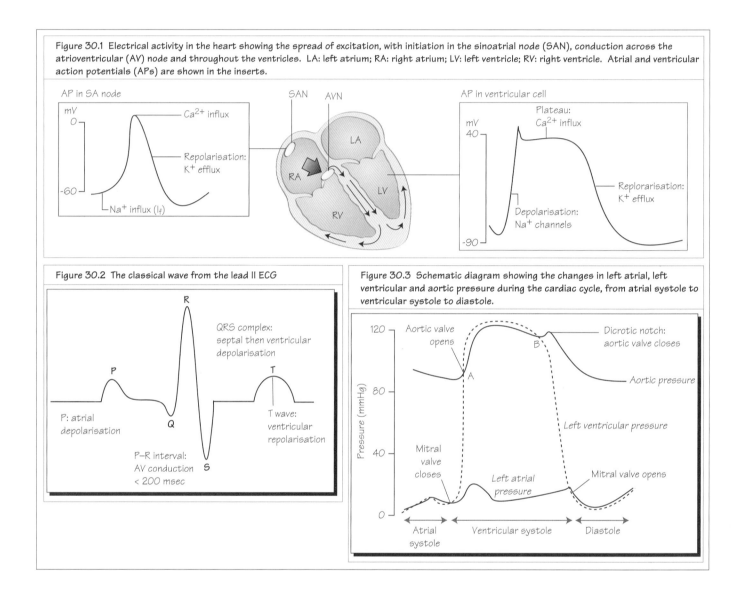

Figure 30.1 Electrical activity in the heart showing the spread of excitation, with initiation in the sinoatrial node (SAN), conduction across the atrioventricular (AV) node and throughout the ventricles. LA: left atrium; RA: right atrium; LV: left ventricle; RV: right ventricle. Atrial and ventricular action potentials (APs) are shown in the inserts.

Figure 30.2 The classical wave from the lead II ECG

Figure 30.3 Schematic diagram showing the changes in left atrial, left ventricular and aortic pressure during the cardiac cycle, from atrial systole to ventricular systole to diastole.

The purpose of the heart is for the **left ventricle** to pump blood around the systemic circulation to perfuse organs and tissues, and for the **right ventricle** to pump blood through the pulmonary circulation to enable gaseous exchange and delivery of oxygenated blood to the left atrium to prime the left ventricle. To achieve this the **cardiac cycle** is a highly coordinated process, which leads to rhythmic and synchronised contractions. **Ventricular systole** is the contractile period and **diastole** is when the heart is not contracting. **Coronary blood flow** supplies the cardiac muscle and only occurs during diastole.

Initiation of the heartbeat

The heartbeat is controlled by the propagation of action potentials leading to coordinated contraction of the cardiac muscle (Figure 30.1).

The heartbeat is initiated by the **sinoatrial node** (SAN), which is the **pacemaker**, as it has the highest intrinsic rate of depolarisation. The pacemaker is set by Na$^+$ influx via the **I$_f$ current**. This leads to an initial depolarization (from −60mV) which takes the membrane to threshold (−45mV) and leads to the opening of voltage-operated Ca^{2+} channels, resulting in slow depolarization as there is no involvement of fast Na$^+$ channels. This is followed by repolarization as the Na$^+$ current switches off and K$^+$ channels open with K$^+$ efflux. The spread of depolarization from the SAN leads to atrial contraction.

To drive the ventricles, depolarisation is conducted across the **atrioventricular (AV) node** and the time required for this to occur leads to a delay (the **AV delay**). The depolarisation then spreads down the **Purkinje fibres** of the **bundle of His**. The Purkinje fibres are specialised conducting fibres that convey the spread of excitation to the ventricular muscle. The **excitation-contraction coupling** starts in the septum and spreads from the apex to the base of the ventricles. The spread of depolarisation is then followed by a wave of repolarisation.

The action potential in ventricular cells is prolonged compared with that in atrial cells and this ensures sufficient time for Ca^{2+} influx to couple to forceful contraction. The initial depolarisation is driven via **voltage-operated ('fast') Na^+ channels** and the plateau of depolarisation lasts typically 200 msec and is associated with Ca^{2+} influx via voltage-operated **L-type Ca^{2+} channels**, which leads to contraction of the ventricular mass. The spread of electrical activity between myocytes is mediated via **gap junctions** composed of connexins at the **intercalated discs** which join the cells.

The electrocardiogram (ECG)

The **ECG** is used to detect the electrical activity of the heart as conducted to the surface of the body via the body's salt solutions. It indicates electrical activity and is not a measure of mechanical events. The recording electrodes can be placed on the limbs and/or on the chest. The 'classical' ECG is referred to as lead II (recorded by an inferior lead, Figure 30.2) and is divided into the following.

• **P-waves**: atrial depolarisation. These are relatively small, reflecting the small mass of the atria.

• **P-R interval** (sometimes referred to as P-Q) (120–200 msec): a period due to conduction delay across the atrioventricular node.

• **QRS complex** an initial dip reflects the septal depolarisation and this is then followed by the spread of depolarisation from the apex to the base.

• **T wave**: ventricular repolarisation.

The ST length corresponds with ejection and the T-P interval corresponds with cardiac filling.

A positive deflection on the ECG reflects a wave of depolarisation towards (or a wave of repolarisation away from) the positive electrode. By comparing the relative magnitudes of ventricular QRS waveforms from different leads (e.g. I, II, III), vectoral analysis determines the 'cardiac axis' of depolarisation. This can be shifted to the right (e.g. pulmonary hypertension) or to the left (e.g. systemic hypertension).

Clinically, the ECG identifies disorders of rate, conduction (e.g. heart block where AV conduction is either slowed or completely blocked), rhythm (e.g. atrial flutter and fibrillation) and ischaemic heart disease (where the ST segment is elevated in myocardial infarction or depressed in ischaemia associated with angina).

Cardiac cycle (Figure 30.3)

The heart is designed to pump blood unidirectionally and to achieve this, intracardiac valves open and close during the cardiac cycle. During atrial systole atrial valves (**mitral** or **bicuspid** in the left atrium and **tricuspid** in the right) are open and allow blood into the ventricles, and as ventricular pressure increases the atrial valves shut. Normally 70% of blood flows directly from the atria to the ventricles and only 30% of flow is due to atrial contraction. Hence the atria act as primers to increase ventricular efficiency.

As the left ventricle fills, the aortic valve is shut as aortic pressure exceeds that in the ventricles. However, as pressure rises in the ventricles, due to contraction, the aortic valves open and blood is ejected into the aorta. As there is **isovolumic relaxation** the aortic pressure then exceeds ventricular pressure and the aortic valve closes. An equivalent process occurs on the right side with the pulmonary valve opening into the pulmonary artery. Only when ventricular pressure is less than atrial pressure do the atrial valves open and the cycle is repeated.

Cardiac haemodynamics

The ventricular ejection of either the left or right ventricle is the **stroke volume**. In the healthy adult, the stroke volume is typically 70 mL and the volume ejected per minute is the **cardiac output**.

Cardiac output = Stroke volume × heart rate

At rest the stroke volume is ~70 mL and heart rate is typically 72 beat per minute and so cardiac output is of the order of 5 L per minute. This is increased according to demand (e.g. exercise) and can reach values of around 20–25 L in highly trained individuals.

Stroke volume is the volume ejected by each ventricle per cycle and is the difference between **end diastolic volume (EDV)** and **end systolic volume (ESV)**. The EDV is determined by the preload on the heart, which is governed by venous return (i.e. the volume of blood returning to the heart from the venous system and is related to venous tone, blood volume and posture). Stroke volume is affected by the contractility of cardiac muscle, which is governed by the **Frank-Starling relationship**. This states that the force of contraction is proportional the initial degree of fibre stretch. Mechanistically, as cardiac muscle is stretched there is an increase in calcium sensitivity of troponin C and so more contractile actin-myosin links are formed in the muscle, and the contractile response is enhanced. As a consequence, as the EDV increases then the force of contraction rises proportionately. This ensures that the stroke volumes of the right and left ventricles are matched.

The stroke volume is also affected by **afterload**, which is the force it has to work against. Afterload is determined by factors such as **peripheral resistance** and **aortic stiffness**. As afterload increases at a constant preload then stroke volume will decrease.

Autonomic control of the heart

Sympathetic: noradrenaline and circulating adrenaline act at β_1-**adrenoceptors**, which are coupled via adenylyl cyclase to an increase in intracellular cAMP. The increase in cAMP, via cAMP-dependent protein kinase, leads to increased Ca^{2+} entry and increased sensitivity of the contractile elements to Ca^{2+}. These changes lead to an increase in the force of contraction (**positive inotropic**). Sympathetic activity increases the Frank-Starling relationship such that an EDV gives an even greater increase in force of contraction. Sympathetic stimulation also increases the rate of pacemaker depolarisation and so increases heart rate (**positive chronotropic**).

Parasympathetic: acetylcholine from the vagus nerve acts on M_2 **muscarinic receptors**, which are negatively coupled to cAMP, and this leads to the activation of hyperpolarising K^+ currents to slow the pacemaker at the SAN and slow AV conduction. This slows the heart rate (**negative chronotropic**).

Michael D Randall

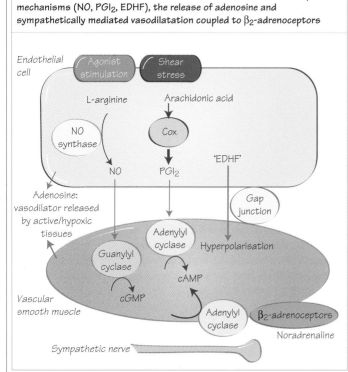

Figure 31.1 Mechanisms of vasodilatation involving endothelium-dependent mechanisms (NO, PGI$_2$, EDHF), the release of adenosine and sympathetically mediated vasodilatation coupled to β$_2$-adrenoceptors

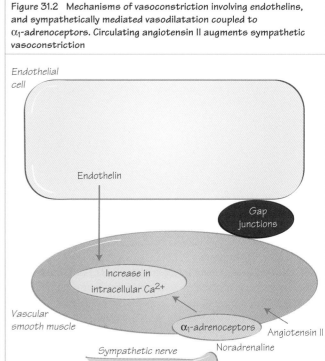

Figure 31.2 Mechanisms of vasoconstriction involving endothelins, and sympathetically mediated vasodilatation coupled to α$_1$-adrenoceptors. Circulating angiotensin II augments sympathetic vasoconstriction

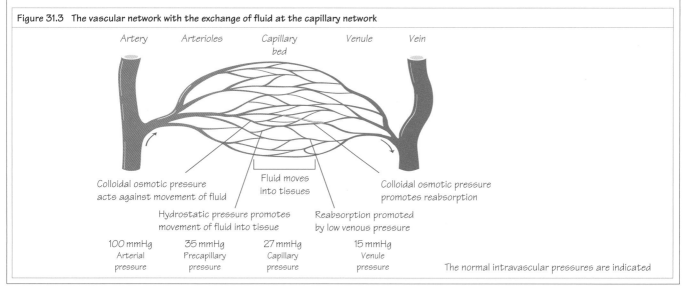

Figure 31.3 The vascular network with the exchange of fluid at the capillary network

The purpose of the cardiovascular system is to ensure perfusion of the tissues with blood, allowing for the delivery of nutrients and oxygen, and the removal of metabolites including CO_2. This is achieved by the **systemic circulation**, which delivers oxygenated blood via arteries and then arterioles (<50 μm in diameter) to the capillary network, where exchange occurs.

Regulation of vascular tone

Blood flow is driven by the increased pressure generated by the heart. Blood readily flows through low-resistance conduit arteries (e.g. the aorta then the superior mesenteric artery) to the tissues and organs. At this point the control of blood flow, and therefore tissue, perfusion is determined by **vascular resistance**. This impedes flow, meaning that blood follows the route of least resistance and is facilitated by vasodilatation and opposed by vasoconstriction.

Vascular resistance is determined by **Poiseuille's law**:

$$\text{Resistance} = \frac{(8 \times \text{viscosity} \times \text{length})}{(\pi r^4)}$$

Therefore vascular resistance is proportional to **1/radius⁴**, meaning that small decreases in radius lead to substantial increases in vascular resistance. Hence, small changes in vessel diameter, governed by vascular tone, have profound effects on blood flow and pressure.

Autonomic control of vascular tone

One of the key regulators of arterial diameter and resistance is the sympathetic nervous system. Sympathetic nerve fibres release noradrenaline, which activates α_1-adrenoceptors on the vascular smooth muscle, leading to an increase in intracellular Ca^{2+} via release from stores and Ca^{2+} influx via L-type calcium channels. This leads to vasoconstriction and increases vascular resistance. Sympathetic innervation and circulating adrenaline also stimulate β_2-adrenoceptors (coupled via adenylyl cyclase to cAMP), largely associated with arteries supplying skeletal muscle, leading to vasodilatation, which results in increased blood flow, for example during exercise (Figures 31.1 and 31.2).

Sympathetic control is also augmented by angiotensin II (AII) (Chapter 32) from the renin-angiotensin system. This system is activated by both indications of low blood pressure and sympathetic stimulation, and results in the release of renin by the juxtaglomerular (granular) cells of the kidney.

Endothelial autacoids and vascular control

The vascular endothelium is now recognised as a key regulator of vascular tone by the release of endothelium-derived autacoids (Figure 31.1). The archetypical endothelium-derived relaxant is the gas **nitric oxide (NO)**, which is derived from L-arginine via NO synthase. There is a tonic release of NO, which helps to modulate vascular resistance and control blood pressure. The release of NO also occurs in response to agonists and shear stress resulting from blood flow. This leads to flow-dependent dilatation to match blood flow to demand. NO acts on the vascular smooth muscle to stimulate guanylyl cyclase, which increases levels of cGMP, resulting in vasodilatation.

The endothelium also releases the prostanoid, **prostacyclin (PGI₂)**, and the so-called **endothelium-derived hyperpolarising factor (EDHF)**, which also causes vasodilatation. The activity of EDHF may, in part, be explained by the transfer of electrical current (hyperpolarisation) via gap junctions to the vascular smooth muscle.

The endothelium also releases peptides of the **endothelin** family, which are the most potent vasoconstrictors known.

Metabolic control

Metabolism may also regulate blood flow. Products of metabolism (e.g. **adenosine** from ATP) are released by very active tissues (e.g. cardiac muscle) to cause local vasodilatation and match blood flow to metabolic demand. When blood flow is transiently stopped to a tissue (e.g. a limb) the restoration of blood flow is at a greater rate, **'reactive hyperaemia'**. This response is due to the release of vasodilator mediators (e.g. prostanoids), metabolites (e.g. adenosine, K^+) and the activation of ATP-sensitive potassium channels.

Capillary exchange (Figure 31.3)

The movement of fluid at the capillary bed is tightly regulated. Arterial pressure provides **hydrostatic pressure**, which is the driving force for fluid (blood components but not red blood cells or large proteins) to move out of the circulation. This is the **precapillary pressure**. The **colloidal osmotic pressure**, generated by the plasma proteins retained in the intravascular compartment, acts against fluid moving out.

Interstitial or tissue fluid is then reabsorbed into the venous circulation and the reabsorption of water is promoted by plasma protein colloidal osmotic pressure. The hydrostatic pressure in the venous circulation acts against reabsorption and so a low venous pressure promotes reabsorption.

The surface area of the capillary bed also plays a role and a large surface area facilitates exchange. For example, as skeletal muscle becomes active there is capillary recruitment to increase the surface area and so increase exchange.

This is summarised by Starling's equation:

$$\text{Fluid flow} \propto (P_c - P_i) - \sigma (\pi_p - \pi_i)$$

where P_c = capillary pressure and P_i = interstitial pressure, and so $(P_c - P_i)$ is the pressure gradient or hydrostatic force; π_p is the colloidal osmotic pressure in the plasma and π_i is the interstitial colloidal osmotic pressure such that $(\pi_p - \pi_i)$ is the colloidal osmotic gradient; σ is the reflection coefficient, which takes account of the difficulty of proteins to pass across the capillary wall.

The tissue pressure in the tissue is normally constant and so has little influence on fluid exchange. However, if it were to increase then it would alter the hydrostatic gradient and limit the movement of fluid into the extravascular compartment.

The reabsorption of fluid is usually less than that entering the interstitium and the lymphatic system plays a role is reabsorbing this excess fluid and also proteins that have escaped from the blood.

Oedema

This is the accumulation of fluid in the tissues and leads to swelling. This is a pathological event and may result from the following.

Low levels of protein (associated with liver disease as the liver is a key site of plasma protein synthesis, or malnutrition): the reduced colloidal osmotic pressure reduces the driving force for retention of fluid on the arterial side and reduces the driving force for reabsorption on the venous side. ***Increased venous pressure*** (associated with heart failure): the increase in venous pressure acts as hydrostatic force, which reduces the reabsorption of fluid in the venous side. In left-sided heart failure this leads to pulmonary oedema and in right-sided heart failure it leads to peripheral oedema. ***Lymphatic obstruction***: this impedes return of fluid and proteins from the tissue via the lymphatic system to the veins. ***Inflammation***: inflammatory mediators such as histamine can increase capillary permeability, leading to extravasation of fluid and oedema. ***Arteriolar vasodilatation*** (e.g. due to calcium channel inhibitors such as amlodipine): this leads to an increase in blood flow with an increase precapillary pressure and so increases the hydrostatic driving force for fluid to move out leading to oedema.

Venous return

The venous circulation is a low-pressure system whose role is to return blood to the heart ('venous return'). The movement of blood through the venous circulation is driven by the following.

Vascular tone: although veins are less muscular then arteries, venoconstriction promotes return to the heart and venodilatation reduces venous return. ***Skeletal muscle pump***: in which leg muscles contract and squeeze blood from superficial veins to deep veins to the vena cava. Movement is facilitated by venous valves, which ensures unidirectional flow. ***Breathing***: inspiration decreases intrathoracic pressure and provides a pressure gradient to promote venous return.

32 Blood pressure

Michael D Randall

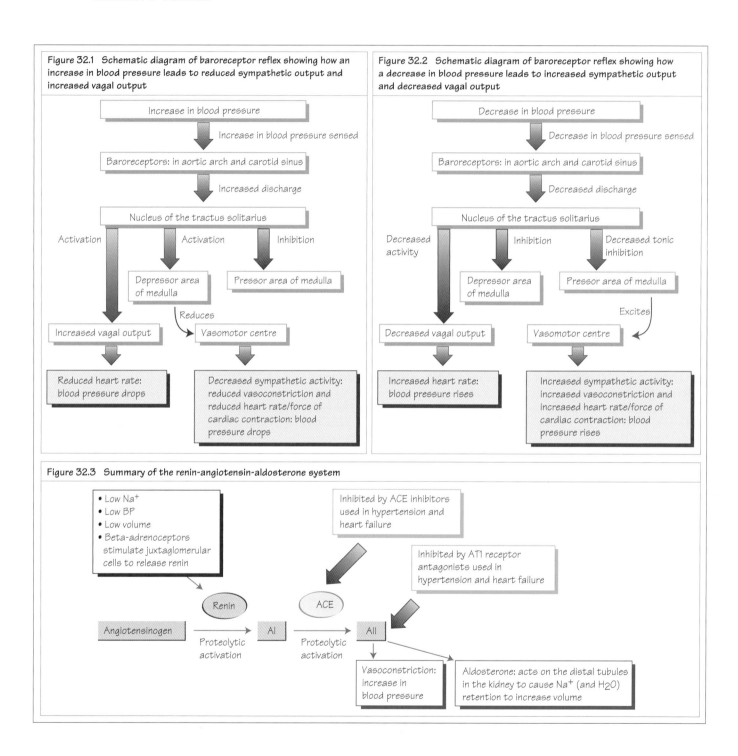

Figure 32.1 Schematic diagram of baroreceptor reflex showing how an increase in blood pressure leads to reduced sympathetic output and increased vagal output

Increase in blood pressure

Increase in blood pressure sensed

Baroreceptors: in aortic arch and carotid sinus

Increased discharge

Nucleus of the tractus solitarius

Activation — Activation — Inhibition

Depressor area of medulla

Pressor area of medulla

Reduces

Increased vagal output

Vasomotor centre

Reduced heart rate: blood pressure drops

Decreased sympathetic activity: reduced vasoconstriction and reduced heart rate/force of cardiac contraction: blood pressure drops

Figure 32.2 Schematic diagram of baroreceptor reflex showing how a decrease in blood pressure leads to increased sympathetic output and decreased vagal output

Decrease in blood pressure

Decrease in blood pressure sensed

Baroreceptors: in aortic arch and carotid sinus

Decreased discharge

Nucleus of the tractus solitarius

Decreased activity — Inhibition — Decreased tonic inhibition

Depressor area of medulla

Pressor area of medulla

Excites

Decreased vagal output

Vasomotor centre

Increased heart rate: blood pressure rises

Increased sympathetic activity: increased vasoconstriction and increased heart rate/force of cardiac contraction: blood pressure rises

Figure 32.3 Summary of the renin-angiotensin-aldosterone system

- Low Na^+
- Low BP
- Low volume
- Beta-adrenoceptors stimulate juxtaglomerular cells to release renin

Inhibited by ACE inhibitors used in hypertension and heart failure

Inhibited by AT1 receptor antagonists used in hypertension and heart failure

Renin

ACE

Angiotensinogen → Proteolytic activation → AI → Proteolytic activation → AII

Vasoconstriction: increase in blood pressure

Aldosterone: acts on the distal tubules in the kidney to cause Na^+ (and H_2O) retention to increase volume

Blood pressure is a measure of the pressure in the systemic cardiovascular system and is reported as central arterial pressure (i.e. equivalent to that in a large artery at the height of the heart). The higher value is the **systolic blood pressure** as the left ventricle contracts and ejects, and the lower value is the **diastolic blood pressure** when the heart is not contracting. In a healthy adult, normal values are 120 mmHg (systolic) and 80 mmHg (diastolic), and mean arterial pressure is reported as:

Mean arterial pressure(MAP)

  = diastolic pressure + 1/3 of the (pulse pressure)

where **pulse pressure** is the difference between systolic pressure and diastolic pressure.

MAP in a healthy adult is approximately 93 mmHg. The mean arterial pressure is the time-averaged pressure experienced by the systemic circulation.

Blood pressure is determined by **cardiac output** (CO) × **total peripheral resistance** (TPR) and is tightly controlled to ensure appropriate tissue perfusion. **Hypertension** is pathological and is a sustained increase in blood pressure at rest, such that diastolic blood pressure is ≥90 mmHg and systolic is ≥140 mmHg. In the healthy adult, blood pressure is tightly regulated by nervous and hormonal mechanisms.

Nervous control of blood pressure and baroreceptor control

Blood pressure is regulated in the short term by the autonomic nervous system, with sympathetic innervation of arterial smooth muscle leading to α_1-adrenoceptor-mediated vasoconstriction and an increase TPR (Chapter 31). To ensure maintenance of blood pressure, **baroreceptors** in the carotid sinus and aortic arch sense pressure, and as pressure increases there are increased impulses to the **nucleus of the solitary tract (nucleus tractus solitarius; NTS)** in the brain. Increases in pressure inhibit the 'pressor' area in the rostral ventrolateral medulla to reduce sympathetic output from the vasomotor centre. Increases in pressure also stimulate the 'depressor' area in the caudal ventrolateral medulla to inhibit sympathetic output from the vasomotor centre (Figure 32.1). This is accompanied by increased vagal output to lower blood pressure. Decreases in blood pressure lead to the 'pressor' centre dominating and decreased vagal output to restore blood pressure (Figure 32.2).

Postural control of blood pressure

Changes in posture lead to alterations in pressure due to the hydrostatic influence on the blood. For example, when changing from lying down to standing up, the change in fluid distribution would tend to cause a reduction in central blood pressure. The reduction in central arterial pressure would tend to lead to less pressure in the cerebral circulation and could lead to 'light headedness'. However, the **baroreceptor reflex** aims to maintain a relatively constant blood pressure with any change in posture. An initial drop in blood pressure would initiate a baroreceptor reflex, resulting in increased sympathetic activity (with peripheral vasoconstriction) and decreased vagal activity to maintain a relatively constant blood pressure. **Autonomic dysfunction** or drug treatments that interfere with volume control (diuretics) or α_1-adrenoceptor-mediated vasoconstriction (α_1-adrenoceptor antagonists) can impair these responses and lead to **postural** or **ortho-static hypotension** (i.e. when systolic blood pressure drops >20 mmHg) when changing from lying or sitting down to standing.

Volume control of blood pressure

In the longer term it is blood volume that has the greater influence on blood pressure, and this is tightly regulated. Volume is linked to Na^+ balance, as water follows Na^+ by osmosis. Blood volume and Na^+ balance are tightly controlled by the kidneys and this is achieved by the **renin-angiotensin-aldosterone system** (RAAS) (Chapter 38) (Figure 32.3). Low levels of Na^+ and low blood pressures are sensed by the **macula densa cells** of the **juxtaglomerular apparatus** in the kidneys, which respond by releasing renin. This is also stimulated by β-adrenoceptor-mediated sympathetic stimulation. **Renin** is a proteolytic enzyme that activates by cleavage of the circulating hormone **angiotensinogen** to form the peptide **angiotensin I (AI)**. Following this, AI is activated by the **angiotensin converting enzyme** (ACE), which is largely located in the lungs, to form **angiotensin II** (AII). AII acts at the angiotensin AT_1 receptor and is a potent vasoconstrictor and also augments sympathetically induced vasoconstriction to increase blood pressure. AII also stimulates the release of the steroid hormone **aldosterone** from the zona glomerulosa of the adrenal cortex. Aldosterone then acts on distal tubular cells of the kidney to increase the number of sodium channels and sodium pumps, and this promotes the reasbsorption of Na^+ (with a concomitant loss of K^+), followed by water.

Vasopressin or the **antidiuretic hormone** (ADH) also plays a role in volume control (Chapter 38). ADH acts on the collecting ducts of the kidney, leading to the activation of **aquaporins** (water channels) and this promotes water reabsorption and volume control.

Hypertension

As defined above, this is the sustained and pathological increase in blood pressure. **Essential hypertension** accounts for 90–95% of cases and its aetiology is multifactorial, with no single identifiable cause. **Secondary hypertension** (5–10%) is when the increase in blood pressure is associated with another pathology, e.g. renal artery stenosis (associated with increased activation of RAAS), Conn's syndrome (associated with increased release of aldosterone), phaeochromocytoma (tumour-secreting catecholamines), or fluid-retaining drugs (e.g. steroids and non-steroidal anti-inflammatory drugs, NSAIDs). Secondary hypertension is usually treated by managing the associated condition. Essential hypertension is managed by lifestyle measures (e.g. weight loss, decreased alcohol consumption, increased physical activity) and may be treated with antihypertensives. As blood pressure is the product of cardiac output and TPR, the principle is to reduce one of these determinants.

Widely used antihypertensives include:
- **angiotensin converting enzyme (ACE) inhibitors** (e.g. ramipril): these reduce the production of AII and so reduce TPR. AT_1 receptor antagonists (e.g. losartan) are also used and inhibit the actions of AII;
- **calcium channel blockers** (e.g. amlodipine): these inhibit voltage-operated Ca^{2+} channels in vascular smooth muscle to cause vasodilatation and so reduce TPR;
- **diuretics** (e.g. thiazide-like agents such as indapamide): act on the distal convoluted tubule cells of the kidney to inhibit NaCl reabsorption (and so water reabsorption). These lead to a reduction in circulating volume and reduction in blood pressure. They also cause vasodilatation.

Michael D Randall

Figure 33.1 Summary of haemopoiesis

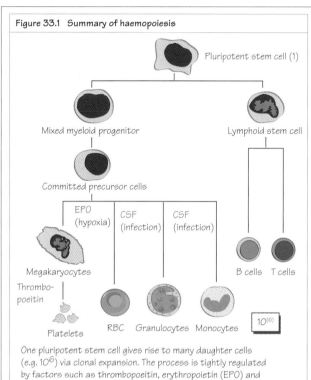

One pluripotent stem cell gives rise to many daughter cells (e.g. 10^6) via clonal expansion. The process is tightly regulated by factors such as thrombopoeitin, erythropoietin (EPO) and colony-stimulating factors (CSFs)

Figure 33.2 Centrifuged blood sample to indicate its normal composition

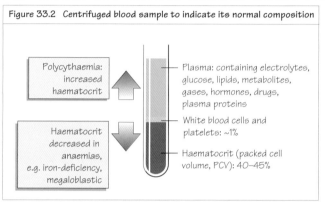

Polycythaemia: increased haematocrit

Haematocrit decreased in anaemias, e.g. iron-deficiency, megaloblastic

Plasma: containing electrolytes, glucose, lipids, metabolites, gases, hormones, drugs, plasma proteins

White blood cells and platelets: ~1%

Haematocrit (packed cell volume, PCV): 40–45%

Table 33.1 Alterations in differential blood cell counts

Cell type	Increased	Decreased
Erythrocytes [Males $4.5–6.5 \times 10^{12}$/L] [Females $3.9–5.6 \times 10^{12}$/L]	Polycythemia • Primary: stem cell defect leading to uncontrolled proliferation • Secondary: (Patho)physiological response to hypoxia associated with ascent to altitude, smoking and COPD	Anaemia • Microcytic associated with iron deficiency • Macrocytic associated with folate and/or vitamin B_{12} deficiency • Normocytic associated with chronic conditions, e.g. renal disease
Leucocytes [Total $4.0–11.0 \times 10^9$/L]	Leucocytosis	Leucopenia
Neutrophils [$2.5–7.5 \times 10^9$/L]	Neutrophilia • Response to infections (bacterial/fungal) • Inflammation • Trauma	Neutropenia • Drug-induced as an adverse drug reaction. Patient may present with increased infections • Infection (viral, malaria)
Eosinophils [$0.04–0.44 \times 10^9$/L]	Eosinophilia • Associated with allergy/atopy • Parasitic infections	
Monocytes [$0.2–0.8 \times 10^9$/L]	Monocytosis • Associated with chronic infections, e.g. tuberculosis	
Lymphocytes [$1.5–3.5 \times 10^9$/L]	Lymphocytosis • Response to infection (bacterial, viral) • Lymphoma – malignancy of lymphatic tissue leading to uncontrolled production	Lymphopenia • Inflammation – depletion of cells • Lymphoma – malignancy of lymphatic tissue impairing production • Steroids – anti-inflammatory actions reducing production
Platelets [$150–400 \times 10^9$/L]	Thrombophilia • Increased risk of thrombosis	Thrombocytopenia • May be drug-induced as an adverse drug reaction • Idiopathic: no identifiable cause

The volume of blood in an adult is around 5 litres and is normally composed of **red blood cells** (RBCs: erythrocytes) for gas transport (Chapter 25), white blood cells (WBCs) (**neutrophils, eosinophils, basophils, monocytes** and **lymphocytes**) for defence/immunology and **platelets** (for clotting). The remainder is plasma, a solution of electrolytes, glucose, lipids, metabolites, gases, hormones, drugs and plasma proteins. **Serum** is coagulated plasma.

Control of blood production

Production of blood cells (**haemopoiesis**) is a tightly regulated process in which a **pluripotent stem cell** is committed to one cell line and undergoes many cell divisions, leading to **clonal expansion**. RBC production is stimulated by the polypeptide **erythropoietin** (EPO), which is released by renal peritubular cells in response to hypoxia. **Colony-stimulating factors** (CSFs), e.g. **G-CSF** (granulocyte CSF), act on the neutrophil cell line and are increased in infections to increase the WBC count (Figure 33.1).

Blood counts

The full blood count is the number of blood cells per volume of blood and is differentiated into RBCs, WBC types and platelets.

The amount of **haemoglobin** (Hb) in blood is expressed as (g) per 100 mL of blood and used to identify **anaemias**.

Haematocrit (packed cell volume, PCV) is the percentage of blood that is made up of RBCs. It is expressed as either a percentage (typically 40–45%) or as a fraction (0.40–0.45).

Mean corpuscular volume (MCV) is the volume (fl) of individual RBCs [normal range = 80–95 fl]. Increased MCV is described as **macrocytosis** and a decreased MCV as **microcytosis**.

Blood groups

These are determined by antigens (glycoproteins) expressed on RBC membranes and antibodies to other antigens may be in plasma. There are more than 400 groups, but **ABO** and **Rhesus** are the clinically important ones. **Group A** (A antigens and b-antibodies), **Group B** (B antigens and a-antibodies), **Group AB** (A and B antigens and no antibodies), and **Group O** (a and b antibodies).

• The **Rhesus D (RhD)** antigen confers the Rhesus status (positive). Patients are identified as being A, B, AB, or O, and are either Rh+ve or Rh–ve. This system is essential to ensure correct cross-matching of blood for transfusions, as exposure to an antigen from a different group leads to life-threatening **transfusion reactions**. This involves antibodies being raised against the foreign antigen, leading to a severe immune response with haemolysis of RBCs.

Blood from the **O Rh–ve** group is regarded as a **universal donor** as it lacks antigens and as such will not provoke an immune response. O–ve blood is therefore used in dire emergencies for transfusions until cross-matched blood is available.

Haemolytic disease of the newborn

Approximately 85% of the population are Rh+ve, consequently mothers who are Rh–ve are likely to carry to a Rh+ve fetus. In a first pregnancy this is unlikely to lead to complications, but at birth the transfer of fetal blood leads to the mother raising antibodies against the D-antigen. These antibodies would then attack a subsequent fetus that was Rh+ve, potentially leading to fetal death. To eliminate this risk the mother receives **anti-D immunisation** after the first birth to bind any D-antigens and so prevent the production of antibodies.

Anaemias

These are common clinical conditions with reduced Hb levels, leading to the symptoms of breathlessness, weakness, lethargy and tachycar-dia. The patient may have pale conjunctiva, and anaemia is also associated with glossitis (painful red tongue) and angular cheilitis (fissures at corner of mouth).

Microcytic

Iron deficiency anaemia is the most common form of anaemia and develops once all of the body's iron stores have been depleted. This is usually secondary to negative iron balance through chronic blood loss due to **gastrointestinal bleeds** or **excessive menstrual bleeding**. The lack of iron results in impaired synthesis of Hb and RBCs, which are smaller than normal, i.e. **microcytic** (reduced MCV).

Normocytic

Anaemia associated with chronic conditions tends to be normocytic. An example of this is **renal anaemia**, in which patients with chronic kidney disease often develop normocytic anaemia due to reduced EPO production from the kidneys. It is managed with injections of EPO.

Macrocytic

The RBCs are macrocytic (increased MCV) and a common cause is **megaloblastic anaemia**. In this condition there is abnormal RBC maturation as a result of defective DNA synthesis, and the bone marrow contains **megaloblasts**. Megaloblastic anaemia is caused by deficiencies of either **vitamin B_{12} or folic acid**. Vitamin B_{12} is an essential cofactor for purine and pyrimidine synthesis (hence the defective DNA synthesis and impaired cell division). Folate is an essential substrate for thymidylate synthesis.

Pernicious anaemia is a version of megaloblastic anaemia in which the body raises antibodies against the **intrinsic factor** released from parietal cells in the stomach. The intrinsic factor normally binds to vitamin B_{12} and is essential for its absorption in the ileum. Therefore, in this condition there is impaired absorption of vitamin B_{12}, leading to deficiencies and megaloblastic anaemia, which is managed by injections of a vitamin B_{12} analogue.

Haemolytic anaemias

Haemolytic anaemias are characterised by increased RBC destruction. These can be acquired, for example through increased destruction associated with transfusion reactions or malaria. They can also be genetic and associated with abnormal forms of Hb that predispose to RBC destruction.

• **Sickle cell anaemia** involves a **single nucleotide polymorphism** in which there is a single amino acid substitution of glutamic acid with valine. This leads to abnormal Hb, which forms insoluble crystals at low O_2 tensions and the RBCs form fragile sickle shapes, which may block microcirculation.

• **Thalassaemias**: these are genetic conditions in which there is reduced rate of α or β globin units production. There are a range of variations, for example deletion of all four of the copies of the α-globin genes results in Hb with 4γ subunits being formed, which is incompatible with life and leads to death of the fetus. The loss of one or two of the α-globin genes is referred to as an α-thalassaemia trait and is not usually associated with anaemia (but MCV is usually low).

Aplastic anaemia

Aplastic anaemia is the lack of production of blood cells and platelets by the bone marrow. Mostly cases are acquired due to viral infection, radiation, or drugs causing damage to the bone marrow. This is a potentially fatal condition and is managed symptomatically by transfusions. Curative treatment is via bone marrow transplantation.

34 Blood: 2

Michael D Randall

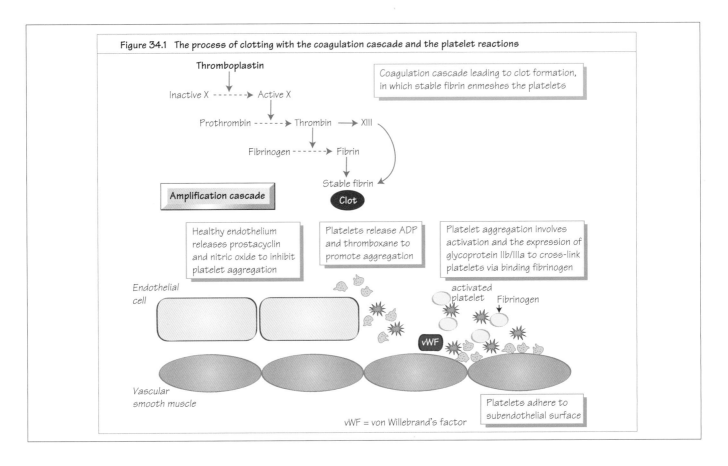

Figure 34.1 The process of clotting with the coagulation cascade and the platelet reactions

Coagulation cascade leading to clot formation, in which stable fibrin enmeshes the platelets

Healthy endothelium releases prostacyclin and nitric oxide to inhibit platelet aggregation

Platelets release ADP and thromboxane to promote aggregation

Platelet aggregation involves activation and the expression of glycoprotein IIb/IIIa to cross-link platelets via binding fibrinogen

Platelets adhere to subendothelial surface

vWF = von Willebrand's factor

Coagulation and thrombosis (Figure 34.1)

The process of haemostasis is the formation of clots at the site of damage to a blood vessel to prevent blood loss. It involves both coagulation (via plasma-borne proteins) and platelet aggregation.

Coagulation

Activation of the coagulation cascade results in the production of insoluble fibrin. This process involves many steps in which precursor coagulation factors are activated by activated factors. As such, the coagulation cascade is an **amplification cascade**, with each step resulting in a substantial activation of the next components. This means that a relatively small event can lead to large biological response. Many of the reactions involve **serine protease** activity cleaving the precursor factor, and the final product is stabilised fibrin, which enmeshes platelet aggregates.

The **initiation phase** (previously termed extrinsic pathway) involves the release of **thromboplastin** (tissue factor) from damaged tissues. Thromboplastin then complexes with activated factor VIIa in the plasma and this leads to the activation of factor X. Factor Xa then leads to the activation of prothrombin to thrombin, which hydrolyses fibrinogen to release fibrinopeptides A and B, which are polymerised to form fibrin. Thrombin also activates factor XIII to form XIIIa, which cross-links the fibrin.

Platelet adhesion and aggregation

In parallel with the coagulation cascade is the **platelet reaction**, in which platelets adhere to subendothelial surface on vessel damage and this is facilitated by binding to **von Willebrand's factor (vWF)**. **Platelet adhesion** then leads to the **release reaction**, in which platelets release **adenosine diphosphate** (ADP) and **thromboxane** (TXA$_2$) to promote platelet aggregation. ADP binds to receptors on platelets and this leads to the expression of **glycoprotein IIb/IIIa** in the platelet membranes and promotes cross-linking by binding vWF and fibrinogen. TXA$_2$ promotes aggregation by reducing intracellular levels of cAMP.

Thrombosis

Thrombosis is the unwanted formation of blood clots. On the venous side of the circulation thrombosis is largely associated with stasis of blood. For example, immobility may lead to the formation of **deep vein thrombosis** (DVTs) in the deep veins of the calf muscles in the legs. The thrombus may break off and enter the circulation where it can become lodged in the lungs. This is a life-threatening **pulmonary embolism** due to blockade of the pulmonary circulation.

Arterial thrombosis usually forms at atherosclerotic sites, in which the plaque may rupture, leading to platelet adhesion and aggregation. The resulting clot formation can lead to an arterial blockage. In the coronary circulation this leads to a **myocardial infarction** and in cerebral vessels formation of the blockage or an embolus results in a **thromboembolic stroke**.

Atrial fibrillation leads to impaired pumping of the blood from the left atrium and the stasis of blood predisposes towards thrombosis. Blood clots form and may then break off and enter the systemic circulation and become lodged in the cerebral circulation leading to a **transient ischaemic attack (TIA)**.

Anticoagulants

To prevent thrombosis the oral anticoagulant **warfarin** is used. Warfarin is a vitamin K antagonist and blocks the **vitamin K epoxide reductase** (VKOR), which is an enzyme in the liver responsible for the post-translational modification of coagulation factors. Warfarin therefore inhibits the synthesis of certain coagulation factors. Clinically, warfarin is a difficult drug to use and has many drug interactions. It requires extensive monitoring of its anticoagulant activity by measuring the **prothrombin time**, expressed as the **international normalised ratio** (INR).

Injectible anticoagulants are the **heparins**, which have immediate actions via activating antithrombin III in the plasma, which inhibits serine protease activities of some of the coagulation factors.

More recently **direct thrombin inhibitors** (e.g. dabigatran) have been introduced and do not require extensive monitoring.

Antiplatelet drugs

Low-dose (75 mg) **aspirin** is highly effective at reducing the risk of myocardial infarction and ischaemic stroke in at risk patients. Aspirin inhibits the cyclooxygenase enzyme responsible for producing prostacyclin in the endothelium (which inhibits platelet aggregation) and TX$_2$ in platelets. The actions of aspirin are irreversible, but since the endothelial cells have a nucleus they are, in time, able to produce new cyclooxygenases and so prostacyclin. However, platelets, which lack a nucleus, are incapable of producing more enzyme and therefore cannot produce TXA$_2$. Consequently aspirin shifts the balance to favour prostacyclin over TXA$_2$ and reduces the chances of platelet aggregation.

Clopidogrel is an ADP (P2Y$_{12}$) receptor antagonist and prevents ADP-induced expression of glycoprotein IIb/IIIa. Therefore, clopidogrel is also used to prevent platelet aggregation.

Problems with haemostasis

Haemophilias are genetic conditions in which affected patients have low or absent levels of Factor VIII (haemophilia A) or IX (haemophilia B) of the clotting cascade. This means that affected patients bleed profusely on minor trauma and require treatment with coagulation factor.

Von Willebrand's disease is an hereditary lack or defect in vWF and results in increased bruising and mucosal bleeding (e.g. nose bleeds).

Thrombocytopenia is a reduction in platelet count due to impaired production of platelets. It may be induced by the toxic or immunological effects of drugs on platelet production. It may also occur in the absence of an identifiable cause (idiopathic). The reduction in platelet count leads to easy bleeding and bruising.

Disseminated intravascular coagulation involves widespread and uncontrolled activation of the coagulant cascade throughout the vascular system. This may occur due to the presence of procoagulant material (e.g. amniotic fluid) in the circulation stimulating coagulation. The uncontrolled production of fibrin leads to the excessive consumption of coagulation factors and the patient is at risk of severe haemorrhage due to depletion of factors and platelets.

Leukaemias and lymphomas
Leukaemias

Leukaemias are haematological malignancies in which abnormal cells accumulate in the bone marrow and this may lead to bone marrow failure. The malignant transformation can result in the increased production of abnormal white blood cells, which increase the patient's susceptibility to infection. Associated bone marrow failure leads to anaemia and thrombocytopenia. There are number of different forms of leukaemia.

• **Acute leukaemias** usually have a short time course between discovery and death if they are untreated. There is failure of cell maturation, and useless cells accumulate in bone marrow and then spill over into the circulation. They are divided into **myeloid** or **lymphoblastic**, depending on which cell line is involved.

• **Chronic myeloid leukaemia** involves the replacement of normal bone marrow cells with cells with an abnormal chromosome (90% of patients have Philadelphia chromosome).

• **Chronic lymphocytic leukaemia** is the most common form and especially affects the elderly. It is characterised by abnormal lymphocytes in lymphoid tissue (including the bone).

Lymphomas

These are malignancies of the lymphatic tissue in which there is replacement of lymphoid tissue with abnormal cells. Depending on the histology, they are divided into either Hodgkin's disease or non-Hodgkin's lymphoma (high or low grade).

Management

Both leukaemias and lymphomas may be managed by anticancer chemotherapy (Chapter 65) and some leukaemias can be cured by bone marrow transplantation with stem cells following destruction of diseased bone marrow by high-dose chemotherapy and irradiation.

Michael D Randall

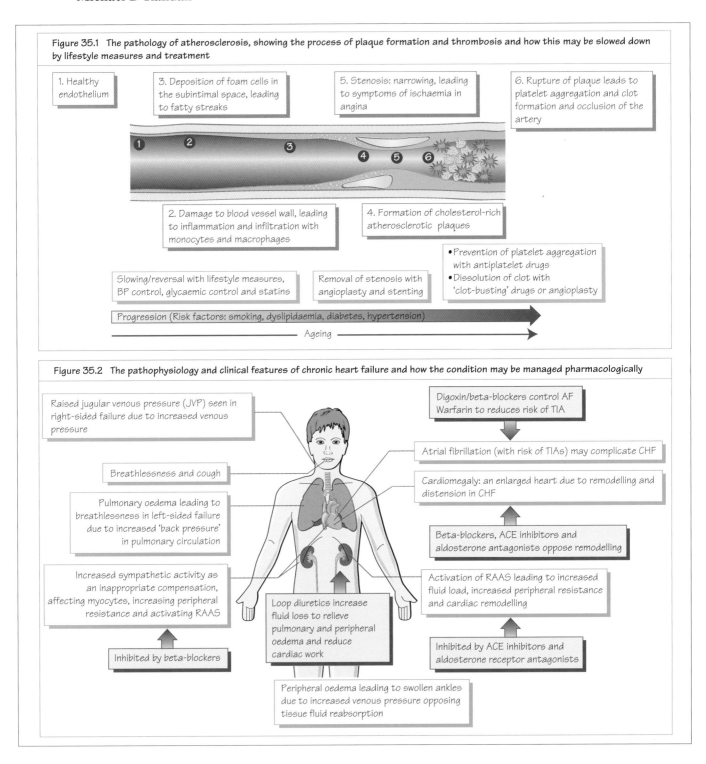

Figure 35.1 The pathology of atherosclerosis, showing the process of plaque formation and thrombosis and how this may be slowed down by lifestyle measures and treatment

1. Healthy endothelium

3. Deposition of foam cells in the subintimal space, leading to fatty streaks

5. Stenosis: narrowing, leading to symptoms of ischaemia in angina

6. Rupture of plaque leads to platelet aggregation and clot formation and occlusion of the artery

2. Damage to blood vessel wall, leading to inflammation and infiltration with monocytes and macrophages

4. Formation of cholesterol-rich atherosclerotic plaques

- Prevention of platelet aggregation with antiplatelet drugs
- Dissolution of clot with 'clot-busting' drugs or angioplasty

Slowing/reversal with lifestyle measures, BP control, glycaemic control and statins

Removal of stenosis with angioplasty and stenting

Progression (Risk factors: smoking, dyslipidaemia, diabetes, hypertension)

Ageing

Figure 35.2 The pathophysiology and clinical features of chronic heart failure and how the condition may be managed pharmacologically

Raised jugular venous pressure (JVP) seen in right-sided failure due to increased venous pressure

Breathlessness and cough

Pulmonary oedema leading to breathlessness in left-sided failure due to increased 'back pressure' in pulmonary circulation

Increased sympathetic activity as an inappropriate compensation, affecting myocytes, increasing peripheral resistance and activating RAAS

Inhibited by beta-blockers

Loop diuretics increase fluid loss to relieve pulmonary and peripheral oedema and reduce cardiac work

Peripheral oedema leading to swollen ankles due to increased venous pressure opposing tissue fluid reabsorption

Digoxin/beta-blockers control AF Warfarin to reduces risk of TIA

Atrial fibrillation (with risk of TIAs) may complicate CHF

Cardiomegaly: an enlarged heart due to remodelling and distension in CHF

Beta-blockers, ACE inhibitors and aldosterone antagonists oppose remodelling

Activation of RAAS leading to increased fluid load, increased peripheral resistance and cardiac remodelling

Inhibited by ACE inhibitors and aldosterone receptor antagonists

Cardiovascular disease is the biggest killer in the Western world. Ischaemic heart disease is the leading cause of death in the UK, with stroke (after cancer) accounting for the third-highest number of deaths. Cardiovascular disease is an inevitable consequence of the ageing process but is accelerated by the following risk factors (male gender, smoking, ethnicity: Indian subcontinent ethnicity is associated with an increased risk, diabetes: especially with poor glycaemic control, dyslipidaemia: high LDL cholesterol, low HDL cholesterol and high triglycerides; there may be a familial tendency, obesity, family history: close relative with premature cardiovascular disease).

Hypertension (Chapter 32)

This is a key cardiovascular disease and is a risk factor for developing ischaemic heart disease and chronic heart failure.

Ischaemic heart disease

Ischaemic heart disease (IHD) may manifest as either angina or myocardial infarction (MI) and is an important cause of chronic heart failure. In both cases, IHD is generally associated with **atherosclerosis** within the coronary arteries, leading to impaired blood flow or thromboembolic occlusion. In angina, the reductions in coronary blood flow mean that perfusion does not match demand, leading to ischaemia, which provokes the symptoms. **Stable angina** is characterised by chest pain (which may radiate down the left arm and to the jaw), which appears on exertion but is relieved by rest and/or the nitrate **glyceryl trinitrate** (**GTN**) given as a spray. Diagnosis may be based on symptoms and on ST-depression on the electrocardiogram (ECG) during an attack. Patients with stable angina receive beta-blockers (or rate-limiting calcium channel blockers), which reduce cardiac work and by increasing the time for diastole (when coronary flow occurs) increase coronary blood flow. GTN is used to relieve attacks and releases nitric oxide, which causes vasorelaxation, specifically venorelaxation, and this decreases venous return to the heart and so reduces cardiac work. Interventions include angioplasty with **stenting** (see below) or **coronary artery bypass grafting (CABG)**, in which a donor artery (e.g. internal mammary artery) is used to surgically restore the blood flow by bypassing the diseased artery.

Unstable angina is generally due to plaque rupture and the formation of a non-occlusive thromboembolism, or, vasospasm.

In **myocardial infarction** (**MI**) there is often **thromboembolic occlusion** of a coronary artery. The cessation of blood flow results in damage or infarction of the cardiac muscle starved of blood. MI may lead to acute left ventricular failure and/or arrhythmias, which are the leading cause of early mortality. The initial management of MI is now emergency angioplasty, in which a balloon is advanced into the coronary atery to open up the blockage and restore blood flow. This is followed by insertion of a **stent** (a metal cage) to prevent reformation of the narrowing (**restenosis**). Other treatments include the use of 'clot-busting' drugs or **thrombolytic** agents that activate the plasma protein plasminogen to plasmin, which degrades fibrin that forms the clot, resulting in reperfusion. Following an MI, patients are often prescribed the combination of a **beta-blocker**, an **ACE inhibitor**, a **statin** and an **antiplatelet drug** (e.g. low-dose aspirin) for **secondary prevention**.

Ischaemic heart disease is often due to **atheroscelerosis** resulting from **atherogenesis** (Figure 35.1). The formation of changes to the intimal wall of the blood vessel begin in early adulthood with the formation of fatty streaks, and this process, over time, leads to the formation of cholesterol-rich atherosclerotic plaques which lead to partial occlusion of the artery (leading to angina) or they may rupture, leading to thrombus formation (leading to an MI in the coronary artery or stroke in the cerebral circulation). Atherogenesis is regarded as an inflammatory process and when injury occurs (as promoted by smoking, hypertension and possibly infection) activated monocytes and macrophages generate free radicals, which oxidise LDL cholesterol, which in turn damages its receptor and this leads to cholesterol being deposited at the point of the lesion. To slow down atherosclerosis the key approach is reduction of cardiovascular risk through lifestyle changes. Patients who have an elevated cardiovascular risk are prescribed statins.

Statins are cholesterol-lowering drugs that inhibit the endogenous production of cholesterol in the liver by inhibiting the enzyme hydroxyl-methylglutaryl coenzyme A reductase (HMG-CoA reductase), which catalyses the first committed step of cholesterol synthesis. This reduces cholesterol levels by reducing its synthesis and also leads to an upregulation of LDL cholesterol receptors, which promotes the uptake of cholesterol into liver cells. In addition to reducing cholesterol levels, statins may also stabilise cholesterol within the plaques, reducing the chances of a cardiovascular event.

Although total cholesterol should ideally be <5 mmol/L, statins are prescribed in relation to overall cardiovascular risk and are of benefit in patients with 'normal' cholesterol levels.

Chronic heart failure (Figure 34.2)

Hypertension and ischaemic heart disease are both key risk factors for the development of **chronic (or congestive) heart failure (CHF)**. Chronic refers to the long-term nature of this condition, in which the pumping ability of the heart is insufficient for the needs of the body. CHF involves a syndrome of neurohormonal adaptations that are inappropriate and exacerbate the condition.

• Activation of **renin-angiotensin-aldosterone system** (RAAS, Chapter 31): underperfusion of kidneys leads to increased activity of RAAS, resulting in AII-mediated vasoconstriction (with further underperfusion of the kidneys and further activation of RAAS) and aldosterone release, which increases Na^+ reabsorption and fluid retention (which increases cardiac workload and exacerbates CHF).

• Increased **sympathetic activity**: to attempt to increase cardiac work (but also results in activation of RAAS and vasoconstriction).

There is also a compensatory increase in the release of natriuretic peptides from the heart and levels of b-type natriuretic peptide (BNP) are used as markers of CHF.

In **left-sided cardiac failure** back pressure builds up in the pulmonary circulation, leading to pulmonary oedema and breathlessness. In **right-sided failure** there is increased venous pressure leading to peripheral oedema, typically swollen ankles.

CHF is diagnosed by reduced ejection fraction on an echocardiogram. It may also be identified by increased levels of BNP and pulmonary oedema observed on a chest X-ray.

CHF is managed by:

• **Loop diuretics** (e.g. furosemide): leading to substantial diuresis, reducing circulating volume and so cardiac work.

• **ACE inhibitors** (e.g. ramipril): to oppose to RAAS "overactivity" if it will.

• **Beta-blockers** (e.g. bisoprolol): low dose, cardioselective agents are used cautiously to oppose the toxic effects of excessive sympathetic stimulation of the heart.

• **Aldosterone receptor antagonists** (e.g. spironolactone): to oppose the toxic effects of aldosterone on the heart.

• **Digoxin:** inhibits the Na^+ pump (Chapter 18); intracellular Na^+ is then exchanged for calcium, resulting in an increase in force of contraction. Digoxin also increases vagal slowing of atrioventricular (AV) node conduction and is used in atrial fibrillation.

Cerebrovascular disease (Chapter 57)

Cerebrovascular disease (stroke) is either **thromboembolic** (about 90% of cases) or **haemorrhagic** (about 10% of cases). Thromboembolic or ischaemic stroke is often due to atherosclerosis in the cerebral circulation resulting in thrombosis, or due to clot formation associated with stasis of blood due to poor atrial ejection in **atrial fibrillation**. Anticoagulants (e.g. warfarin) or antiplatelet drugs are given for prophylaxis in atrial fibrillation.

Deborah Merrick

Figure 36.1 Anatomy of the renal system, highlighting the relative positions of the kidneys, ureters and bladder

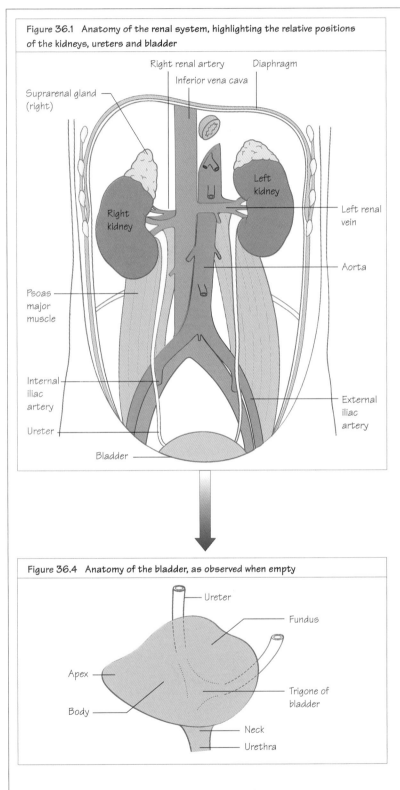

Right renal artery
Diaphragm
Inferior vena cava
Suprarenal gland (right)
Left kidney
Right kidney
Left renal vein
Aorta
Psoas major muscle
Internal iliac artery
Ureter
External iliac artery
Bladder

Figure 36.2 The kidney, showing the renal artery, renal vein and ureter at the hilum

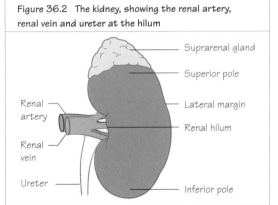

Suprarenal gland
Superior pole
Lateral margin
Renal artery
Renal hilum
Renal vein
Ureter
Inferior pole

Figure 36.3 Internal structure of the kidney

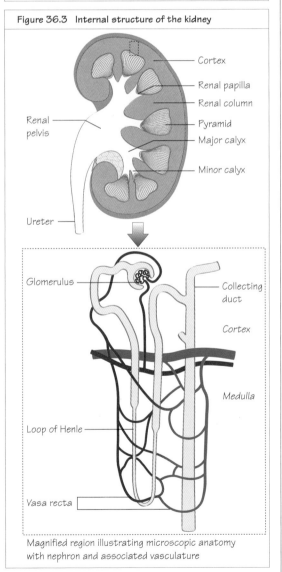

Cortex
Renal papilla
Renal column
Pyramid
Major calyx
Minor calyx
Renal pelvis
Ureter

Glomerulus
Collecting duct
Cortex
Medulla
Loop of Henle
Vasa recta

Magnified region illustrating microscopic anatomy with nephron and associated vasculature

Figure 36.4 Anatomy of the bladder, as observed when empty

Ureter
Fundus
Apex
Trigone of bladder
Body
Neck
Urethra

The renal system is involved in the removal of waste products, excess water and salts from the blood in the form of urine. It controls the level of water and electrolytes within the body and maintains the acid-base balance of blood. The renal system comprises the kidneys, ureters, bladder and urethra.

Kidneys and ureters
Kidneys
The kidneys are retroperitoneal organs located on the posterior abdominal wall at the level of T12-L3 vertebrae (Figure 36.1). Occupying a region either side of the vertebral column, the right kidney lies slightly lower than the left. The kidneys have some mobility, being able to move up to 2–3 cm during respiration and as a result of changes in body positioning (e.g. moving from erect to supine position). The kidneys have anterior and posterior surfaces, medial and lateral margins, and also superior and inferior poles (Figure 36.2). On the medial concave margin is a vertical slit called the renal hilum, which is the region where vessels, nerves and the renal pelvis enter/leave the kidney. The superomedial aspect of each kidney makes contact with the suprarenal (adrenal) gland. These two organs function independently, with a fascial septum separating them. The kidneys and suprarenal glands are surrounded by a protective layer of fat (perinephric fat), which in turn is enclosed by a layer of renal fascia. The kidneys receive their blood supply directly from the abdominal aorta, via the renal arteries (Figures 36.1 and 36.2). Close to the hilum, the right and left renal arteries divide into approximately five segmental arteries to supply the kidney. Venous blood drains through the renal veins to empty into the inferior vena cava (Figure 36.1). Lymphatic drainage of the kidney is to the lumbar lymph nodes. Innervation is from sympathetic, parasympathetic and visceral afferent fibres via the renal plexus.

Each kidney is composed of an **outer cortex** and an **inner medulla**. The medulla is composed of **renal pyramids** (approximately 10–18), which have an apex and base. The cortex extends to the base of the pyramid and between the pyramids, forming the renal columns (Figure 36.3). The cortex and medulla are composed of nephrons, which are the functional units of the kidney. Each **nephron** has a **glomerulus** (situated in the cortex) and a long tubule (**loop of Henle**) that extends into the medulla of the kidney, before uniting with a collecting tubule. Numerous blood vessels (**vasa recta**) are also found in the medulla (Figure 36.3).

Ureters
These are retroperitoneal muscular ducts (~25 cm in length) that carry urine from the kidneys to the bladder. The superior distended end of the ureter is called the renal pelvis, which is formed by the union of two to three major calices (Figure 36.3). A major calyx is formed by the union of two to three minor calices. Each minor calyx is indented by the renal papilla (apex of the renal pyramid), which has a perforated tip where large collecting ducts open to deliver urine into a major calyx. The ureters descend through the abdomen, running along the transverse processes of the lumbar vertebrae before crossing the pelvic brim by passing over the external iliac artery (Figure 36.1). The ureters descend along the lateral walls of the pelvis before entering the bladder. During their route from the kidney to the bladder the ureters are constricted at three sites: ureteropelvic junction, crossing external iliac artery (pelvic brim) and traversing the bladder wall (Figure 36.1). Arteries supplying the ureters are numerous, including branches from the renal arteries, abdominal aorta, testicular/ovarian arteries and branches of the internal iliac arteries. Veins draining the ureters accompany the arteries and are similarly named; lymphatic drainage is to the lumbar, common iliac, external iliac and internal iliac lymph nodes.

Bladder and urethra
Bladder (Chapter 40)
The bladder is a subperitoneal hollow muscular organ located in the pelvis. It functions to collect urine and then expel the waste fluid into the urethra during the process of micturition. When empty, the bladder has an apex, body, neck and fundus, lying posterior to the pubic bones (Figure 36.4). The bladder extends superiorly as it fills, reaching as high as the level of the umbilicus when full. The bladder wall is composed predominantly of the detrusor muscle. The **trigone muscle** of the bladder is a smooth triangular region of the mucosa between the ureteric orifices and the internal urethral orifice (Figure 36.4). Branches of the internal iliac arteries supply the bladder; namely, superior vesical arteries supply the anterosuperior aspects of the bladder, and inferior vesical arteries (male) or vaginal arteries (female) supply inferoposterior aspects. Veins draining the bladder correspond to the arteries they accompany, acting as tributaries to the internal iliac vein. Lymph from the bladder drains to the external iliac (superior surface of bladder), internal iliac (fundus) and sacral or common iliac (neck) lymph nodes. Parasympathetic fibres innervating the bladder arise from the sacral spinal cord levels, conveyed by the pelvic splanchnic nerves and inferior hypogastric plexuses. Sympathetic innervation is conveyed from T11-L2/L3 spinal cord levels to pelvic plexuses through the hypogastric plexuses and nerves. Sensory fibres (visceral afferents) transmitting sensations (e.g. pain from overdistention) follow the course of the parasympathetic (from inferior bladder) or sympathetic (from superior bladder) fibres.

Urethra
This is a muscular tube passing from the internal urethral orifice of the bladder to the external urethral orifice of the glans penis (male) or vestibule of the vagina (female). The urethra functions as an exit route for urine out of the body, varying in length in males (~20 cm) compared with females (~4 cm). Blood supply to the urethra is from the branches of the internal iliac arteries, including internal pudendal arteries and vaginal arteries (female) or prostatic branches of the inferior vesical and middle rectal arteries (male). Veins accompanying the arteries are named accordingly. Most lymph draining from the urethra enters the internal iliac nodes and to a lesser extent the inguinal lymph nodes.

37 Renal physiology: filtration and tubular function

Sue Chan

Figure 37.1 Kidney nephron

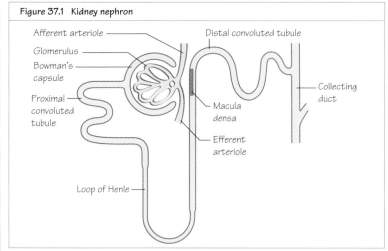

Figure 37.2 Starling forces and filtration

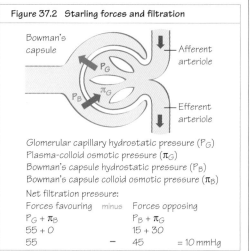

Glomerular capillary hydrostatic pressure (P_G)
Plasma-colloid osmotic pressure (π_G)
Bowman's capsule hydrostatic pressure (P_B)
Bowman's capsule colloid osmotic pressure (π_B)
Net filtration pressure:

Forces favouring	minus	Forces opposing	
$P_G + \pi_B$		$P_B + \pi_G$	
55 + 0		15 + 30	
55	−	45	= 10 mmHg

Figure 37.3 Proximal convoluted tubule (PCT)

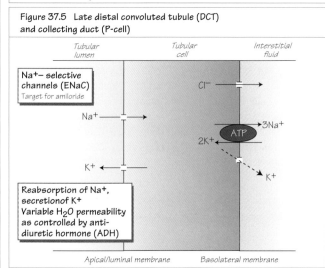

Na⁺/H⁺ antiporter
Secretion of H⁺ into tubule lumen

Na⁺/glucose symporter
Also Na⁺/ AA symporter

Na⁺/K⁺ ATPase
3 Na⁺ out, 2K⁺ in

Figure 37.4 Early distal convoluted tubule (DCT)

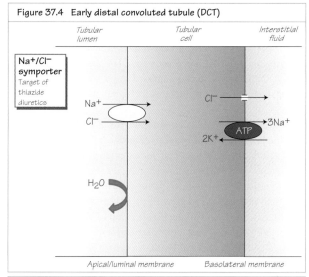

Na⁺/Cl⁻ symporter
Target of thiazide diuretics

Figure 37.5 Late distal convoluted tubule (DCT) and collecting duct (P-cell)

Na⁺- selective channels (ENaC)
Target for amiloride

Reabsorption of Na⁺, secretionof K⁺
Variable H₂O permeability as controlled by anti-diuretic hormone (ADH)

Figure 37.6 Late distal convoluted tubule (DCT) and collecting duct (I-cell)

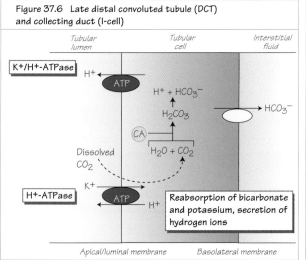

K⁺/H⁺-ATPase

H⁺-ATPase

Reabsorption of bicarbonate and potassium, secretion of hydrogen ions

Each nephron consists of a cup-shaped Bowman's capsule surrounding the glomerulus, which then passes to the proximal convoluted tubule, the loop of Henle, with the distal convoluted tubule draining into the collecting duct (Figure 37.1). There are two types of nephron: cortical (70–80%), with short loop of Henle and a network of peritubular capillaries supplying the tubular system; and juxtamedullary (20–30%), with long loop of Henle and specialised peritubular capillaries consisting of long vascular loops (vasa recta).

Filtration

The excretion of substances in urine is dependent on three processes: **filtration, reabsorption** and **secretion**. Urine formation begins with **filtration** of large amounts of fluid through the glomerular capillaries into the Bowman's space. Blood enters the network of glomerular capillaries via an afferent capillary, and leaves through an efferent arteriole, rather than a venule. Vasoconstriction of the afferent arteriole creates high hydrostatic pressure inside the glomerular capillaries to force the movement of water and solutes across the capillary wall. The glomerular capillary membrane is comprised of three layers (instead of the usual two): capillary endothelial cells form a layer with 70 nm pores or fenestrae; a basement membrane of negatively charged collagen and glycoproteins; then the epithelial visceral layer of the Bowman's capsule, known as **podocytes**, having long, foot-like projections that interdigitate to give filtration slits (slit pores, 25–65 nm). This **glomerular filter**, with each of the three layers having a negative charge, limits the filtration of a substance on both its molecular charge and size. The ultrafiltrate therefore consists of water, electrolytes, small molecules (<70 kDa) such as glucose, urea and amino acids, and is virtually protein-free.

Starling forces (Chapter 31) determine the movement of fluid between plasma and interstitium (tubule), summarised in Figure 37.2. **Renal blood flow** and **glomerular filtration rate** (**GFR**) are maintained at a relatively constant level, a process known as **autoregulation**. This involves two feedback mechanisms: an intrinsic **myogenic** property of blood vessels to resist stretching during increased arterial pressures; and the **tubuloglomerular feedback** involving the **macula densa**, a short segment of tubular cells (at the end of the ascending limb of the loop of Henle), which together with vascular **granular** cells (medial layer of the afferent arteriole adjacent to the vascular poles of the glomerulus) form the **juxtaglomerular apparatus**. The macula densa cells sense changes in tubular fluid NaCl concentration and volume/flow rate in volume delivery in the distal tubule, secreting vasoactive substances that control the vascular tone of blood vessels (such as adenosine, prostaglandins) and the control of renin release from the granular cells (see Chapter 39).

GFR can provide an estimate of the efficiency of renal filtration and hence renal function. In clinical medicine, creatinine (a metabolite of skeletal muscle creatine phosphate breakdown) is used to **estimate GFR** as it is almost completely cleared from the body by glomerular filtration.

The ultrafiltrate passes along the nephron tubule where its volume and content are altered by the processes of **reabsorption** (movement of filtered substance from tubular lumen to tubular capillaries) and **secretion** (movement of substances from vascular compartment to tubular fluid).

Proximal convoluted tubule (PCT)

Continuous with the Bowman's space, the proximal convoluted tubule lies entirely in the cortex. The first part of the tubule is highly convoluted with the second straighter part leading on to the loop of Henle.

Reabsorption

This is the predominant site of solute and water reabsorption: approximately 65% of filtered water, Na^+, K^+, Cl^- and other solutes, together with almost all of the glucose and amino acids in the ultrafiltrate. The tubular epithelial cells have a large apical membrane surface area due to the presence of many microvilli, together with a large number of mitochondria, to support the active transport process. Tubular reabsorption of all solutes is dependent, either directly or indirectly, on the **Na^+/K^+-ATPase pump**, present on the basolateral membrane (Figure 37.3). Active extrusion of Na^+ creates a low Na^+ concentration within the tubular cell, providing a concentration and electrical gradient for luminal Na^+ to move into the tubular cell, driving reabsorption of glucose and amino acids (co-transporters via secondary active transport) and the secretion of H^+ (Na^+/H^+ antiporter), with concomitant indirect reabsorption of filtered bicarbonate (via carbonic anhydrase) (Figure 37.3). Water is reabsorbed, driven by the tubular osmotic gradient established by solute reabsorption, by osmosis across 'leaky' tight junctions and via aquaporin water channels.

Secretion

The PCT is an important site for the secretion of organic acids and bases such as bile salts, oxalates and catecholamines. In addition to waste products of metabolism, the kidney also removes a large number of drugs and their metabolites (including thiazide-like diuretics, furosemide, penicillins, opioids) and toxins. Secretion is mainly an active process.

Loop of Henle

The loop of Henle extends into the medulla (descending thin limb), with the thick segment of the ascending limb responsible for the reabsorption of a further 25% of the filtered Na^+ load. The countercurrent multiplier system for the production of the hyperosmotic renal medulla, a key element in concentration of urine, is described in Chapter 38.

Distal convoluted tubule (DCT)

The early DCT reabsorbs Na^+, K^+ and Cl^- but is virtually impermeable to water and urea, thus diluting the tubular fluid (Figure 37.4). Sodium is reabsorbed together with chloride ions via the Na^+/Cl^- co-transporter, the Na^+ gradient for this Na^+ ion movement created by, once again, the basolateral Na^+/K^+-ATPase pump.

Late DCT and cortical collecting duct

These segments have similar functional characteristics, comprising of two distinct cell types with different transport properties.

Principal or P-cells

Sodium reabsorption and potassium secretion depends on the activity of the basolateral Na^+/K^+-ATPase pump. The hormone aldosterone can upregulate the expression of the Na^+/K^+-ATPase pump and the epithelial Na^+ channel, promoting increased sodium (and hence water) reabsorption together with increased potassium elimination (Figure 37.5). Additionally, vasopressin (or antidiuretic hormone) can cause increased transepithelial water transport.

Intercalated or I-cells

These cells are highly abundant with mitochondria, and are involved in active secretion of H^+ ions (via H^+-ATPase and K^+/H^+-ATPase) and reabsorption of bicarbonate and potassium ions (Figure 37.6). Thus, these cells play a key role in acid-base balance.

Sue Chan

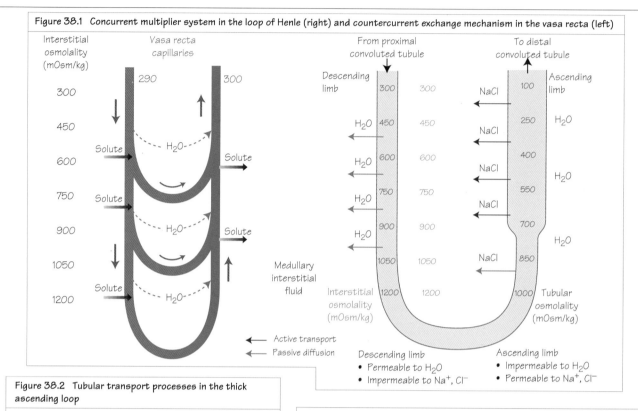

Figure 38.1 Concurrent multiplier system in the loop of Henle (right) and countercurrent exchange mechanism in the vasa recta (left)

Descending limb
• Permeable to H_2O
• Impermeable to Na^+, Cl^-

Ascending limb
• Impermeable to H_2O
• Permeable to Na^+, Cl^-

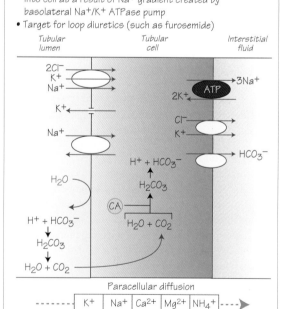

Figure 38.2 Tubular transport processes in the thick ascending loop

$Na^+/K^+/2Cl^-$ symporter
• Movement of Na^+, K^+ and $2Cl^-$ from apical membrane into cell as a result of Na^+ gradient created by basolateral Na^+/K^+ ATPase pump
• Target for loop diuretics (such as furosemide)

Table 38.1 Permeability properties of nephron segments involved in urine concentration and dilution

Tubule segment	Permeability			Effects of ADH
	NaCl	Urea	Water	
Loop of Henle				
Thin descending limb	Very low ↑	Very low ↑	High	
Thin ascending limb	Very high	Moderate	Impermeable	
Thick ascending limb	Moderate	Very low ↑	Impermeable	NaCl reabsorption
Distal convoluted tubule	Moderate	Very low ↑	Variable	Water resorption late DCT
Collecting duct				
Cortical	Low ↑	Very low ↑	Variable	Water resorption
Medullary	Low ↑	Moderate	Variable	Water and urea resorption

The loop of Henle and the distal nephron are involved in the process of urine concentration. There are two key basic requirements: a **hyperosmotic renal medullary interstitium**, which provides the osmotic gradient for water reabsorption; and actions of **antidiuretic hormone (ADH)** (or vasopressin), which increase the water permeability in the late distal convoluted tubule and the collecting duct.

The loop of Henle consists of three functionally distinct segments: the **thin descending limb** and the **thin ascending limb** (only present in long loops of Henle of juxtamedullary nephrons) have thin epithelial membranes with poorly developed brush borders, few mitochondria and hence metabolic activity; the epithelial cells of the **ascending limb of Henle** have highly invaginated apical membranes and an abundance of mitochondria.

Tubular fluid entering the descending limb of the loop of Henle is isotonic with plasma/interstitial fluid (~290 mOsm/kg). The thin descending limb is highly permeable to water with very low permeability to solutes (such as NaCl and urea). Much of the water reabsorption in the loop of Henle (~20% of the filtered water) occurs along this segment. Thus, tubular fluid moving towards the tip of the loop becomes more solute concentrated (Figure 38.1). Meanwhile, the ascending segments are impermeable to water (an important feature in the process of concentration of urine). The thin segment has much lower solute reabsorptive capacity than that of the thick segment. As in the proximal convoluted tubule, the basolateral **Na⁺/K⁺-ATPase pump** maintains a low intracellular Na⁺ concentration and this provides a favourable gradient for the reabsorption of tubular Na⁺ ions, primarily via the apical **Na⁺/K⁺/2Cl⁻ symporter**, with the apical K⁺ channel enabling K⁺ transported via Na⁺/K⁺/2Cl⁻ transporter to be recycled back (Figure 38.2). This creates a slight positive charge in the tubular lumen, sufficient to force cations (such as Ca^{2+} and Mg^{2+}) to diffuse paracellularly into the interstitial fluid. There is also a Na⁺-H⁺ antiporter in apical membrane that enables Na⁺ reabsorption and H⁺ secretion (with HCO_3^- reabsorption) (Figure 38.2). The tubular fluid in the ascending limb becomes more dilute (hypo-osmotic) as it flows towards the distal convoluted tubule due to this high solute reabsorption (Figure 38.1).

Countercurrent multiplication

This mechanism is dependent on both the form and the function of the loop of Henle: the two parallel limbs of the descending and ascending limbs with the flow of tubular fluid running in opposite directions (**countercurrent flow**) increases or 'multiplies' the osmotic gradient between tubular fluid and interstitial space.

The most important element in the development and maintenance of the high medullary osmolality is the active transport of Na⁺ and co-transport of other ions from the thick ascending limb into the interstitium. The active pump mechanism allows a gradient of 200 mOsm/kg to be created across the tubular walls along the length of the tubule (Figure 38.1). As the **ascending limb** is impermeable to water, solute reabsorption occurs in the absence of accompanying water reabsorption, with high solute concentration in the renal medulla. As the **descending limb** is very permeable to water, the tubular fluid osmolality quickly becomes equal with that of the renal medullary interstitium, increasing as the tubular fluid flows towards the tip of the loop of Henle (Figure 38.1).

At the junction of the medulla with the cortex, the interstitium osmolality is ~300 mOsm/kg, virtually all of this is due to NaCl. The osmolality of the medullary interstitial fluid increases progressively to about 1200 mOsm/kg in the pelvic tip of the medulla, with NaCl and urea contributing equally to the hyperosmotic interstitium here. Approximately 50% of filtered urea is reabsorbed in the proximal convoluted tubule. However, the lack of permeability to urea in the thick ascending limb of the loop of Henle and the distal convoluted tubule results in the increased concentration of urea as it passes along the tubule, as water and other solutes are reabsorbed. The medullary collecting duct is relatively permeable to urea and so urea diffuses down its concentration gradient (via UT-A transporters) into the medulla, where some of urea passes back into the thin segments of the loop of Henle. Thus, the different permeability of segments (Table 38.1) of the nephron leads to the **'recycling' of urea**.

The medullary capillaries, in particular the **vasa recta**, are highly permeable to solutes and water. The parallel configuration of the long vascular loops of the vasa recta means that although a large amount of fluid and solute exchange occurs across the capillary walls (between the plasma and the medullary interstitium), there is little net dilution of the concentration of the interstitial fluid at each level of the renal medulla (Figure 38.1). This **countercurrent exchange** process minimises dissipation of the built-up solute gradient by diffusion into the capillary system, preserving hyperosmolality of the renal medulla.

Distal nephron and actions of antidiuretic hormone, ADH

The water permeability of the late distal tubule and the collecting duct is dependent on the plasma concentration of antidiuretic hormone, ADH (Table 38.1). In the absence of ADH, the P-cells are almost impermeable to water and fail to reabsorb water while continuing to reabsorb solute, thus dilute urine is excreted. At high levels of ADH, water permeability is greatly enhanced, particularly in the cortical collecting duct, with a large amount of water reabsorbed into the renal cortex, where it is quickly taken away by peritubular capillaries. ADH also increases the transport of urea out of the medullary collecting duct, further increasing the renal medullary hyperosmolality, thus promoting the gradient for water reabsorption and the production of concentrated urine.

39 Regulation of body fluids

Sue Chan

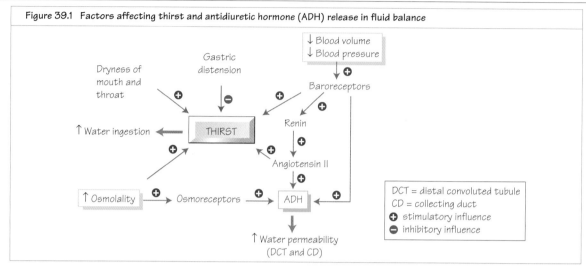

Figure 39.1 Factors affecting thirst and antidiuretic hormone (ADH) release in fluid balance

DCT = distal convoluted tubule
CD = collecting duct
⊕ stimulatory influence
⊖ inhibitory influence

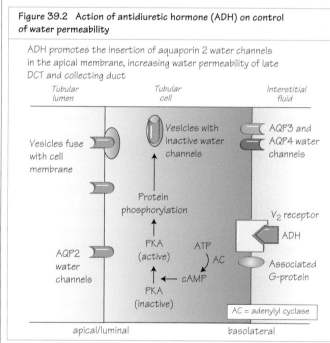

Figure 39.2 Action of antidiuretic hormone (ADH) on control of water permeability

ADH promotes the insertion of aquaporin 2 water channels in the apical membrane, increasing water permeability of late DCT and collecting duct

AC = adenylyl cyclase

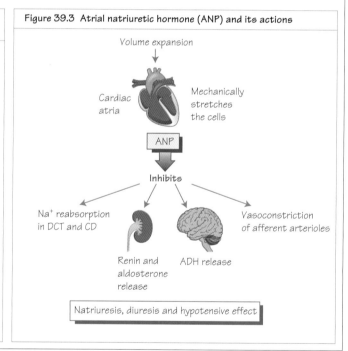

Figure 39.3 Atrial natriuretic hormone (ANP) and its actions

Water constitutes approximately 60% of the healthy human body, with the water in the intracellular and extracellular (interstitial fluid and blood plasma) compartments in osmotic equilibrium. Sodium and chloride ions are abundant in extracellular fluid, while in intracellular fluid, these ions are at low levels with a high concentration of potassium ions. The osmotic effect of these solutes acting across cell membranes determines the distribution of fluid between extracellular and intracellular compartments. Alterations to extracellular fluid osmolality can cause cell swelling or shrinking, which can lead to cell death. The kidney plays a key role in the close regulation of extracellular fluid osmolality via two primary mechanisms: the osmoreceptor-antidiuretic hormone (ADH, or vasopressin) system; and the thirst mechanism.

 Medical Sciences at a Glance, First Edition. Edited by Michael D Randall. © 2014 John Wiley & Sons, Ltd. Published 2014 by John Wiley & Sons, Ltd.

Antidiuretic hormone

The secretion of **antidiuretic hormone** (ADH, also known as vasopressin, Chapter 45) from the posterior pituitary is influenced by the osmolality of body fluids (osmotic), and the volume and pressure of the vascular system (Figure 39.1). **Osmotic control** of ADH secretion is highly sensitive, with a change of 1% being sufficient to alter ADH release. Shrinkage of **osmoreceptor cells** located in the anterior hypothalamus (close to supraoptic nuclei) in response to an increase in extracellular fluid osmolality (due to water deficit, for example) leads to nerve signals being sent to hypothalamic ADH-producing neuroendocrine cells (Chapter 45), culminating in the release of ADH from axon termini in the posterior pituitary. At the kidney, ADH interact with V_2 receptors on principal (P) cells, promoting the translocation of **aquaporin-2 water channels** to the apical membrane, which results in increased water reabsorption and excretion of a small volume of concentrated urine (Figure 39.2). The water conserved dilutes extracellular solutes, thereby correcting the initial hyperosmotic extracellular fluid. The opposite sequence of events occurs with hypo-osmotic extracellular fluid (such as with excess water ingestion).

Haemodynamic control of ADH release involves receptors in low pressure (left atrium and large pulmonary vessels) and high pressure (aortic arch and carotid sinus) regions of the circulation, which detect changes in blood volume and pressure, with afferent signals leading to appropriate control of ADH release to restore blood volume/pressure to normal (Figure 39.1). This is a much less sensitive mechanism than that of osmotic control; change of 5–10% reduction in blood volume is required for plasma ADH levels to change appreciably.

Fluid intake is regulated by the **thirst response**, the conscious desire to drink water. Neural centres involved in regulating water intake (thirst centre) located in the hypothalamus (in regions similar to those in control of ADH release) respond to a number of stimuli (Figure 39.1). It seems that the ADH and thirst systems work in concert to maintain water balance (Figure a), although with regard to body fluid osmolality, ADH secretion is secreted at a lower threshold than that for thirst. Thus, an increase in plasma osmolality evokes thirst with water ingestion and secretion of ADH with resultant conservation of water, while a fall in plasma osmolality leads to suppressed thirst and a lack of ADH release with enhanced renal water excretion.

Other hormones in renal excretion of salt and water

The **renin-angiotensin-aldosterone system** (Chapter 32) plays an important role in regulating sodium and water reabsorption. **Renin** is secreted by granular cells (juxtaglomerular apparatus, Chapter 37) in response to activation of sympathetic nervous system (via β_2-adrenoceptors), reduced renal perfusion pressure (afferent arteriole baroreceptors), or a fall in tubular fluid [NaCl] sensed by tubular macula densa cells – usually due to a decrease in glomerular filtration rate resulting in slower filtrate movement through the proximal tubule and thus more time for reabsorption, leading to a lower [NaCl] in the tubular fluid at the macula densa; tubuloglomerular feedback (Chapter 37). **Angiotensin II** stimulates release of aldosterone, arteriolar vasoconstriction (efferent more than afferent), ADH secretion and thirst, and enhances renal NaCl reabsorption. **Aldosterone** is secreted by zona glomerulosa cells of the adrenal cortex (Chapter 48); it promotes Na^+ (and hence water) reabsorption, with K^+ elimination, by upregulation of the expression of Na^+/Cl^- co-transporter (early DCT), the epithelial Na^+ channel and basolateral Na^+/K^+-ATPase pump in principal (P) cells of the late DCT and collecting duct. Overall, activation of the renin-angiotensin-aldosterone system results in increased total peripheral resistance, thus increasing blood pressure and raising GFR, together with Na^+ and water reabsorption.

A number of natriuretic hormones contribute to volume regulation. **Atrial natriuretic peptide** (ANP) is released from cardiac atrial muscle fibres in response to atrial stretching as a result of increased blood volume. The combined actions of ANP lead to increased excretion of NaCl and water, which helps to compensate for the excess blood volume (Figure 39.3).

Disorders

• **Diabetes insipidus (DI)**: arises from lack of ADH production (central or pituitary DI), or ADH insensitivity in the kidney (nephrogenic DI). Excessive volume of dilute urine is produced (polyuria), due to lack of antidiuresis activity of ADH.

• **Syndrome of inappropriate antidiuretic hormone secretion (SIADH)**: may arise from many causes (central nervous system pathology, malignancy, drugs). Reduced water excretion (small volume of highly concentrated urine) with hyponatraemia (<135 mmol/L, due to dilution effect of water retention).

• **Hyperaldosteronism**: (primary, such as aldosterone-secreting adrenal adenoma [**Conn's syndrome**]; secondary, such as renin-producing tumour or reduced blood supply as in renal artery stenosis): presents with hypertension (water retention), hypernatraemia and hypokalaemia.

• **Hypoaldosteronism** (low aldosterone levels, with primary adrenal insufficiency as in Addison's disease or common form of congenital adrenal hyperplasia [Chapter 48]): leads to hyponatraemia and hyperkalaemia; patients may experience postural hypotension and muscle weakness.

Diuretics

• **Osmotic diuretics** (such a mannitol): freely filtered, increasing the osmolality of the tubular fluid, thus reducing water reabsorption. Used in management of cerebral oedema.

• **Loop diuretics** (such as furosemide): block the **$Na^+/K^+/2Cl^-$ symporter** of the thick ascending limb of loop of Henle, thus reducing the hyperosmolality of the renal medullary interstitium required for urine concentration. Also, reduction of NaCl entry into macula densa, with resultant increase in renin release from granular cells. Used in management of chronic heart failure (Chapter 35) and in renal failure (to improve diuresis).

• **Thiazide-like diuretics** (such as chlortalidone): inhibit **Na^+/Cl^- co-transporter** in early DCT. Ineffective in moderate renal impairment as renal secretion by the PCT weak acid transporter is required prior to acting on DCT.

• **Potassium-sparing diuretics** include aldosterone receptor antagonist spironolactone and sodium channel blockers such as amiloride. Weak diuretics may be used to offset hypokalaemia often seen with thiazide-like and loop diuretics.

40 Bladder function and dysfunction

Michael D Randall

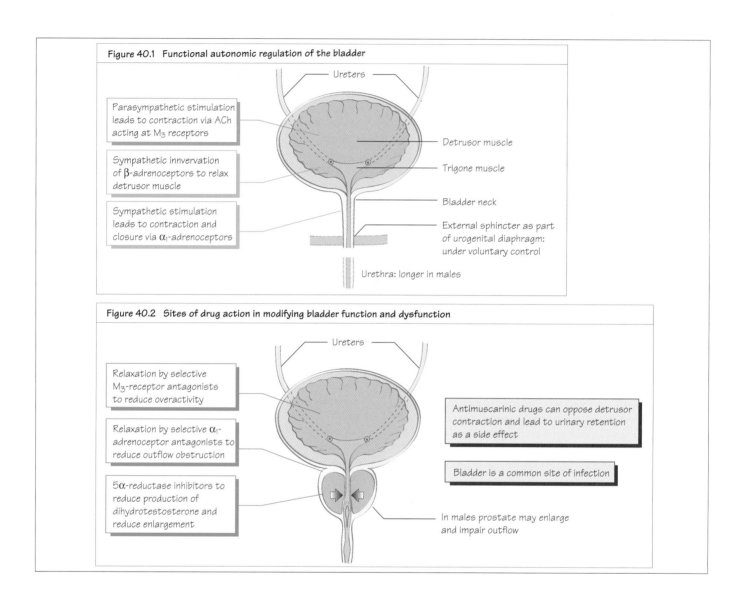

Figure 40.1 Functional autonomic regulation of the bladder

Ureters

Parasympathetic stimulation leads to contraction via ACh acting at M_3 receptors

Sympathetic innervation of β-adrenoceptors to relax detrusor muscle

Sympathetic stimulation leads to contraction and closure via α_1-adrenoceptors

Detrusor muscle

Trigone muscle

Bladder neck

External sphincter as part of urogenital diaphragm: under voluntary control

Urethra: longer in males

Figure 40.2 Sites of drug action in modifying bladder function and dysfunction

Ureters

Relaxation by selective M_3-receptor antagonists to reduce overactivity

Relaxation by selective α_1-adrenoceptor antagonists to reduce outflow obstruction

5α-reductase inhibitors to reduce production of dihydrotestosterone and reduce enlargement

Antimuscarinic drugs can oppose detrusor contraction and lead to urinary retention as a side effect

Bladder is a common site of infection

In males prostate may enlarge and impair outflow

The urinary bladder is a muscular organ in the pelvis that stores normally sterile urine prior to **micturition**. In the healthy adult, the volume of the bladder is typically 300–500 mL. The bladder receives urine (at approximately 1 mL/min) from the kidneys via two muscular **ureters** (Chapter 36) that enter the bladder low down near the neck. The ureters drain into the bladder via **vesico-ureteric junction**, which ensures that flow is unidirectional and that there is no reflux of urine from the bladder to the kidneys, which could lead to infection. The bladder then stores urine prior to its elimination through the external sphincter and then via the **urethra** (Chapter 36).

The bladder is made up of the following.
• **Detrusor muscle**: this is smooth muscle in the body of the bladder. When relaxed, it enables the bladder to hold urine and when it contracts there is an increase in internal pressure and so urine is voided.
• **Trigone muscle**: this is triangular smooth muscle at the base of the bladder at the urethral opening.
• **Urothelium**: the inner transitional epithelial layer of the bladder, which may release mediators (such as ATP) to regulate tone.

Autonomic control (Figure 40.1)
The key innervation of the detrusor muscle is **parasympathetic** via acetylcholine acting at muscarinic M_3 receptors, which leads to contraction and micturition. Sympathetic innervation results in noradrenaline acting at β_2- and β_3-adrenoceptors to relax the detrusor muscle, resulting in the bladder relaxing and storing urine. Noradrenaline also acts at α_1-adrenoceptors to contract the neck of the bladder and urethra to facilitate the storage of urine.

Somatic control
The external sphincter is made up of skeletal muscle associated with the **urogenital diaphragm** and is regulated via the somatic nervous system such that acetylcholine acts at nicotinic receptors to cause contraction of the urethra.

Micturition
Once the internal pressure reaches a certain level this stretches sensory fibres and initiates the **micturition reflex**, which is autonomic but regulated by the brain, which either facilitates or inhibits the reflex. The micturition reflex leads to bladder emptying via contraction of the detrusor muscle, leading to an increase in pressure and relaxation of the external sphincter.

Disorders of bladder function
Cystitis
Irritation of the bladder by chemicals or due to infection leads to the common symptoms of discomfort and an urge to pass urine. **Urinary tract infections** (**UTI**) are relatively common, especially in females, who have a shorter urethra compared with males. UTIs may present with increased frequency of urination, often with a burning sensation. *Escherichia coli* is the commonest cause of UTIs and readily managed by antibiotic therapy (trimethoprim as a first choice agent).

Benign prostatic hypertrophy (BPH)
BPH is characterised by enlargement of the prostate gland around the urethra in males and is common over the age of 50 years. The enlarged prostate impairs urinary outflow and so leads to a frequent desire to pass urine with hesitancy, poor outflow and incomplete emptying. The stagnation of urine may also predispose towards infections. The obstruction of urinary outflow also poses a risk of renal failure.

Selective α_1-**adrenoceptor antagonists** (e.g. tamsulosin) are used to relax smooth muscle in the prostate and the neck of the bladder to aid urine flow. Prostatic enlargement is also testosterone-dependent and **inhibitors of 5α-reductase** (e.g. finasteride), the enzyme that converts testosterone to the more potent dihydrotestosterone, are also used (Figure 40.2).

Overactive bladder
This involves increased bladder contractility with increased urge to pass urine, leading to increased frequency, and there may or may not be incontinence or leakage. Common pharmacological management involves use of **selective muscarinic receptor antagonists** (e.g. oxybutynin) to inhibit involuntary contractions of the detrusor muscle which are responsible for the increased activity.

Stress incontinence
This is common in women and is caused by either sphincter weakness or urethral hypermobility. This is common following pregnancy and associated with weakness of the pelvic floor.

Stones
The urinary tract is susceptible to the formation of stones rich in calcium salts such as calcium oxalate. These can lead to obstruction and severe pain in the ureters. In the bladder, stone formation can become the focus of infection.

Side effects of drugs
Drugs that have antimuscarinic side effects (such as tricyclic antidepressants) are associated with urinary retention because they impair parasympathetically mediated voiding of the bladder.

Structure of the gastrointestinal system

Deborah Merrick

Figure 41.1   Anatomy of the digestive system, illustrating the relative positions of the digestive tract and accessory organs of digestion

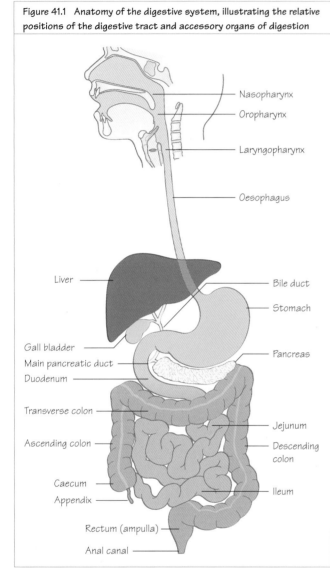

Figure 41.2   The pharynx, visualised during deglutition

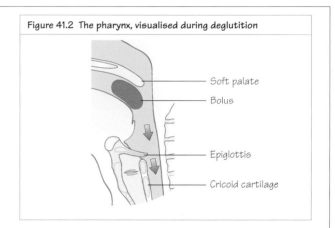

Figure 41.3   The stomach and duodenum, highlighting rugae and plicae circulares

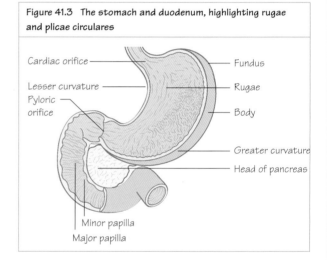

Figure 41.4   The Jejunum and ileum, with differences illustrated

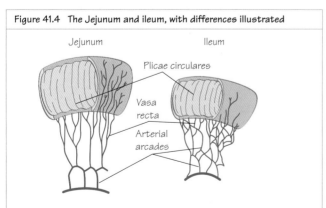

Figure 41.5   The rectum and anal canal

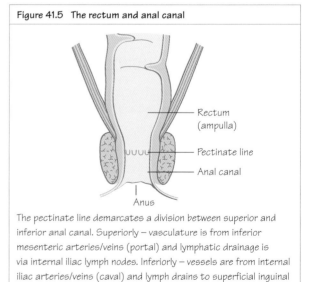

The pectinate line demarcates a division between superior and inferior anal canal. Superiorly – vasculature is from inferior mesenteric arteries/veins (portal) and lymphatic drainage is via internal iliac lymph nodes. Inferiorly – vessels are from internal iliac arteries/veins (caval) and lymph drains to superficial inguinal lymph nodes

The digestive system extends from the lips to the anus and consists of a series of organs and glands. The digestive tract is a tube-like passageway that conducts the food we eat, allowing absorption of vital nutrients along most of its length. Accessory organs (e.g. pancreas) secrete substances that aid digestion.

Digestive tract

Mucosa lines the hollow organs of the digestive tract. In the mouth, stomach and small intestines the mucosa contains glands that produce secretions to help digest food. Contraction of the smooth muscle within the walls of the digestive tract helps move food along its length.

Oral cavity: consists of the oral vestibule and the oral cavity proper. Food entering the oral cavity is chewed (mastication) and mixed with saliva to form a ball (bolus) of food. The tongue pushes the bolus upwards and backwards against the hard palate to enter the oropharynx (Figures 41.1 and 41.2).

Pharynx: a funnel-shaped muscular structure situated posterior to the nasal cavity (nasopharynx), oral cavity (oropharynx) and larynx (laryngopharynx). During the process of swallowing (deglutition), the nasopharynx becomes shut off from the oropharynx by elevation of the soft palate. The larynx and laryngopharynx are pulled upwards, while the epiglottis prevents food from entering the airways (Figure 41.2). Successive waves of contraction of the pharyngeal constrictor muscles move the bolus into the oesophagus.

Oesophagus: a muscular tube connecting the pharynx superiorly to the stomach inferiorly (~25 cm in length). It passes from the level of cricoid cartilage (opposite C6 vertebrae), running posterior to the trachea. It descends through the thorax, entering the abdomen by piercing the diaphragm at vertebral level T10. During its descent the oesophagus is compressed by three structures: the arch of aorta, left main bronchus and diaphragm.

Stomach: dilated portion of the digestive tract located in the upper abdomen. The stomach has two orifices (cardiac and pyloric), two curvatures (greater and lesser), a fundus, body, pyloric antrum and pylorus. The inner mucosal lining is thrown into multiple longitudinal folds (rugae) which become obliterated when the stomach becomes distended (Figure 41.3).

Small intestines: the major site of absorption within the digestive tract. Its longitudinal muscle forms a continuous layer around the gut. Its outer wall is smooth, whereas the internal mucous membrane is thrown into multiple folds called plicae circulares.

• *Duodenum*: ~25 cm in length, beginning at the pyloric sphincter and is C-shaped, curving around the head of the pancreas. Secretions from the accessory organs of digestion enter the duodenum at the major and minor papilla (Figure 41.3).

• *Jejunum and ileum*: ~6 m in length, the jejunum commences at the duodenojejunal flexure and the ileum terminates by joining the large intestines at the ileocaecal junction. There is no distinct dividing feature separating the jejunum and ileum, but some subtle differences are noted. For example, the jejunum has a wider diameter, thicker walls and contains increased number of plicae circulares (Figure 41.4).

Large intestines: function to absorb water and to store undigested food before excretion from the body as faeces (defecation). The longitudinal muscle of the large intestines is arranged in three bands called the teniae coli, and its walls, unlike the small intestines, are sacculated.

• *Caecum and appendix*: the caecum is a blind-ended pouch that joins the ileum and ascending colon. Attached to its posteromedial surface is the appendix.

• *Ascending colon*: extends from the caecum to the right lobe of the liver (hepatic flexure or right colic flexure), where it turns and becomes continuous with the transverse colon.

• *Transverse colon*: passes to the left colic flexure (splenic flexure), then turns and continues at the descending colon.

• *Descending colon*: descends from the left colic flexure to the pelvic brim where it becomes continuous with the sigmoid colon.

• *Sigmoid colon*: named according to its S-shaped appearance; continuous with the rectum at vertebral level S3.

Rectum and anal canal: the rectum passes inferiorly, following the curvature of the sacrum and coccyx. It dilates (rectal ampulla) before piercing the pelvic floor to become continuous with the anal canal. The short anal canal (~4 cm) passes posteroinferiorly to open at the anus. Halfway along its length is the pectinate line, which demarcates a distinct change in innervation and vascular supply of the anal canal (Figure 41.5). The lateral walls of the canal are kept in apposition by levator ani and the anal sphincters muscles until defecation.

Vasculature of the digestive tract

Arterial supply is predominantly from branches of the external carotid arteries (oral cavity and pharynx), inferior thyroid arteries and descending thoracic aorta (oesophagus), abdominal aorta (inferior oesophagus through to superior half of the anal canal) and internal iliac arteries (inferior anal canal). Veins draining the digestive tract correspond to the arteries they accompany. Likewise, deep lymphatic vessels also accompany the major blood vessels, traversing one or more lymph nodes before draining predominantly into the thoracic duct or right lymphatic duct.

Innervation of the digestive tract

This is by the autonomic nervous system (including enteric nervous system) as well as visceral afferents. In general, sympathetic innervation reduces blood flow (vasoconstrictor) and decreases secretions and motility (peristalsis) of the digestive tract. Parasympathetic stimulation increases motility and secretion. The enteric system, found within the tract walls, is principally composed of myenteric (Auerbach's) and submucosal (Meissner's) plexuses controlling movement and secretion.

Accessory organs of digestion

Pancreas: exocrine function produces pancreatic enzymatic juices to aid digestion. The pancreatic secretions pass into the main and accessory pancreatic ducts to enter the duodenum via the major and minor papilla respectively.

Liver and gall bladder: the liver produces bile, which is stored and concentrated in the gall bladder. Bile leaves the gall bladder via the cystic duct and then the bile duct to enter the duodenum at the major papilla (Figures 41.1 and 41.3).

Michael D Randall

Figure 42.1 The control of saliva production

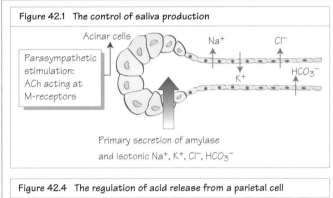

Acinar cells

Parasympathetic stimulation: ACh acting at M-receptors

Primary secretion of amylase and isotonic Na^+, K^+, Cl^-, HCO_3^-

Na^+ Cl^-

K^+ HCO_3^-

Figure 42.4 The regulation of acid release from a parietal cell

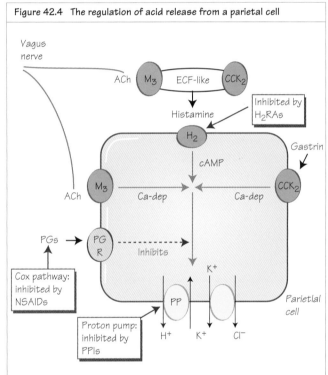

Vagus nerve

ACh M_3 ECF-like CCK_2

Histamine

Inhibited by H_2RAs

H_2

cAMP   Gastrin

M_3 Ca-dep   Ca-dep CCK_2

ACh

PGs →   PG R

Inhibits

Cox pathway: inhibited by NSAIDs

K^+

PP

Proton pump: inhibited by PPIs

H^+ K^+ Cl^-

Parietlal cell

Figure 42.2 Cephalic and gastric phases of gastric acid secretion

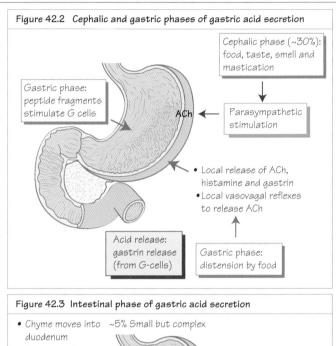

Cephalic phase (~30%): food, taste, smell and mastication

Parasympathetic stimulation

Gastric phase: peptide fragments stimulate G cells

ACh

• Local release of ACh, histamine and gastrin
• Local vasovagal reflexes to release ACh

Acid release: gastrin release (from G-cells)

Gastric phase: distension by food

Figure 42.3 Intestinal phase of gastric acid secretion

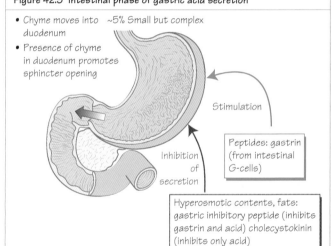

• Chyme moves into duodenum
• Presence of chyme in duodenum promotes sphincter opening

~5% Small but complex

Stimulation

Inhibition of secretion

Peptides: gastrin (from intestinal G-cells)

Hyperosmotic contents, fats: gastric inhibitory peptide (inhibits gastrin and acid) cholecystokinin (inhibits only acid)

Salivation

The process of digestion starts in the mouth with mastication, in which the physical breakdown of food is combined with saliva. Salivation occurs as saliva is produced by the parotid, submandibular and sublingual glands, and saliva lubricates the mouth, aids dental hygiene, adds fluid to the food and initiates the breakdown of starches by addition of amylase. **Acinar cells** secrete amylase and electrolytes with similar tonicity to plasma, and striated and excitatory ducts modify secretions. A healthy human produces about 1–1.5 L of saliva per day.

Control of salivation (Figure 42.1)

This process is under autonomic control with parasympathetic nerves releasing acetylcholine (ACh) to act at muscarinic receptors to increase the production of saliva and increase blood flow to promote fluid movement. Parasympathetic nerves also release vasoactive intestinal polypeptide (VIP), which causes vasodilatation to enhance saliva secretion. Parasympathetic control makes the saliva watery (hypotonic relative to plasma), while sympathetic control increases its viscosity. Drugs with antimuscarinic side effects may block the production of saliva as a side effect, leading to a dry mouth.

Gastric physiology

The food is then swallowed, which is largely a reflex action (controlled via the swallowing centre in the medulla and lower pons), and the bolus of food then passes down the oesophagus via peristalsis, through the lower oesophageal sphincter and into the stomach. Food is retained in the stomach for several hours, during which time the gastric mucosa releases acid (pH of the gastric contents is pH1–1.5) and proteolytic enzymes to initiate the breakdown of proteins. **Chief cells** of gastric mucosa release **pepsinogens** and the acid environment activates these to form **pepsins**. This is also an autocatalytic process as the newly formed pepsin activates further pepsinogens, which are endopeptidases and so act within peptide chain. The acidic environment is also the optimum pH for pepsin activity.

Gastric acid secretion (Figures 42.2, 42.3 and 42.4)

The production of gastric acid is a tightly regulated process. Parietal cells of the gastric mucosa contain H^+/K^+ ATPases (**proton pumps**) on their lumenal surfaces and these antiport H^+ out of the cell in exchange for K^+. Gastric acid secretion is under **cephalic control** (central control stimulated by the presence of food in the mouth and chewing), which involves direct parasympathetic vagal stimulation and indirect parasympathetic control via the release of histamine from enterochromaffin (ECF)-like cells. For direct control, ACh acts at muscarinic M_3 receptors, which couple via increasing intracellular calcium to activate the proton pump. **Histamine** released from the ECF-like cells acts on histamine H_2 receptors to increase cAMP, which also activates the proton pump via phosphorylation. The final stimulatory pathway is via the hormone gastrin. Gastrin is released by G-cells of the antrum and leads to the **gastric phase**. The release of gastrin is stimulated by the presence of the food in the stomach, passes via the bloodstream to act on the stomach and the **gastrin** acts at cholesytokinin CCK_2 receptors to stimulate histamine release from the ECF-like cells and also directly on parietal CCK_2 receptors to cause calcium-dependent proton pump activation. The final phase of control is the **intestinal phase**, in which protein digestion products stimulate the release of gastrin from G-cells.

Cytoprotection

The acidic and proteolytic secretions of the gastric mucosa are likely to cause erosion and so the local production of prostaglandins (PGE_2 and PGI_2) stimulates bicarbonate and mucus secretion by superficial epithelial cells. These prostaglandins also act on the parietal cells to inhibit the proton pump.

Roles of the stomach

Food is retained in the stomach for a number of hours and so the stomach acts as a storage site. Fatty foods tend to float to the top and solid foods are retained for longer periods of time. During this time the acidic environment sterilises the contents and activated pepsin digests protein, to give the end product chyme. Some absorption of small molecules occurs from the stomach.

Parietal cells also release an **intrinsic factor** (**IF**), a glycoprotein that binds to vitamin B_{12}, and this complex enables this vitamin to be absorbed in the small intestines. A lack of IF due to surgical loss of the stomach or autoimmune disease is associated with vitamin B_{12} deficiency and leads to megaloblastic anaemia (Chapter 33).

Dyspepsia

This is a common complaint that affects the upper gastrointestinal tract and encompasses:
- **gastro-oesophageal reflux disease**: acidic gastric contents reflux up and damage the oesophagus;
- **gastritis**: inflammation of the stomach;
- **peptic ulceration**: damage and erosion of the stomach or duodenum such that an ulcer forms; this may lead to bleeding.

Peptic ulceration

The principal cause of peptic ulceration is due to infection with *Helicobacter pylori*, which can lead inflammation and ulceration. About 70% of gastric ulcers and 90% of duodenal ulcers are associated with *H. pylori* infection. The second most important cause of ulceration is due to non-steroidal anti-inflammatory drugs (NSAIDs) which inhibit the production of cytoprotective prostanoids and so promote acid secretion and reduce gastric protection.

Pharmacology of dyspepsia

Symptoms of dyspepsia may be relieved by antacids such as magnesium hydroxide, which neutralise the acid. Suppression of acid release is a far more effective approach and involves either the use of **histamine H_2 receptor antagonists (H₂RAs)** (e.g. ranitidine), which block histamine-induced acid secretion, or **proton pump inhibitors (PPIs)** (e.g. omeprazole), which irreversibly block the proton pump (and therefore the final common pathway of acid secretion).

The most appropriate treatment for *H. pylori*-dependent ulceration is the use of 'triple therapy', with two antibiotics (from clarithromycin, amoxicillin and metronidazole) to eradicate the infection, and a PPI.

43 Lower gastrointestinal physiology

Michael D Randall

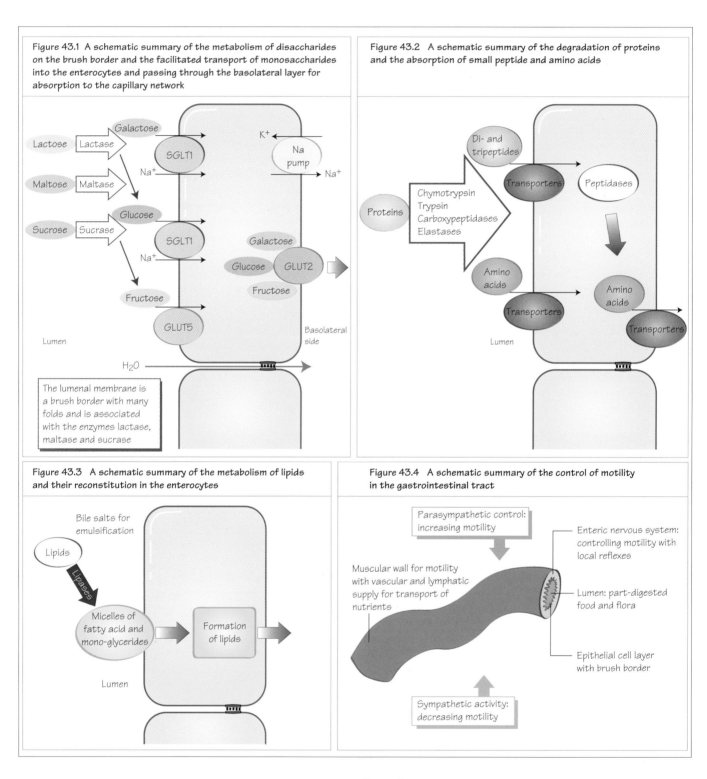

Figure 43.1 A schematic summary of the metabolism of disaccharides on the brush border and the facilitated transport of monosaccharides into the enterocytes and passing through the basolateral layer for absorption to the capillary network

Figure 43.2 A schematic summary of the degradation of proteins and the absorption of small peptide and amino acids

Figure 43.3 A schematic summary of the metabolism of lipids and their reconstitution in the enterocytes

Figure 43.4 A schematic summary of the control of motility in the gastrointestinal tract

The principal role of the lower gastrointestinal tract is to provide a large volume for the processes of digestion and a large surface area for the absorption of nutrients.

Duodenum

As **chyme** passes from the stomach into the duodenum, it is acted on by pancreatic secretions that contain **lipases** to digest lipids, **pancre-**

atic amylases to break down carbohydrates, nucleases to break down nucleic acids and precursors to proteolytic enzymes (chymotrypsinogen, trypsinogen, procarboxypeptidases A and B and proelastases), which are activated by trypsin (to chymotrypsin, trypsin, carboxypeptidases A and B and elastases respectively) to break down a variety of proteins. This process of activation is to prevent autodigestion.

The pancreatic secretions are also rich in bicarbonate to neutralise the stomach acid and inhibit the activity of pepsins, and the pH in the small intestines is ~ 5.3. The pancreatic enzymes are made by the acinar cells of the exocrine pancreas feeding into epithelium-lined ducts. The secretion of enzymes is stimulated via cholecystokinin (CCK) in response to the presence of fats and protein in the duodenum. The epithelial cells in the secretory ducts release bicarbonate and this is promoted by the hormone secretin, released by the duodenal cells in response to acid entering the duodenum.

Hepatic products are also released from the gall bladder at this site, and they contain bile salts, which emulsify fat. The bile salts are efficiently recycled (90–95% are reabsorbed in the terminal ileum and this is referred to as enterohepatic cycling (Chapter 44)).

Jejunum and ileum

The duodenum leads into the jejunum and ileum, which provide a muscular wall for peristalsis and large surface area for absorption of nutrients. Structurally the lumenal side is made up of villi and the epithelial cells have a brush border of microvilli to increase the surface area.

Absorption of monosaccharides (Figure 43.1)

This occurs predominantly in the duodenum and jejunum. Carbohydrates are broken down to monosaccharides, and the brush borders contain disaccharidases to break down disaccharides (maltase breaks down maltose to glucose; sucrose breaks down sucrose to glucose and fructose; and lactase breaks down lactose to galactose and glucose). The monosaccharides are then co-transported into the epithelial cells (enterocytes) of the villi via a sodium co-transporter (e.g. SGLT1: the sodium-glucose transporter protein-1, which transports either glucose or galactose) driven by the concentration gradient for sodium created by the basolateral sodium pump. The monosaccharides then pass out of the basolateral membrane via the GLUT2 transporter into the dense capillary network to complete absorption into the body.

Absorption of peptides and amino acids (Figure 43.2)

Di- and tri-peptides from protein degradation, including those formed by the brush border peptidases, are transported efficiently across the cell membranes. This is driven via the electrochemical difference for protons across the membrane, generated via $Na^+{:}H^+$ exchange. Inside the cell, peptides are then further broken down by peptidases to amino acids, which are then absorbed systemically.

Amino acids are transported, predominantly in the ileum, by specific amino acid transporters.

Absorption of lipids (Figure 43.3)

Emulsified fat is broken down by lipases to liberate free fatty acids and monoglycerides, which form micelles with hydrophobic cores and hydrophilic shells. These micelles promote the delivery of lipids to the microvilli membranes and the hydrophobic core can then pass into the epithelial cells. Once inside the cells, fats are formed and these are transported by the lymphatic system to enter the blood at the thoracic duct.

Absorption of electrolytes

The passage of Na^+ is driven by the sodium pump in the basolateral membrane, which keeps intracellular Na^+ low and generates a diffusion gradient from the lumen so that Na^+ enters via both transporters and channels.

Potassium is taken up in the small intestines but its movement in the colon depends on it electrochemical gradient from the lumen to the epithelial layer. Hence large volumes associated diarrhoea may promote secretion of potassium, leading to hypokalaemia.

Calcium balance is regulated via activated vitamin D (calcitriol), which increases the amount of a calcium-binding protein in the brush border. This occurs largely in the duodenum and jejunum.

Absorption of water

In health, some 99% of ingested (~2 L/day) and secreted (~7 L/day) water is reabsorbed in the gastrointestinal tract and this occurs predominantly in the small intestines. Epithelial cells are connected by tight junctions. These are more permeable to water in the duodenum and this decreases down the lower gastrointestinal tract. Therefore, in the upper areas, substantial amounts of water are reabsorbed by the paracellular route, and this is driven by osmotic gradients generated via electrolyte absorption, largely driven by the Na^+ pump.

Large intestines

The colon, which leads to the rectum and anus, forms the final section of the lower intestinal tract. The role of the colon is the final absorption of water and electrolytes to form more solid faeces.

Motility (Figure 43.4)

The lower gastrointestinal tract is made up of muscular tubes that are responsible for propelling the contents through the tract via peristalsis. This is a highly regulated process, as too rapid a transit limits the time for absorption of water and may lead to diarrhoea, while too slow a transit can lead to constipation. The gastrointestinal tract is under autonomic control, where, broadly speaking, parasympathetic stimulation enhances motility and sympathetic activation inhibits motility. The enteric nervous system (made up of submucosal and myenteric plexuses) is a well-developed arrangement of local neurones that coordinate local motor and secretory activity. The enteric nervous system can work in the absence of autonomic control and provides local reflex control in response to stimuli via sensory afferents from chemo and mechanoreceptors.

Pathophysiology

The lower gastrointestinal tract is affected by a number of pathologies. Viral and bacterial infections are common occurrences and can lead to secretory diarrhoea.

The primary treatment of diarrhoea is oral rehydration therapy, in which a solution of glucose and electrolytes is given. The uptake of glucose is coupled to Na^+ and this leads to the update of Na^+, which is followed osmotically by water, leading to rehydration.

In other conditions, motility may be affected, and reduced smooth muscle activity leads to constipation. Reduced smooth muscle activity can be a side effect of opioid drugs, which act at opioid receptors to cause presynaptic inhibition of parasympathetic activity (Chapter 20), and so constipation is a common side effect of opioids.

Inflammatory bowel diseases (ulcerative colitis and Crohn's disease) are autoimmune diseases that result in severe inflammation within the gastrointestinal system.

Michael D Randall

Figure 44.1 A schematic summary of the physiological roles of the liver

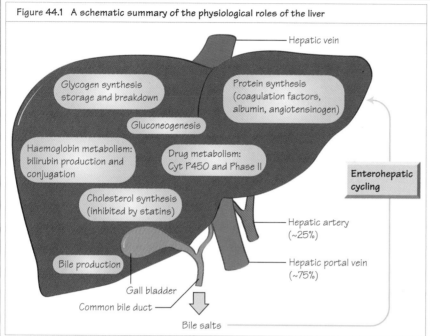

- Hepatic vein
- Glycogen synthesis storage and breakdown
- Protein synthesis (coagulation factors, albumin, angiotensinogen)
- Gluconeogenesis
- Haemoglobin metabolism: bilirubin production and conjugation
- Drug metabolism: Cyt P450 and Phase II
- Cholesterol synthesis (inhibited by statins)
- Enterohepatic cycling
- Hepatic artery (~25%)
- Hepatic portal vein (~75%)
- Bile production
- Gall bladder
- Common bile duct
- Bile salts

Figure 44.2 A functional unit of the liver

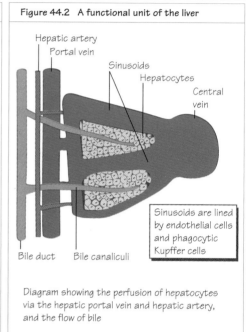

- Hepatic artery
- Portal vein
- Sinusoids
- Hepatocytes
- Central vein
- Bile duct
- Bile canaliculi

Sinusoids are lined by endothelial cells and phagocytic Kupffer cells

Diagram showing the perfusion of hepatocytes via the hepatic portal vein and hepatic artery, and the flow of bile

---

Table 44.1 Key liver function tests and their significance.
Typical normal ranges are given but these can vary between different assays and laboratories

Marker	Typical normal ranges	Clinical significance
Bilirubin	3–17 µmol/L	• Increased if there is increased red blood cell breakdown (haemolysis), intrahepatic dysfunction or cholestasis • Accumulation of bilirubin in the blood leads to jaundice (yellow colouration of the skin and sclera)
Aminotransferases, e.g. Alanine aminotransferase (ALT)	ALT: 5–45 iu/L	• These may leak out of damaged hepatocytes • Elevated levels are consistent with ongoing hepatocellular damage
Alkaline phosphatase (ALP)	40–120 Iu/L	• Produced by a number of tissues including the liver, placenta and bone • ALP is excreted by the bile ducts which is impaired in cholestasis, leading to increased plasma levels
Gamma glutamyl transpeptidase (γGT)	<70 iu/L (males) <40 iu/L (females)	• Elevated levels may indicate alcohol abuse or induction of drug metabolism • Levels are also raised in cholestasis
Albumin	35–50 g/L	• Levels decrease as the synthetic activity of the liver is reduced in liver disease • Indicates impaired synthetic activity of liver
International normalised ratio	1–1.2	• Coagulation of the blood takes longer when the synthesis of coagulation factors is impaired in liver disease • Indicates impaired synthetic activity of liver

---

The liver is the central biochemical (and largest) organ, playing many roles to ensure homeostasis (Figure 44.1). In the adult, the liver weighs approximately 1.5 kg and receives approximately 25% of cardiac output. Seventy five per cent of liver blood flow is derived from the **hepatic portal vein**, which drains the gastrointestinal tract and so delivers nutrients to the liver, and toxins, which may be metabolised before entering the systemic circulation. The remaining blood flow is from the hepatic artery.

The liver is made up of thousands of functional units called lobules, which feed into a central vein. The hepatocytes are bathed in sinusoids, which receive blood from the hepatic portal vein and the hepatic arteries. The sinusoids are surrounded by an endothelium and also contain **phagocytic Kupffer cells**. The hepatocytes then form and feed into bile canaliculi, leading to bile ductules and then bile ducts, taking the bile to the gall bladder for storage (Figure 44.2).

Metabolic roles
The liver is a key store of energy in the form of glycogen and is active in both glycogen synthesis from glucose, and glyogenolysis to liberate glucose. The synthesis of glycogen is promoted by insulin, following the cellular uptake of glucose from the blood derived from the gastrointestinal tract. The liver also plays a role in **gluconeogenesis**, in which glucose is synthesised from non-carbohydrates such as certain amino acids, glycerol (from lipids), pyruvate and lactate (Chapter 12).

Synthesis of proteins
Many **plasma-borne proteins** are synthesised in the liver. These include coagulation factors (all except factor VIII), transport albumins (present in the plasma and contribute towards oncotic pressure), angiotensinogen (the precursor to the renin-angiotensin-aldosterone system [RAAS] pathway) and thrombopoietin (a peptide that regulates platelet production).

Lipid metabolism
Some 75% of cholesterol in the body is made endogenously by the liver and the remainder is from the diet. **Cholesterol** is synthesised from acetyl-CoA, which forms 3-hydroxy-3-methyl-glutaryl-CoA that is then acted on by enzyme **HMG CoA reductase** to form mevalonate and, ultimately, 27-carbon atom cholesterol. HMG CoA reductase is the first committed step in the pathway and is inhibited by cholesterol-lowering drugs (statins; Chapter 35).

The liver synthesises triglycerides from esterification of fatty acid acyl-Co-As with glycerol-3-phosphate.

Lipids are transported around the body by lipoproteins, and hepatocytes express low-density lipoprotein (LDL) receptors for the uptake of cholesterol derived from cellular degradation around the body. The liver also produces very-low-density lipoprotein (VLDL) for the transport of cholesterol and triglycerides and LDL cholesterol.

Haemoglobin and bilirubin
Red blood cells are broken down by the reticuloendothelial system of the liver, spleen and bone marrow. The iron is efficiently recycled and the porphyrin moiety of haem derived from haemoglobin is converted in the spleen and hepatocytes to bilirubin. Bilirubin is highly water insoluble and is conjugated in the liver to form water-soluble conjugates.

Bile
The liver produces 400–800 mL of bile per day and is made up of water, electrolytes, bile salts (derived from cholesterol), conjugated bilirubin, cholesterol, lecithin and some amino acids. It is stored in the gall bladder and excreted down the bile duct into the duodenum. The release of bile is principally stimulated by cholecystokinin as a consequence of food entering the duodenum. Bile is a detergent used to emulsify fats prior to digestion by lipases. Accordingly, bile will also promote the absorption of fat-soluble vitamins (A, D, E and K). Some 95% of bile salts are reabsorbed by **enterohepatic cycling**, in which constituents are reabsorbed in the ileum.

Drug metabolism
The liver plays a central role in drug metabolism and usually results in the production of an inactive compound that is more readily excreted (into the bile or via the kidneys), although in some cases drugs (in the form of **prodrugs**) are activated by hepatic metabolism. Drug metabolism is divided into **phase I** and **phase II**. Phase I generally involves oxidation (but may also involve reduction or hydrolysis) and this often involves hepatic oxidation via the **cytochrome P450** (CYP450) family. These reactions involve reduced NADP, molecular oxygen and CYP450 isoenzymes. Phase II involves a transferase reaction and conjugation (glucuronidation, methylation, sulphation, acetylation, glutathione conjugates, amino acid conjugates, mercapturic acid formation) to promote elimination. Phase I and phase II reactions usually happen sequentially.

Hormone metabolism
A number of steroid hormones (oestrogens, testosterone, aldosterone, cortisol), peptide hormones (insulin, growth hormone) and thyroxine are metabolised in the liver. In the cases of cortisol, oestrogens and testosterone, their metabolism involves conjugation to promote excretion.

Cholestasis
This is the inability of the liver to either produce or excrete bile. It may be due to intrahepatic problems, leading to the inability of the intrahepatic biliary ductules to produce bile, or may be extrahepatic due to blockage of the bile duct, e.g. due to gall stones.

Liver function tests (LFTs)
These are standard biochemical tests that measure a number of markers in the blood which may suggest altered liver biochemistry (Table 44.1). The battery of tests should be analysed to 'build up a picture' of possible pathologies and changes.

Liver disease
Liver disease may be acute (for example due to viral infection in hepatitis) or chronic (for example alcoholic liver disease). Liver failure has many pathophysiological effects, including the following.
- **Hyperbilirubinaemia**: with jaundice, nausea and itching as toxic effects of bilirubin.
- **Ascites**: fluid accumulation in the peritoneal cavity, partly associated with increased levels of aldosterone (due to impaired hepatic metabolism) leading to Na⁺ and fluid retention. Acites is be managed by draining and/or diuretics (Chapter 39).
- **Increased bleeding**: due to impaired synthesis of coagulation factors.
- **Oesophageal varices**: increased portal pressure may lead to pathological dilation of veins in the oesophagus. These may rupture and lead to severe blood loss.
- **Encephalopathy:** impaired metabolism of nitrogenous toxins from gut flora may lead to altered neurotransmitter production in the brain, leading to changes in personality and behaviour.

45 Hypothalamus and pituitary

Sue Chan

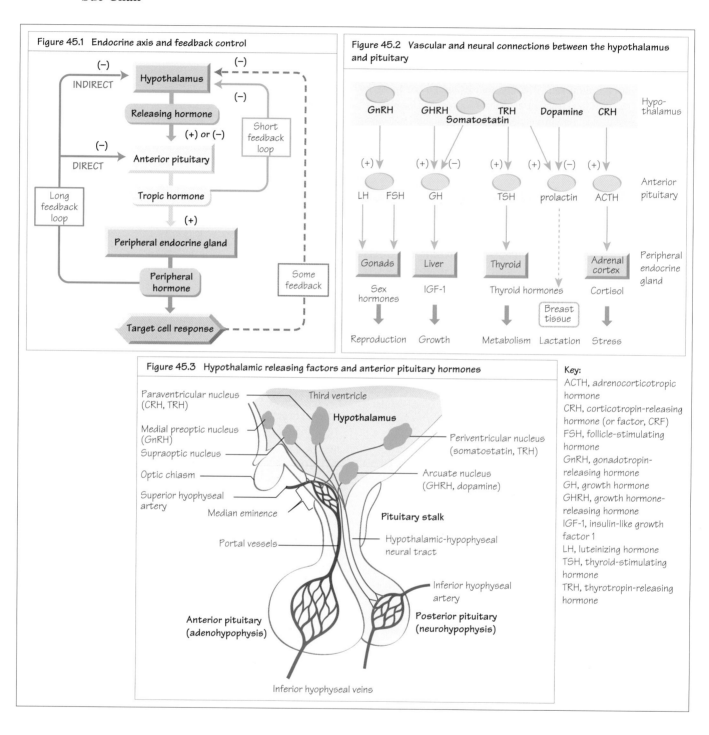

Figure 45.1 Endocrine axis and feedback control

Figure 45.2 Vascular and neural connections between the hypothalamus and pituitary

Figure 45.3 Hypothalamic releasing factors and anterior pituitary hormones

Key:
ACTH, adrenocorticotropic hormone
CRH, corticotropin-releasing hormone (or factor, CRF)
FSH, follicle-stimulating hormone
GnRH, gonadotropin-releasing hormone
GH, growth hormone
GHRH, growth hormone-releasing hormone
IGF-1, insulin-like growth factor 1
LH, luteinizing hormone
TSH, thyroid-stimulating hormone
TRH, thyrotropin-releasing hormone

The endocrine system is composed of several ductless glands that secrete chemical messengers known as **hormones** directly into the bloodstream. At target tissues, hormones interact with specific high-affinity receptors located on the plasma membrane, as in the case of protein (peptide) hormones or amines, or intracellularly (nuclear, cytosolic) as with thyroid and steroid hormones. Hormones exert their functions in four broad physiological areas: maintenance of internal environment, energy balance, growth and development, and reproduction.

Regulation of endocrine secretion

This involves feedback loop control systems that are tuned to set-points, which may be modified by circadian rhythm, seasonal cycles, age and other influences such as stress. Many hormones function as

Table 45.1 Secretory cells of the anterior pituitary

Cell type	% of endocrine population	Hormone	Structure
Acidophil cells somatotroph	~50	Growth hormone (GH)	Single-chain polypeptides with disulphide bonds
Lactotroph	~10–25	Prolactin (PRL)	
Basophil cells gonadotroph	~20	Follicle-stimulating hormone (FSH) Luteinising hormone (LH)	Glycoproteins
Corticotroph	~10	Adrenocorticotropic hormone (ACTH)	Peptide
Thyrotroph	5–10	Thyroid-stimulating hormone (TSH)	Glycoprotein

part of a cascade (**endocrine axis**, Figure 45.1), where secretions of the hypothalamus-pituitary-target gland permit signal amplification, flexibility of response to a variety of physiological stimuli and fine regulation of the end hormone product.

The core of the **neuroendocrine system** is represented by the **hypothalamic–pituitary complex**. Within the **hypothalamus**, reside important collections of neuronal cell bodies (termed nuclei) involved in endocrine function (Figure 45.2). A funnel-shaped stalk, the infundibulum, extends from the floor of the hypothalamus to connect with the **pituitary gland** (**hypophysis**), which lies in a bony cavity (sella turcica) in the sphenoid bone. An important anatomical relation to the pituitary gland is the optic chiasm (Figure 45.2); therefore any expanding lesion of the pituitary or hypothalamus can present with visual field defects.

The pituitary gland is composed of two main lobes: the **anterior lobe** (**adenohypophysis**) and the **posterior lobe** (**neurohypophysis**). Developmentally, the anterior gland derives from the ectodermal Rathke's pouch, an extension of the roof of the primitive oral cavity. The posterior gland forms from a neural down-growth of the di-encephalon. The two tissues migrate and fuse to give rise to the pituitary gland.

Hormones of the hypothalamus and pituitary gland

Hypothalamic releasing hormones

Peptide hormones synthesised in the cell bodies of small **parvocellular** neurones are released from axonal endings into capillary loops at the median eminence (Figure 45.2). They are transported via the **hypothalamic-hypophyseal portal vessels** to the capillary plexus within the anterior pituitary, where they act to stimulate or inhibit the release of hormones of specific cell types (Figure 45.3). Damage to the pituitary stalk (physical trauma, surgery, or disease) impairing blood flow to the pituitary can lead to disrupted control of anterior pituitary hormone release.

Anterior pituitary hormones

The anterior pituitary is composed of five different secretory cell types, each of which secretes a different peptide hormone (Table 45.1). These hormones act on peripheral endocrine glands to stimulate hormone secretion (**tropic** effect) or on non-endocrine tissue to exert direct effects (e.g. prolactin on mammary tissue). **Negative feedback**

control, whereby the release of hormone leads to events that inhibit further secretion, at several points in the endocrine axis allows for the maintenance of plasma hormone levels close to the set-point. Additionally, secretion of hypothalamic releasing hormones may be modulated by neuronal input from higher levels of the brain. Note that, unlike other anterior pituitary hormones, prolactin secretion is under tonic inhibitory control by the hypothalamus.

Posterior pituitary hormones

Vasopressin (also called arginine vasopressin [AVP] or antidiuretic hormone [ADH; Chapter 38] because of its main physiological effects) and **oxytocin** are synthesised in the hypothalamus, in the cell bodies of **magnocellular** neurones, located in the supraoptic and paraventricular nuclei (Figure 45.2). Different subsets of the neurones produce either vasopressin or oxytocin. The hormones are transported down the neuronal axons (which comprise the **hypothalamic-hypophyseal neural tract**) to the posterior pituitary, where they are stored (Figure 45.2). The stimuli for release of the posterior hormones are neural signals (**neuroendocrine reflex**).

• Vasopressin release is regulated by plasma osmolality (detected by hypothalamic osmoreceptors) and also blood pressure/volume (detected by baroreceptors), with neural signals sent to hypothalamic nuclei to modulate the secretion of vasopressin from the posterior pituitary accordingly. The main effects of vasopressin in humans are increased renal water reabsorption (via V_2-receptors, Chapter 38) and vasoconstriction (V_1-receptors).

• Oxytocin: suckling or stimulation of the cervix (copulation or parturition) generates neural signals that are relayed to the oxytocinergic neurones in the hypothalamus, with action potentials to the posterior pituitary resulting in the release of oxytocin into the bloodstream; oxytocin acts to stimulate the contraction of the myoepithelial cells that eject milk from the breast, and to stimulate the contraction of the uterus (myometrium). This is a rare example of **positive feedback**.

Endocrine disorders

These can results from hormone deficiency, hormone excess, or hormone resistance. Along with baseline hormone levels, feedback relationships within an endocrine axis form the basis of diagnostic testing (dynamic or provocative testing) in determining where the defect lies. Defects at the level of the peripheral endocrine gland, the anterior pituitary, or the hypothalamus are referred to as **primary**, **secondary** and **tertiary** endocrine disorders respectively.

Pituitary disease: the most common cause is **pituitary tumours**. Pituitary tumours represent ~10% of all intracranial neoplasms and over 99% are benign (non-invasive) tumours known as adenomas. These tumours can either be microadenomas (less than 10 mm in diameter) or macroadenomas. Pituitary adenomas can cause problems in a number of ways:

• hyper-secretion of a pituitary hormone;
• inadequate production of other remaining pituitary hormones;
• exert local effects on anatomically related structures (e.g. headaches, visual disturbances).

Approximately 75% of the adenomas are endocrinologically active, with prolactin-producing adenomas (prolactinomas) being the most common (approximately 40%). Growth hormone-producing adenomas produce acromegaly (adult).

Hypopituitarism: an underproduction of pituitary hormones. The term pan-hypopituitarism refers to the situation when all the pituitary hormones are underproduced. In the clinical situation, hypopituitarism usually varies depending on the dominant hormone that is deficient.

46 Endocrine pancreas

Sue Chan

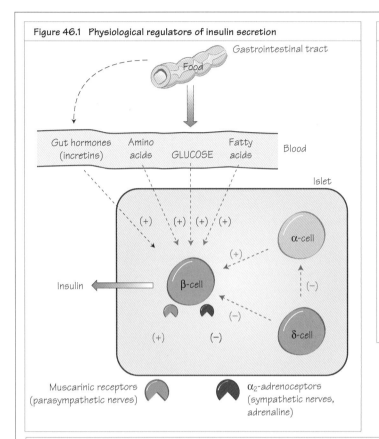

Figure 46.1 Physiological regulators of insulin secretion

Gastrointestinal tract
Food

Gut hormones (incretins) | Amino acids | GLUCOSE | Fatty acids | Blood

Islet

(+) (+) (+) (+)

α-cell

(+)

Insulin

β-cell

(−)

δ-cell

(−)

(+)   (−)

Muscarinic receptors (parasympathetic nerves)

α₂-adrenoceptors (sympathetic nerves, adrenaline)

Table 46.2 Diagnostic criteria for diabetes mellitus (WHO)

Diagnostic criteria

The patient has symptoms, and one of the following:
- Fasting plasma glucose ≥ 7.0 mmol/L (after 8-hour overnight fast)
- Random plasma glucose ≥ 11.1 mmol/L
- Plasma glucose concentraton > 11.1 mmol/L, 2-hour after 75 g glucose in an oral glucose tolerance test (OGTT)
- HbA1c > 6.5 % or 48 mmol/ mol*

If the patient is asymptomatic, two independent plasma glucose measurements (with values in the diabetes range) on separate days are required for a diagnosis of DM

Further categories and impaired glucose regulation:

Impaired glucose tolerance, if
Fasting ≤ 7.0 mmol/L
and
Random or OGTT > 7.8 but < 11.0 mmol/L

Impaired fasting glycaemia, if
Fasting ≥ 6.1 mmol/L but < 7.0 mmol/L

*HbA1c glycated haemoglobin correlates with average blood glucose level over the last 8–12 weeks (life span of red blood cells)

Table 46.1 Cell types within an islet of Langerhans (typical human adult islet)

Cell type		% of the islet	Hormone(s)	Function	Paracrine effects
α	A	30–40	Glucagon	Counter-regulatory hormone to insulin. Increases blood glucose	(+) Insulin secretion
β	B	50–60	Insulin, amylin	Lowers blood glucose (amylin delays gastric emptying)	(−) Glucagon secretion
δ	D	5–10	Somastatin	Inhibitory effects on digestive processes, islet hormone secretions?	(−) Islet cell secretions
PP	F	1–5	Pancreatic polypeptide	Inhibition of exocrine secretion?	(−) Islet cell secretions
ε		< 1	Ghrelin	Promote cell growth and maturation in developing pancreas?	(−) Insulin secretions

Glucose represents an essential energy substrate for many tissues and the maintenance of narrow-controlled blood glucose concentrations (**glucose homeostasis**) is central for a constant provision of glucose to the brain. Glucose homeostasis is dependent on three co-ordinated and simultaneously ongoing processes involving insulin secretion by the pancreas, hepatic glucose output, and glucose uptake by splanchnic (liver and gut) and peripheral tissues (muscle and fat). This involves a complex interplay of hormonal and neural mechanisms in the CNS, the autonomic nervous system and the endocrine pancreas.

Islets of Langerhans

The endocrine pancreas in the adult human consists of approximately one million islets of Langerhans (diameter 50–300 μm), scattered throughout the pancreas and constituting approximately 1–2% of the total pancreatic mass. As well as being highly vascularised (~10% pancreatic blood flow), the islets are richly innervated with nerve fibres of the autonomic nervous system and of the gastrointestinal neuroendocrine system. Within an islet, at least five peptide hormone-producing cells have been identified: α, β, δ, PP, ε (also called A, B, D, F, epsilon) (Table 46.1). The majority of islets are composed of insulin-secreting β-cells, intermingled with fewer α-cells and δ-cells. Islets located in the posterior portion of the head of the pancreas are pancreatic polypeptide-rich, with PP-cells representing 80% of the islet cells. More recently, ghrelin-secreting ε-cells have been described in fetal islets; the expression of this cell type becomes rare soon after birth. Islet cells can influence each other through **paracrine** (between adjacent cells) and **autocrine** (act on original secretory cell) communication. Additionally, islets also contain bioactive agents (e.g. neuropeptide Y, galanin) that have been shown to influence exocrine function.

Insulin

Insulin is a 51-amino acid peptide hormone, synthesised initially as the prohormone precursor proinsulin, with subsequent cleavage of the internal C-peptide to give rise to the mature insulin molecule, which comprises an A-chain (21 amino acids) connected to a B-chain (30 amino acids) by two disulfide bonds. The main physiological regulator of insulin release is plasma glucose, influenced by other nutrients, gastrointestinal hormones (**incretins**, e.g. **glucagon-like peptide 1, GLP-1**) and nervous input (Figure 46.1). Insulin, like other peptide **hormones**, has a short plasma half-life of several minutes. At target tissues, the binding of insulin to its receptor results in autophosphorylation via the **receptor's intrinsic tyrosine kinase activity**. This initiates a series of interactions with docking proteins, leading to a cascade of phosphorylation/dephosphorylation reactions. Insulin lowers blood glucose levels by:
- increasing glucose uptake in adipose and skeletal muscle;
- increasing glycogen synthesis, inhibiting glycogenolysis;
- increasing protein synthesis, inhibiting protein breakdown;
- increasing lipogenesis, inhibiting lipolysis;
- inhibiting gluconeogenesis.

Other effects of insulin include uptake of cellular K^+ ions (via Na^+/K^+ ATPase), growth regulation and control of vascular function.

Glucagon

A 29-amino acid peptide, as the primary counter-regulatory hormone to insulin, glucagon increases blood glucose levels by stimulating hepatic glucose output (elevated glyogenolysis and gluconeogenesis) and lipolysis. Glucagon is rapidly secreted when plasma glucose levels fall, and is inhibited by elevated glucose concentrations. Other stimuli include amino acids (such as protein-rich meal), activation of both sympathetic and parasympathetic nervous input.

Somatostatin

Exists in two forms, a 14-amino acid and a 28-amino acid peptide. Its release is glucose dependent. Its physiological role is unclear; suggestions include regulation of the nutrient flow via control of digestion (endocrine) and a tonic inhibitory influence on insulin and glucagon secretion (paracrine).

Diabetes mellitus (DM)

Diabetes mellitus is a metabolic disorder characterised by **chronic hyperglycaemia**. Signs and symptoms include glucosuria (plasma glucose concentration exceeds the transport maximum for renal absorption, with glucose appearing in the urine), polyuria and thirst (due to osmotic diuresis), and fatigue/malaise. The diagnostic criteria are given in Table 46.2. There are two broad categories of DM.

Type 1 (T1DM): an autoimmune condition causing specific destruction of the islet β-cells, with absolute insulin deficiency. Approximately 70–90% β-cell loss occurs before clinical disease is observed. Genetic factors (~30% susceptibility, association with human leucocyte antigen [HLA] haplotypes DR3 and DR4) and environmental triggers (such as viral, toxins) are thought to be important in the aetiology of T1DM. Autoantibodies to glutamic acid decarboxylase (GAD), insulin and insulinoma-associated protein (IA-2) may be detected. Lack of insulin action can lead to excessive hepatic fatty acid β-oxidation with the abnormal production of ketone bodies, causing metabolic acidosis (ketoacidosis). Patients with T1DM require exogenous insulin. This form accounts for 5–15% of all DM, depending on the population.

Type 2 (T2DM): a heterogeneous condition caused by impaired insulin secretion, decreased insulin sensitivity in target tissues (**insulin resistance**), or both. A strong genetic component, together with other risk factors such as obesity and sedentary lifestyle, contribute to the disorder. The mechanisms underlying insulin resistance are not fully established: defects in insulin signalling and abnormal secretion of adipose-derived factors (**adipokines**) such as **resistin** and **tumour necrosis factor-alpha (TNF-α)** may be involved. It is thought that β-cell function progressively declines as the elevated insulin demands exhaust β-cell insulin secretory capacity to overcome peripheral insulin resistance; the resultant hyperglycaemia then manifests with the symptoms of DM described above. The primary treatment for insulin resistance involves diet and lifestyle recommendations: exercise (increases insulin sensitivity of peripheral tissues) and weight loss (if patient is overweight/ obese). Pharmacological management involves drugs to increase β-cell output, including **sulphonylureas** (inhibitors of ATP-sensitive K-channel on β-cells) and meglitinides (post-prandial glucose regulators), while drugs to improve insulin action include **metformin** (a biguanide; activator of AMP kinase) and glitazones (or **thiazolinediones; PPAR-γ agonists**). Incretin-based medicines (such as GLP-1 analogues and dipeptidyl peptidase IV [DPP-IV] inhibitors [gliptins]) which increase insulin release, promote satiety and delay gastric emptying have recently been included in the pharmacotherapy of T2DM. In advanced T2DM, where the patient's insulin secretory response is severely compromised, then exogenous insulin is required. T2DM accounts for 85–95% of cases of DM.

Chronic diabetic complications may be micro- or macrovascular. **Microvascular** complications include retinopathy, nephropathy and neuropathy. Neuropathy is specific to patients with DM due to damage of small vessels (capillary pathology) by hyperglycaemia (e.g. sorbitol) and glycation of proteins. **Macrovascular** complications include ischaemic heart disease, stroke and peripheral vascular disease due to accelerated atherosclerosis.

47 Thyroid gland

Sue Chan

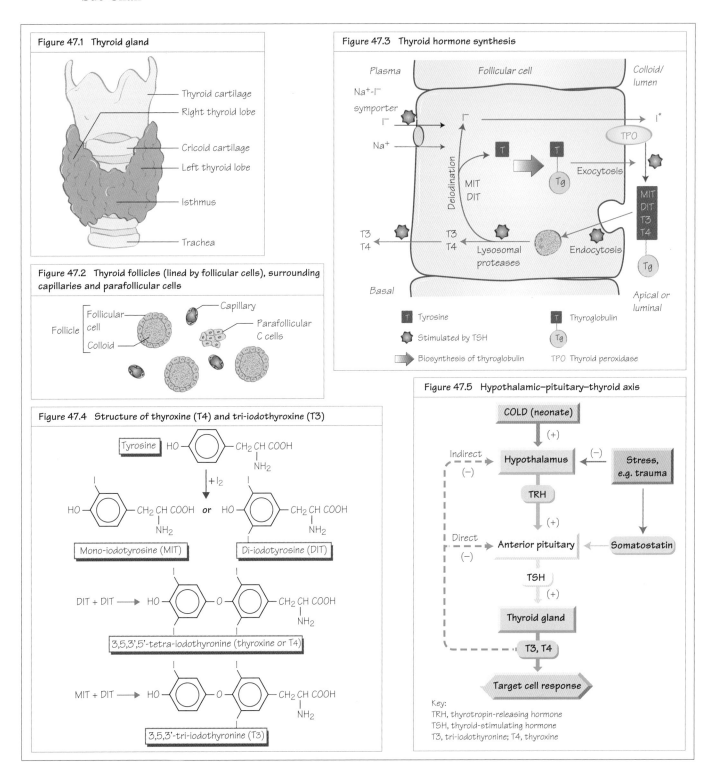

Figure 47.1 Thyroid gland

Figure 47.2 Thyroid follicles (lined by follicular cells), surrounding capillaries and parafollicular cells

Figure 47.3 Thyroid hormone synthesis

Figure 47.4 Structure of thyroxine (T4) and tri-iodothyroxine (T3)

Figure 47.5 Hypothalamic–pituitary–thyroid axis

Anatomy

The **thyroid gland** is located anterior to the cricoid cartilage in the anterior neck, composed of two lobes connected by a branch of tissue known as the isthmus (Figure 47.1), which lies over the second and third tracheal rings. The thyroid is a very vascular organ; in conditions of severe hyperplasia, greater blood flow rates may become audible as a noise (bruit). Two pairs of **parathyroid glands** are located on the posterior surface of the thyroid gland.

Histology

The thyroid gland is composed of a large number of **follicles** (Figure 47.2). Each follicle is formed by a single layer of cuboidal epithelial cells (**follicular cells**), which secrete into the interior of the follicle; the lumen is filled with a proteinaceous, viscous material called **colloid**, which acts as a store for thyroid hormones (on the glycoprotein **thyroglobulin**). Scattered around the follicles are larger **parafollicular** or **C cells** that produce **calcitonin**. Within the parathyroid gland, **parathyroid hormone** (**PTH**) is secreted by chief cells, while the function of oxyphil cells remains unknown.

Parathyroid hormone and calcitonin

Parathyroid hormone

Secretion of PTH is stimulated by low plasma calcium levels. PTH acts to raise plasma calcium levels by stimulating calcium resorption of bone, stimulating calcium uptake from the gastrointestinal tract, enhancing renal excretion of phosphate. PTH is required for renal 'activation' of vitamin D into 1,25-dihydroxycholecalciferol, which acts to promote calcium reabsorption from the gut.

Calcitonin

Calcitonin is released in response to high plasma calcium levels. Calcitonin lowers plasma calcium by inhibiting bone resorption and inhibiting reabsorption in the kidney.

Thyroid hormones: thyroxine (T4) and tri-iodothyronine (T3)

Synthesis

Thyroid hormones are the only hormones that require an essential trace element, iodine, for the production of active hormone. The follicular cell actively accumulates iodide (I^-) ions via the Na^+-I^- symporter (driven by the inward Na^+ gradient), expressed on the basement membrane (this process is also called **iodide trapping**, Figure 47.3). At the apical (or luminal) membrane, I^- is transported into the follicle lumen by a transporter called 'pendrin'. I^- is oxidised into an active intermediate by the enzyme **thyroid peroxidase** (or thyroperoxidase, TPO). TPO also catalyses the iodination of tyrosine residues (**organification**) on thyroglobulin (a glycoprotein rich in tyrosine residues), to produce **mono-iodotyrosine** (MIT) and **di-iodotyrosine** (DIT); and the coupling of two DIT molecules to form **thyroxine** (T4), or one MIT with one DIT to give **tri-iodothyronine** (T3) (Figure 47.4). The thyroid hormones are stored as part of the thyroglobulin molecule (colloid), with sufficient amount to supply the body with its normal requirements for 2–3 months.

Release

Small portions of colloid are taken up by endocytosis into the cell. These vesicles fuse with lysosomes, which contain protease enzymes that digest the thyroglobulin to release T4 and T3 (Figure 47.3); the thyroid hormones are then released into the bloodstream (exact mechanism(s) unclear). Approximately 95% of thyroid hormone secreted is T4, the remainder is T3, with negligible amounts of reverse T3 (rT3, formed by coupling of DIT with MIT). As lipophilic molecules, thyroid hormones are poorly soluble in blood plasma and are highly bound (99.9%) to plasma-binding proteins (thyroxine-binding globulin, transthyretin and albumin). **De-iodinase** enzymes in the plasma and peripheral tissues metabolise T4 to the more biological active T3 (about four to five times more potent) and the inactive rT3; in effect, T4 acts as a pro-hormone to T3.

Regulation of thyroid function

The thyroid gland is regulated by thyroid-stimulating hormone (TSH), with thyroid hormones exerting negative feedback control of the endocrine axis (hypothalamic-pituitary-thyroid axis; Figure 47.5). Other stimuli include inhibitory (stress, somatostatin, glucocorticoids) and stimulatory (cold exposure in infants) factors. TSH acts to stimulate the synthesis and release of thyroid hormones, including thryoglobulin synthesis (Figure 47.5). TSH also exerts a 'trophic' (to nourish, promote growth) effect, stimulating thyroid growth with hyperplasia (increased size) and hypertrophy (increased number) of follicular cells; excess plasma TSH levels can lead to the development of a **goitre** (enlarged thyroid gland).

Actions of thyroid hormones

In tissues, thyroid hormones diffuse across the plasma membrane into cells, and interact with specific nuclear receptors, which are members of the superfamily of ligand-dependent transcription factors, leading to altered gene expression. Non-genomic actions include direct effects on Na^+/K^+-ATPase and Ca^{2+}-ATPase.

- Metabolism: increase basal metabolic rate, oxygen consumption and heat production; stimulate anabolic and catabolic processes of protein, fat and carbohydrate metabolism.
- Cardiovascular system: increase heart rate, cardiac output, blood pressure. As well as direct effects, thyroid hormones act synergistically with catecholamines by upregulating β-adrenoceptors.
- Growth and development: an essential role in normal development and maturation of the brain, and skeletal growth and bone maturation. Thyroid hormones promote growth hormone release from the pituitary, and act in a permissive manner on the actions of growth hormone in growth and development. Lack of thyroid hormone in the developing newborn leads to cretinism (stunted growth and mental retardation).

Thyroid disorders

Hypothyroidism

Thyroid hormone deficiency is a common disorder, estimated to affect 1–2% of all adults in their lifetime. The most common cause worldwide is iodine deficiency, and it may also arise following radioactive iodine therapy or thyroid surgery. Primary failure of the thyroid gland is usually caused by autoimmune destruction or attack of the thyroid gland; Hashimoto's thyroiditis, which accounts for 90% of all hypothyrodism, is a slowly developing chronic autoimmune disease where there is an immune reaction to thyroglobulin and other components of the thyroid gland. Typical symptoms include lethargy, cold intolerance, weight gain and constipation. Treatment is with synthetic thyroid hormones (such as levo-thyroxine).

Hyperthyroidism

Also known as thyrotoxicosis, hyperthyroidism is characterised by elevated plasma T3 and T4 levels, with sweating, tremor, tachycardia and weight loss. There are several causes, the most common of which is Graves' disease, where autoantibodies against the TSH receptor are generated. The thyroid-stimulating immunoglobulins (TSI) activate the TSH receptor, stimulating the thyroid gland to produce and secrete more T3 and T4. Patients present with a goitre. Lymphocytic infiltration and fluid deposition in the orbital soft tissue causes protrusion of the eyeballs (proptosis, exophthalmos). Treatment may include β-blockers for rapid sympathetic relief of β-adrenoceptor-mediated effects (e.g. tremor, tachycardia), antithyroid drugs (e.g. carbimazole; which inhibit TPO activity and hence thyroid hormone synthesis), surgical removal, or radioactive ^{131}I-iodine to destroy the gland.

48 Adrenal glands and steroid hormones

Sue Chan

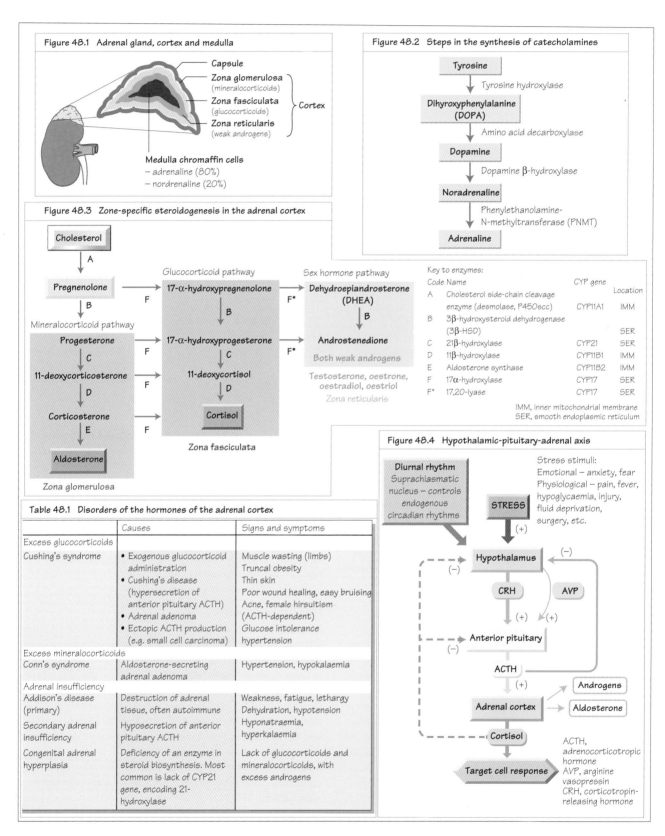

Figure 48.1 Adrenal gland, cortex and medulla

- Capsule
- Zona glomerulosa (mineralocorticoids)
- Zona fasciculata (glucocorticoids) } Cortex
- Zona reticularis (weak androgens)
- Medulla chromaffin cells
  – adrenaline (80%)
  – nordrenaline (20%)

Figure 48.2 Steps in the synthesis of catecholamines

Tyrosine
↓ Tyrosine hydroxylase
Dihyroxyphenylalanine (DOPA)
↓ Amino acid decarboxylase
Dopamine
↓ Dopamine β-hydroxylase
Noradrenaline
↓ Phenylethanolamine-N-methyltransferase (PNMT)
Adrenaline

Figure 48.3 Zone-specific steroidogenesis in the adrenal cortex

Cholesterol → A → Pregnenolone

Glucocorticoid pathway
Pregnenolone → F → 17-α-hydroxypregnenolone

Sex hormone pathway
17-α-hydroxypregnenolone → F* → Dehydroepiandrosterone (DHEA)

Mineralocorticoid pathway
Pregnenolone → B → Progesterone
Progesterone → F → 17-α-hydroxyprogesterone
17-α-hydroxyprogesterone → F* → Androstenedione

Progesterone → C → 11-deoxycorticosterone
11-deoxycorticosterone → F → 11-deoxycortisol
17-α-hydroxyprogesterone → C → 11-deoxycortisol

DHEA → B → Androstenedione
Both weak androgens
Testosterone, oestrone, oestradiol, oestriol
Zona reticularis

11-deoxycorticosterone → D → Corticosterone
11-deoxycortisol → D → Cortisol

Corticosterone → F → Cortisol
Corticosterone → E → Aldosterone

Zona fasciculata
Zona glomerulosa

Key to enzymes:

Code	Name	CYP gene	Location
A	Cholesterol side-chain cleavage enzyme (desmolase, P450scc)	CYP11A1	IMM
B	3β-hydroxysteroid dehydrogenase (3β-HSD)		SER
C	21β-hydroxylase	CYP21	SER
D	11β-hydroxylase	CYP11B1	IMM
E	Aldosterone synthase	CYP11B2	IMM
F	17α-hydroxylase	CYP17	SER
F*	17,20-lyase	CYP17	SER

IMM, inner mitochondrial membrane
SER, smooth endoplasmic reticulum

Figure 48.4 Hypothalamic-pituitary-adrenal axis

Diurnal rhythm
Suprachiasmatic nucleus – controls endogenous circadian rhythms

Stress stimuli:
Emotional – anxiety, fear
Physiological – pain, fever, hypoglycaemia, injury, fluid deprivation, surgery, etc.

STRESS
(+)

Hypothalamus (−)
(−)
CRH   AVP
(+) (+)
Anterior pituitary
(−)
ACTH
(+)
Adrenal cortex → Androgens
→ Aldosterone
Cortisol
Target cell response

ACTH, adrenocorticotropic hormone
AVP, arginine vasopressin
CRH, corticotropin-releasing hormone

Table 48.1 Disorders of the hormones of the adrenal cortex

	Causes	Signs and symptoms
Excess glucocorticoids		
Cushing's syndrome	• Exogenous glucocorticoid administration • Cushing's disease (hypersecretion of anterior pituitary ACTH) • Adrenal adenoma • Ectopic ACTH production (e.g. small cell carcinoma)	Muscle wasting (limbs) Truncal obesity Thin skin Poor wound healing, easy bruising Acne, female hirsuitism (ACTH-dependent) Glucose intolerance hypertension
Excess mineralocorticoids		
Conn's syndrome	Aldosterone-secreting adrenal adenoma	Hypertension, hypokalaemia
Adrenal insufficiency		
Addison's disease (primary)	Destruction of adrenal tissue, often autoimmune	Weakness, fatigue, lethargy Dehydration, hypotension Hyponatraemia, hyperkalaemia
Secondary adrenal insufficiency	Hyposecretion of anterior pituitary ACTH	
Congenital adrenal hyperplasia	Deficiency of an enzyme in steroid biosynthesis. Most common is lack of CYP21 gene, encoding 21-hydroxylase	Lack of glucocorticoids and mineralocorticoids, with excess androgens

 Medical Sciences at a Glance, First Edition. Edited by Michael D Randall. © 2014 John Wiley & Sons, Ltd. Published 2014 by John Wiley & Sons, Ltd.

The adrenal glands are situated on the superior pole of the kidney, embedded in the perirenal fat. The **outer cortex**, which is derived from mesodermal tissue, secretes **steroid hormones**, while the **inner medulla**, derived from neuroectodermal tissue, secretes the **catecholamines adrenaline** and **noradrenaline** (Figure 48.1). The adrenal gland is a highly vascular organ, where the arteriolar network gives rise to a small number of medullary arteries that pass directly through the cortex to the medulla, and an abundance of tiny thin-walled blood vessels called sinusoids, into which cortical cells secrete steroid hormones. Consequently, secretions of the adrenal cortex bathe the cells of the medulla before leaving the gland via the venous system.

Hormones of the adrenal medulla

The adrenal medulla can be described as a modified ganglion of the sympathetic nervous system (Chapter 21); **chromaffin cells** secrete adrenaline and noradrenaline into the bloodstream, innervated by nerve fibres of the splanchnic nerve with acetylcholine (ACh) as the neurotransmitter. ACh acts on nicotinic receptors on the chromaffin cell membrane to increase the rate of catecholamine synthesis and release. The expression of the enzyme that converts noradrenaline to adrenaline, phenylethanolamine-N-methyltransferase (Figure 48.2), is maintained by glucocorticoids, so the vascular arrangement within the adrenal gland ensures that chromaffin cells bathed in steroid-rich blood secrete adrenaline as the primary hormonal product of the adrenal medulla.

Hormones of the adrenal cortex

The adrenal cortex is made up of three zones (Figure 48.1), each zone expressing a distinct complement of enzymes involved in steroidogenesis of a different type of steroid hormones (**zone-specific steroidogenesis**, Figure 48.3).
• Outer **zona glomerulosa**, a thin layer of cells lying underneath the capsule, which secretes **aldosterone**.
• Middle **zona fasciculata**, the widest band of cells, which secretes the glucocorticoids (such as **cortisol**) and small amounts of adrenal androgens.
• Inner **zona reticularis** secretes the adrenal androgens **dehydroepiandrosterone** (**DHEA**) and **androstenedione**.
Many of the enzymes belong to the cytochrome P450 (CYP) monooxidase family. The steroid hormones are synthesised from **cholesterol**, which is mainly derived from plasma low-density lipoprotein (LDL), with smaller amounts from *de novo* synthesis from cellular acetate. The rate-limiting step in steroidogenesis is the transfer of the cholesterol from the outer mitochondrial membrane to the inner mitochondrial membrane; this is where cholesterol side-chain cleavage enzyme (desmolase, P450scc) is located, the enzyme involved in conversion of cholesterol to the first steroid, pregnenolone. Steroidogenic acute regulatory (StAR) protein is thought to play a key role as a cholesterol-shuttling protein. Pregnenolone then exits the mitochondria and is transferred into the microsomal compartment, to be converted to a variety of other steroids, each steroid shuttling between the two subcellular compartments as it progresses along its biosynthetic pathway (Figure 48.3). As lipophilic molecules, steroid hormones are not stored; levels of circulating hormone are controlled primarily by its rate of synthesis. A deficiency of an enzyme involved in steroid biosynthesis can lead to the deficiency of products downstream of the enzyme, with corresponding accumulation of precursors upstream; the most common form of congenital adrenal hyperplasia (CAH, >90%) affects 21-hydroxylase (Figure 48.3, Table 48.1).

Glucocorticoids

Cortisol is the primary glucocorticoid in humans, and also has mineralocorticoid activity. Its metabolic effects generally oppose those of insulin, exerting catabolic effects in muscle and adipose, while in liver it stimulates glycogen synthesis. Cortisol causes elevation in plasma glucose levels, primarily by stimulating hepatic gluconeogenesis and, to a lesser extent, decreasing glucose uptake in skeletal muscle and adipose. At high levels, glucocorticoids exert an anti-inflammatory/immunosuppressive action; synthetic steroids (such as prednisolone) with relatively low mineralocorticoid potencies have thus been developed, and are used to control inflammatory or immune conditions. Cortisol is permissive on the actions of catecholamines on carbohydrate metabolism, and on cardiovascular regulation.

Cortisol production and release is controlled by the hypothalamus and pituitary, forming the **hypothalamic-pituitary-adrenal axis** (Figure 48.4). Superimposed on this basic negative-feedback control are two additional factors that influence plasma cortisol levels by changing the set-point, **diurnal rhythm** and **stress**, which both act on the hypothalamus (Figure 48.4). The diurnal pattern of **adrenocorticotrophic hormone (ACTH)** release dictates the diurnal rhythm of cortisol levels: at its lowest concentration at midnight, rising to a peak between 6am and 8am, and falling throughout the rest of the day. In response to stressors (emotional, e.g. anxiety, or physiological, e.g. fluid deprivation or injury), cortisol and sympathetic nervous activity act together to adapt to the stress situation, with mobilisation of biochemical resources (energy molecules), preparing the body to a state of physical and behavioural readiness. However, chronic activation of the stress response can lead to harmful states, with muscle-wasting, immune suppression, gastric ulcers and hyperglycaemia. ACTH also acts in a trophic manner, where elevated ACTH levels can lead to hypertrophy of the zona fasiculata and reticularis (e.g. CAH), and atrophy of the adrenal cortex with low ACTH levels (adrenal insufficiency, adrenal suppression with chronic use if high-dose steroid medication). Conditions of excess (**Cushing's syndrome**) and deficient (**Addison's disease**) glucocorticoids are described in Table 48.1.

Aldosterone

Aldosterone is produced exclusively by adrenal glomerulosa cells, due to their expression of aldosterone synthase (Figure 48.3). Aldosterone production is primarily controlled by levels of angiotensin II, part of the **renin-angiotensin system** (Chapter 32), and plasma K^+ levels, with minor influence by ACTH. Aldosterone regulates renal Na^+, and hence water, reabsorption with K^+ excretion, acting on late distal tubule and collecting duct (Chapter 39). Dysregulation of aldosterone production may lead to systemic hypertension and hypokalaemia (**Conn's syndrome**; Table 48.1).

Adrenal androgens

DHEA and its sulphated form, with a small amount of androstenedione, are weak androgens. Secretion begins at age 5–6, at very low level, with a surge at puberty, peaking at ages 25–30 years, then slowly tapers off. In women, it contributes to 50% of circulating active androgens, influencing pubic and axillary (arm pit) hair growth, and also sex drive. Under conditions of androgen excess (such as ACTH-dependent Cushing's syndrome, CAH), masculinisation of females can occur (*in utero*: ambiguous external genitalia; adult: excessive facial/body hair [hirsutism], acne). In men, adrenal androgens contribution is negligible against the background of testosterone secretion from the testes. Adrenal androgen production is regulated by ACTH, but the androgens do not exert any feedback control on the endocrine axis (Figure 48.4).

49 The genital system

Deborah Merrick

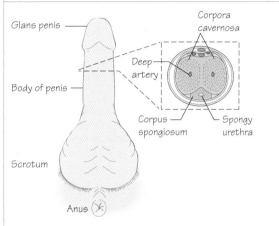

Figure 49.1   Male external genitalia, surface anatomy with associated cross-section through the body of the penis inset

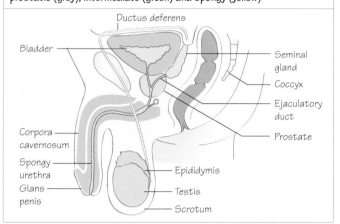

Figure 49.2   Male external and internal genitalia, median section showing the four parts of the male urethra: preprostatic (orange), prostatic (grey), intermediate (green) and spongy (yellow)

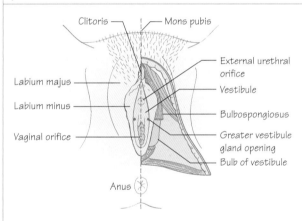

Figure 49.3   Female external genitalia, surface anatomy and perineal musculature shown with vestibule orifices illustrated

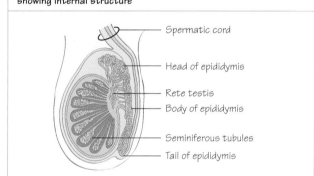

Figure 49.4   Testis and epididymis, lateral view of left testis showing internal structure

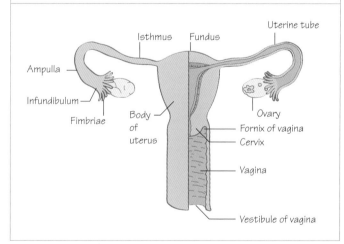

Figure 49.6   Female internal genitalia, illustrating relative positions of the vagina, uterus, uterine tubes and ovaries

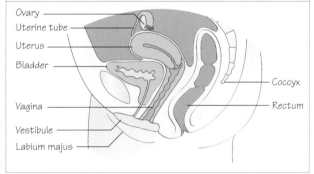

Figure 49.5   Female external and internal genitalia, median section showing relative position of vagina, uterus (anteverted and anteflexed) and ovaries

 Medical Sciences at a Glance, First Edition. Edited by Michael D Randall. © 2014 John Wiley & Sons, Ltd. Published 2014 by John Wiley & Sons, Ltd.

The reproductive system comprises a series of organs that are involved in the production and maturation of gametes. The organs also function to unite the gametes, during sexual reproduction. Anatomically, the reproductive system can be divided into external and internal genitalia.

External genitalia
Male
Penis: organ permitting the exit of urine and semen from the body. It is the principal organ of copulation and is anatomically described in its erect position. It has a fixed root, body and glans penis, and is composed of three bodies of erectile tissue: the paired **corpora cavernosa** and the **corpus spongiosum** (Figure 49.1). The root is composed of the **crura** and **bulb** (containing erectile tissues) along with **ischiocavernosus** and **bulbospongiosus muscles**. Distally the corpus spongiosum expands to form the glans penis. The prepuce (foreskin) covers the glans penis to a variable extent.

Urethra: a muscular tube conveying urine and semen to the external urethral orifice at the tip of the glans penis. The urethra in males is long and subdivided into four distinct regions (Figure 49.2):
• preprostatic (intramural): extends through neck of bladder;
• prostatic: descends through prostate;
• membranous (intermediate): passes through perineal membrane;
• spongy (penile): courses through corpus spongiosum.

Scrotum: a cutaneous sac containing the **testes** and **epididymides**, located posteroinferior to the penis. The dartos muscle attaches to the skin of the scrotum, causing it to wrinkle when cold. The cremaster muscle elevates the testes, holding them closer to the body to minimise heat loss.

Female
The terms vulva and pudendum are terms often used to describe the female external genitalia as a whole, and include the following.

Mons pubis: fatty eminence covered with pubic hair extending anterior to the pubic symphysis, tubercle and superior rami.

Labia majora and minora: paired folds of skin. The more prominent labia majora pass from the mons pubis towards the anus (Figure 49.3). They are filled predominantly with subcutaneous fat, the terminal part of the round ligament of the uterus, and are covered in pubic hair. The smaller labia minora are hairless, consisting of spongy connective tissue containing erectile tissue. The labia minora unite anteriorly to form the prepuce and frenulum of the **clitoris** (Figure 49.3). The clitoris is an erectile organ composed of a root (two crura), body (two corpora cavernosa) and glans.

Vestibule: the space bounded by the labia minora containing the openings of the vagina, urethra, and ducts of the greater and lesser vestibular glands (Figure 49.3). The bulbs of the vestibule are paired erectile masses located beneath the bulbospongiosus muscles either side of the vaginal orifice.

Vasculature of the external genitalia: arterial supply is from branches of the internal and external pudendal arteries. Venous drainage accompanies the arteries and the veins are named accordingly. Lymphatic drainage is via the superficial inguinal, deep inguinal, internal iliac and external iliac lymph nodes.

Internal genitalia
Male
Testes and epididymides: suspended in the scrotum by the spermatic cords (Figure 49.4). The testes are oval shaped, producing sperm and hormones (e.g. testosterone). Sperm is formed in the seminiferous tubules, which connect to the epididymis via the rete testis (Figure 49.4). The epididymis is located on the posterior aspect of the testis; it has a head, body and tail. It appears as a solid structure, but is in fact formed from a single elongated duct with multiple convolutions. The tail of the epididymis is continuous with the **ductus deferens**, which ascends in the spermatic cord to enter the pelvis (Figure 49.2). Before termination, the ductus deferens enlarges (ampulla) before joining the duct of the seminal gland to form the ejaculatory duct.

Seminal glands (vesicles): secrete a thick alkaline fluid that mixes with sperm as it enters the ejaculatory duct and urethra. The glands are located superior to the prostate (Figure 49.2).

Prostate: surrounds the prostatic urethra and is composed of fibromuscular and glandular parts, which secrete a thin milky fluid that plays a role in sperm activation. It provides approximately 20% of the volume of semen (fluid containing secretions from the testes, seminal glands, prostate and **bulbourethral glands**). The bulbourethral glands produce mucus-like secretions, which enter the spongy urethra during sexual arousal (Figure 49.2).

Female
Vagina: a musculomembranous tube connecting the vestibule of the vagina inferiorly to the cervix of the uterus superiorly (Figure 49.5). The vaginal walls are usually collapsed with anterior and posterior walls in close contact; with the exception of the superior aspect, where the cervix holds the walls apart. The vaginal fornix is the recess surrounding the protruding cervix. The vagina functions to receive the penis during intercourse, acts as the inferior portion of the birth canal and is a passageway for menstrual fluid.

Uterus: a muscular, hollow, pear-shaped organ possessing a body and cervix inferiorly. The body comprises the fundus, isthmus and the uterine horns (Figure 49.6). The uterine body wall is composed of three layers: perimetrium (outer-serous), myometrium (middle-muscular) and endometrium (inner-mucous). The cervix is narrow and cylindrical in shape, composed of supravaginal and vaginal parts (Figures 49.5 and 49.6). In non-gravid (non-pregnant) women, the body of the uterus lies on the urinary bladder and the cervix lies between the bladder and rectum. This position can change in relation to the fullness of the bladder/rectum and also during pregnancy.

Uterine tubes: extend from the uterine horns to open into the peritoneal cavity, in close proximity to the ovaries (Figure 49.6). Each tube has four parts: infundibulum (distal), ampulla, isthmus and uterine (proximal). The **ovaries** are almond-shaped structures that expel the oocyte into the peritoneal cavity during ovulation. It is the distal portion of the uterine tubes (fimbriae) that captures the oocyte before passing it to the ampulla.

Vasculature of the internal genitalia: the testes and ovaries receive their blood supply via the testicular and ovarian arteries respectively, which arise from the abdominal aorta. The remaining internal genitalia receive blood supply from branches of the internal iliac arteries. Veins accompany these arteries and have similar names. Lymphatic drainage is chiefly into the lumbar (caval/aortic), internal iliac and external iliac lymph nodes.

50 Reproductive physiology

Michael D Randall

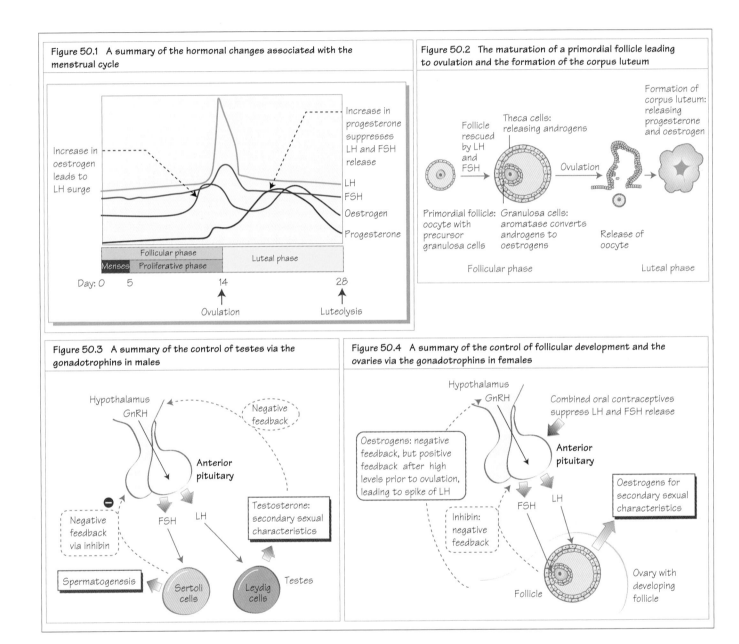

Figure 50.1 A summary of the hormonal changes associated with the menstrual cycle

Figure 50.2 The maturation of a primordial follicle leading to ovulation and the formation of the corpus luteum

Figure 50.3 A summary of the control of testes via the gonadotrophins in males

Figure 50.4 A summary of the control of follicular development and the ovaries via the gonadotrophins in females

Reproductive physiology is tightly regulated via hormonal control by the steroidal sex hormones. The process starts with puberty at around 10–13 years in females and slightly later in males.

In males, puberty is associated with maturation of the reproductive organs, with enlargement of the testes and penis. This is regulated via the release of glycoprotein **gonadotrophins** from the anterior pituitary gland in response to **gonadotrophin-releasing hormone (GnRH)** from the hypothalamus (Figure 50.1). The gonadotrophin, **luteinising hormone (LH)** acts on **Leydig cells** of the testes to stimulate the release of the androgens, including testosterone. The release of testosterone leads to the development of secondary sexual characteristics in males (body and facial hair, voice, muscular physique) and libido. Another gonadotrophin, **follicle-stimulating hormone (FSH)**, acts on the **Sertoli cells** in the semininferous tubules of the testes to promote spermatogenesis. Testosterone also feeds back to inhibit both the hypothalamus and the anterior pituitary. The Sertoli cells exert negative feedback on FSH release via the release **inhibin**, which acts at the anterior pituitary.

In females, adrenache is the maturation of the adrenals, leading to the production of various steroid hormones (e.g. dehydroepiandrostone [DHEA] and androstenedione), which sensitise towards gonadotrophin stimulation. This then leads to gonarche with breast bud development in response to oestradiol. Puberty in females is similarly regulated via LH and FSH, such that increased pulses of the hormones lead to the initiation of the **menstrual cycle** with the regular development and release of ova (Figure 50.2). The female sex hormones lead to the development of secondary sexual characteristics in females, such as breast development.

Hormonal regulation of the menstrual cycle

The human female reproductive cycle is characterised by the **menstrual cycle**, which typically lasts 28 (+/−4) days and coordinates ovulation at its midpoint (Figures 49.3 and 49.4). The cycle is under tight hormonal regulation and divided into four phases.

• **Follicular phase** (from the start of menstrual bleeding to day 14): during this time there is maturation of a **primordial follicle**. Many primordial follicles are present in the ovaries from the fetal stage of the female and they contain an **ovum or oocyte**, arrested in meiosis and surrounded by a single epithelial cell layer (precursor granulosa cells). Many of the primordial follicles undergo atresia but some are rescued by **pulses of LH and FSH**. Follicles mature during the reproductive years and this is influenced by LH, which acts on outer theca cells of the developing follicles, which then release androgens. The androgens are then converted by **aromatase** in the **granulosa cells** to oestrogens, and these levels rise throughout the phase. The maturation process is supported by FSH acting on the granulosa cells. The maturation leads to the formation of a **Graafian follicle**, one of which per cycle becomes dominant.

• **Ovulation**: the Graafian follicle grows substantially and ruptures mid-cycle to release the single oocyte into the peritoneal cavity to enter the oviduct. Ovulation is preceded by the appearance of LH receptors on the granulosa cells and by a surge in LH release due to oestradiol, which at high levels has a positive feedback effect.

• **Luteal phase** (day 14–28): post-ovulation the ruptured follicle becomes the **corpus luteum**, in which the granulosa cells respond to LH by producing progesterone and the theca cells produce oestrogen to provide the optimal conditions for implantation for a fertilised ovum. The progesterone causes negative feedback on GnRH, so that LH and FSH levels become minimal and there is no further follicular development.

• **Luteolysis** (day 28): in the absence of fertilisation the corpus luteum starts to break down, with decreased production of progesterone. This leads to menstruation with the breakdown of the vascular uterine wall, which is shed and leads to menstrual period bleeding.

Conception

Ejaculation during sexual intercourse results in the deposition of spermatozoa in the female genital tract. The spermatozoa undergo capacitation, which results in their ability to fertilise the released oocyte. **Capacitation** involves removing glycoproteins from the spermatozoa to increase membrane permeability in preparation for fertilisation. Once a spermatozoon fuses with an oocyte then fertilisation occurs, in which the maternal and paternal chromosomes are combined. The fertilised zygote then undergoes several cell divisions prior to implantation as a blastocyst in the endometrium.

Pregnancy

If fertilisation occurs the corpus luteum must be retained to maintain pregnancy. This is achieved by the hormone **human chorionic gonadotrophin (hCG)**, which is released initially by the trophoblast cells of the blastocyst and then the placenta and continues to be produced until around three months of gestation. Implantation is favoured by the increased levels of oestrogen, which prepare the uterus.

Maintenance of pregnancy is dependent on the establishment of the **placenta**, which supplies the fetus with nutrients, oxygen and acts as an immunological barrier. The trophoblast secretes large amounts of progesterone to maintain pregnancy and the placenta releases oestrogens to prepare the mother (e.g. increase in breast size). The levels of oestrogens and progesterone increase throughout pregnancy until birth.

Parturition

The signal for birth includes increased levels of DHEA from the fetal adrenal glands. After nine months of gestation birth is initiated by increased uterine contractions in response to increasing oestrogen levels. There is ripening of the cervix in preparation for birth. The electrical activity coupled to contraction is also conducted via gap junctions connecting the myometrial cells. The process of labour also stimulates the release of oxytocin from the posterior pituitary and this also promotes uterine contractions.

Oral contraceptives

These provide effective contraception.

• **Combined oral contraceptives** contain oestrogens and a progestogen, and prevent follicular development, ovulation and luteinisation by suppressing the release of LH and FSH.

• **Progestogen-only containing** pills increase the viscosity of cervical mucus and so prevent penetration by spermatozoa.

51 Human embryology

Deborah Merrick

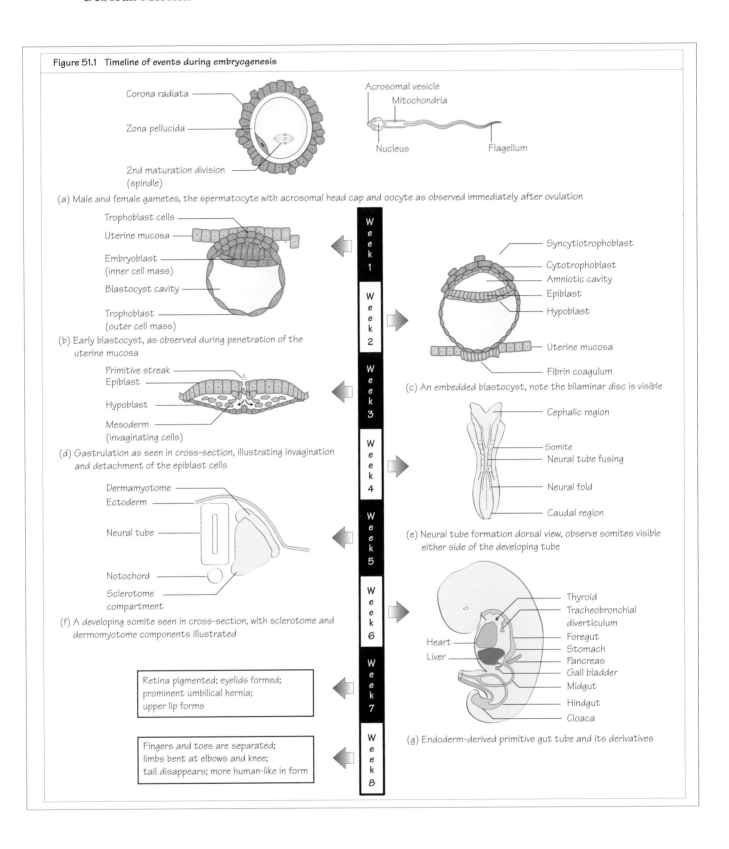

Figure 51.1 Timeline of events during embryogenesis

(a) Male and female gametes, the spermatocyte with acrosomal head cap and oocyte as observed immediately after ovulation

Corona radiata
Zona pellucida
2nd maturation division (spindle)

Acrosomal vesicle
Mitochondria
Nucleus
Flagellum

(b) Early blastocyst, as observed during penetration of the uterine mucosa

Trophoblast cells
Uterine mucosa
Embryoblast (inner cell mass)
Blastocyst cavity
Trophoblast (outer cell mass)

(c) An embedded blastocyst, note the bilaminar disc is visible

Syncytiotrophoblast
Cytotrophoblast
Amniotic cavity
Epiblast
Hypoblast
Uterine mucosa
Fibrin coagulum

(d) Gastrulation as seen in cross-section, illustrating invagination and detachment of the epiblast cells

Primitive streak
Epiblast
Hypoblast
Mesoderm (invaginating cells)

(e) Neural tube formation dorsal view, observe somites visible either side of the developing tube

Cephalic region
Somite
Neural tube fusing
Neural fold
Caudal region

(f) A developing somite seen in cross-section, with sclerotome and dermomyotome components illustrated

Dermamyotome
Ectoderm
Neural tube
Notochord
Sclerotome compartment

(g) Endoderm-derived primitive gut tube and its derivatives

Thyroid
Tracheobronchial diverticulum
Foregut
Stomach
Pancreas
Gall bladder
Midgut
Hindgut
Cloaca
Heart
Liver

Retina pigmented; eyelids formed; prominent umbilical hernia; upper lip forms

Fingers and toes are separated; limbs bent at elbows and knee; tail disappears; more human-like in form

Week 1
Week 2
Week 3
Week 4
Week 5
Week 6
Week 7
Week 8

Medical Sciences at a Glance, First Edition. Edited by Michael D Randall. © 2014 John Wiley & Sons, Ltd. Published 2014 by John Wiley & Sons, Ltd.

Embryology is the developmental study of the embryo during the **first eight weeks following fertilisation**. During the process of fertilisation, male and female gametes fuse to produce a diploid **zygote**. In the days and weeks that follow this remarkable event, tissues and organs of the embryo are derived from three primitive germ layers.

Fertilisation

Fertilisation is the process by which a female oocyte (egg) and male spermatozoa (sperm) fuse. For fertilisation to occur, the spermatozoa must undergo capacitiation and the acrosomal reaction. **Capacitiation** occurs in the female genital tract by the removal of proteins and glycoproteins from the plasma membrane overlying the acrosomal region. Capacitated spermatozoa can then pass through the corona radiate cells freely (Figure 51.1a). The **acrosomal reaction** occurs after the spermatozoa bind to the zona pellucida and involves the release of enzymes required to penetrate this layer, facilitating fusion of the gametes. Once a spermatozoon enters the oocyte the egg responds by preventing other spermatozoa entering, resuming meiotic division and becoming metabolically active. **Cleavage** is a series of mitotic division that occur once the zygote has reached the two-cell stage. The cells, known as **blastomeres**, become compacted, forming an inner and outer cell mass. The inner cell mass will develop as the embryo proper, while the outer cell mass will form the **trophoblast** (which contributes to the placenta). Fluid penetrates the inner cell mass forming the blastocyst cavity; at this stage the embryo is referred to as a **blastocyst**. By the end of week 1, the blastocyst has begun to **implant** into the uterine mucosa (Figure 51.1b). By the end of week 2, it has become completely embedded and a **primitive uteroplacental circulation** is evident. The inner cell mass (**embryoblast**) differentiates into two layers (epiblast and hypoblast) forming a bilaminar disc (Figure 51.1c).

Gastrulation

This is the process that establishes the three germ layers: **ectoderm, mesoderm** and **endoderm** (Figure 51.1d). It begins with the formation of the primitive streak on the surface of the epiblast. Epiblast cells migrate towards the streak, becoming flask-shaped and detaching, before moving below the epiblast cell layer (a process called invagination). Some invaginating cells displace the hypoblast layer and become the endoderm germ layer. Cells remaining in the epiblast layer form the ectoderm and those cells occupying the region between the endoderm and ectoderm become the embryonic mesoderm. The three germ layers are now established.

Organogenesis

This occurs from week 3 to week 8 of development. During this developmental period the three germ layers give rise to all the organs and tissues of the human body.

Ectoderm derivatives: the ectoderm overlying the **notochord** and **prechordal mesoderm** thickens to form the neural plate. This in turn folds and fuses to form the neural tube, a process that is completed at approximately day 25 (Figure 51.1e). This tube represents the primitive central nervous system. It possesses an extended cephalic region characterised by dilations (vesicles) that will develop into the brain and a thinner caudal part that will become the spinal cord. Other derivatives from the ectoderm germ layer include structures that make contact with our surrounding environment, including the peripheral nervous system, skin and sensory epithelium of the ear, nose and eye. **Neural crest cells** are often referred to as the fourth germ layer. The cells arise at the lateral borders of the neural folds as they fuse; they then migrate and enter the underlying mesoderm. The neural crest cells subsequently give rise to numerous structures, including melanocytes (skin and hair follicles), Schwann cells, connective tissue, and bones of the face and skull.

Mesoderm derivatives: mesodermal cells close to the midline proliferate and form a thickened plate called the **paraxial** mesoderm. Located lateral to this is a thinner region of **lateral plate** mesoderm, which is temporarily connected to the paraxial mesoderm by **intermediate** mesoderm. At the beginning of week 3, the paraxial mesoderm becomes organised into segments called the somitomeres. Cells of the somitomeres contribute to the mesenchyme of the head, forming a large proportion of the neurocranium and voluntary muscles of the craniofacial region. In the occipital region and caudally, the somitomeres further organise into somites at around day 20. Approximately three new somites appear in a craniocaudal sequence every day until 42-44 pairs are present by the end of week 5. After receiving signals from surrounding structures such as the neural tube and notochord, each somite differentiates into a sclerotome and dermomyotome component (Figure 51.1f). Cells derived from the sclerotome give rise to cartilage and bone (e.g. vertebrae) and those cells derived from the dermomyotome form the precursors to muscle and the dermis of the skin. The intermediate mesoderm differentiates into urogenital structures, including nephrotomes, which form an important component of the primitive kidney system. The lateral plate mesoderm splits into somatic and splanchnic layers. Mesodermal cells from the somatic layer give rise to the bones and connective tissue of the limbs, and together with the overlying ectoderm, form the lateral body walls. The splanchnic layer gives rise to the walls of the gut tube in association with cells of endodermal origin. The mesodermal embryonic germ layer also gives rise to the circulatory system, including the heart, arteries, veins, lymph vessels, blood and lymph cells. The spleen and cortex of the suprarenal glands are also mesoderm derivatives.

Endoderm derivatives: the main organ system derived from the endoderm germ layer is the gastrointestinal tract (GI tract), which is formed from a primitive gut tube. The formation of the gut tube is a passive event, caused by embryonic growth and folding. The gut tube is divided into the foregut, midgut and hindgut. The endoderm germ layer provides the epithelial lining of the GI tract, respiratory tract and urinary bladder. Other derivatives include the liver, pancreas and parenchyma of the thyroid (see Figure 51.1g).

Fetal period

This is four times the length of the embryonic period, commencing at week 9. This period is characterised by rapid growth and maturation of the multiple tissues and organ systems. For example, the urogenital system differentiates further between males and females during this period.

Deborah Merrick

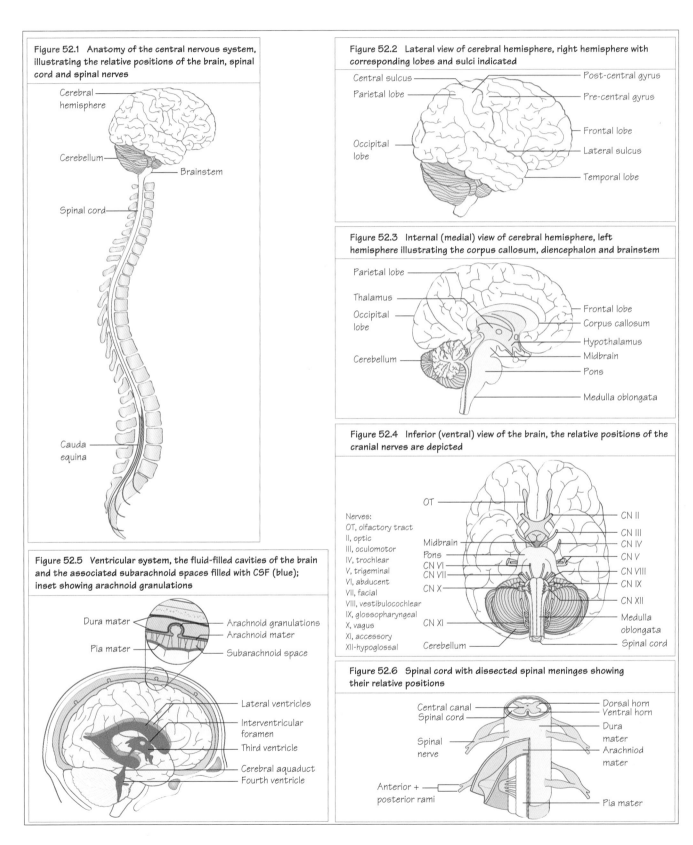

Figure 52.1 Anatomy of the central nervous system, illustrating the relative positions of the brain, spinal cord and spinal nerves

Cerebral hemisphere
Cerebellum
Brainstem
Spinal cord
Cauda equina

Figure 52.2 Lateral view of cerebral hemisphere, right hemisphere with corresponding lobes and sulci indicated

Central sulcus
Parietal lobe
Post-central gyrus
Pre-central gyrus
Frontal lobe
Occipital lobe
Lateral sulcus
Temporal lobe

Figure 52.3 Internal (medial) view of cerebral hemisphere, left hemisphere illustrating the corpus callosum, diencephalon and brainstem

Parietal lobe
Thalamus
Occipital lobe
Cerebellum
Frontal lobe
Corpus callosum
Hypothalamus
Midbrain
Pons
Medulla oblongata

Figure 52.4 Inferior (ventral) view of the brain, the relative positions of the cranial nerves are depicted

Nerves:
OT, olfactory tract
II, optic
III, oculomotor
IV, trochlear
V, trigeminal
VI, abducent
VII, facial
VIII, vestibulocochlear
IX, glossopharyngeal
X, vagus
XI, accessory
XII-hypoglossal

OT
Midbrain
Pons
CN VI
CN VII
CN X
CN XI
Cerebellum
CN II
CN III
CN IV
CN V
CN VIII
CN IX
CN XII
Medulla oblongata
Spinal cord

Figure 52.5 Ventricular system, the fluid-filled cavities of the brain and the associated subarachnoid spaces filled with CSF (blue); inset showing arachnoid granulations

Dura mater
Pia mater
Arachnoid granulations
Arachnoid mater
Subarachnoid space
Lateral ventricles
Interventricular foramen
Third ventricle
Cerebral aquaduct
Fourth ventricle

Figure 52.6 Spinal cord with dissected spinal meninges showing their relative positions

Central canal
Spinal cord
Spinal nerve
Anterior + posterior rami
Dorsal horn
Ventral horn
Dura mater
Arachniod mater
Pia mater

The central nervous system (CNS) allows the coordination and integration of neural signals that control activities of the body, such as respiration. The CNS is also involved in **higher cognitive functions** such as memory and learning. The CNS comprises the brain and spinal cord (Figure 52.1), which are composed of a large number of excitable nerve cells (**neurones**) and specialised tissue (**neuroglia**). Neuronal cell bodies are located within grey matter and the processes of the neurones occupy white matter of the CNS.

Brain

The brain and its membranous coverings are protected by the surrounding neurocranium. The brain is composed of an inner core of white matter surrounded by grey matter. Some specialised grey matter masses (nuclei) are located deep within the white matter.

Cerebrum

The left and right cerebral hemispheres form the largest component of the brain. The cerebral surfaces are thrown into multiple folds (gyri), grooves (sulci) and clefts (fissures). The major sulci separate each hemisphere into frontal, parietal, temporal and occipital lobes, named according to the bones they lie beneath (Figure 52.2). The pattern of gyri and sulci is anatomically important, as some demarcate functional areas of the cortex. For example, the pre-central gyrus corresponds to the primary motor area (Chapter 54) and the post-central gyrus is associated with the primary sensory area of the cortex (Chapter 53). The left and right hemispheres are connected by a large mass of white matter, the corpus callosum. The diencephalon forms the central core of the cerebrum and includes the thalamus and hypothalamus (Figure 52.3 and Chapter 55).

Brainstem

The brainstem is composed of the midbrain (rostral), pons and medulla oblongata (caudal). Cranial nerves III–IV (midbrain), V (pons), VI–VII (pons-medulla junction) and VIII–XII (medulla oblongata) are associated with the brainstem (Figures 52.3 and 52.4).

Cerebellum

This lies posterior to the pons and medulla and is composed of two hemispheres, thrown into folds (folis) united by the vermis (Figure 52.3 and 52.4). The cerebellum connects to the midbrain, pons and medulla oblongata via large bundles of nerve fibres called the superior, middle and inferior cerebellar peduncles, respectively.

Vasculature of the brain

The brain receives approximately one-sixth of the cardiac output via the vertebral and internal carotid arteries. These blood vessels form a collateral circulation by anastomosing at the base of the brain (**circle of Willis**). Cerebral veins draining the brain empty into a series of venous sinuses (Figure 52.5) before returning to the heart via the internal jugular vein.

Meninges and cerebrospinal fluid

Meninges

The meninges are three membranous layers called **pia mater**, **arachnoid mater** and **dura mater** (Figure 52.6). These coverings are termed either cranial meninges (those associated with the brain) or spinal meninges (associated with the spinal cord). The pia mater closely adheres to the surface of the brain and spinal cord (Figures 52.5 and 52.6). The arachnoid mater forms a cobweb-like covering that is separated from the pia mater by the subarachnoid space, which contains **cerebrospinal fluid (CSF)**. The external cranial dura mater is a thick, two-layered membrane. The outer (periosteal) layer closely associates with the internal aspect of the cranium and the inner (meningeal) layer forms dural infoldings (e.g. falx cerebri). The dural venous sinuses form between the two dural layers where the dural infoldings attach (Figure 52.5). The dura mater surrounding the spinal cord is separated from the vertebral bodies by adipose tissue in the epidural (extradural) space. The meninges form a supporting network for vessels and form a fluid-filled cavity that surrounds and protects the brain and spinal cord.

Ventricular system

This comprises two lateral ventricles and midline third and fourth ventricles (Figure 52.5). Choroidal epithelial cells of the choroid plexuses located within the ventricles secrete CSF (400–500 mL/day). The lateral ventricles connect with the third ventricle via interventricular foramina (of Monro). The third ventricle is continuous with the cerebral aqueduct (of Sylvius), which opens into the fourth ventricle. The fourth ventricle then tapers to become the central canal of the spinal cord. A median aperture (of Magendie) and two lateral apertures (of Luschka) allow CSF to enter the subarachnoid space. CSF is reabsorbed into the venous system via arachnoid granulations (Figure 52.5).

Spinal cord

The spinal cord is continuous with the **medulla oblongata** (Figure 52.1). It is located within the vertebral canal of the vertebral column, surrounded by the spinal meninges and CSF in the subarachnoid space (Figure 52.6). The spinal cord is shorter than the vertebral canal, terminating in the lumbar region in adults (intervertebral disc between L1 and L2 vertebrae). Close to its termination, the roughly cylindrical cord tapers to a cone-shaped structure called the conus medullaris. At its apex, the filum terminale descends to attach to the coccyx, helping to anchor the spinal cord. Thirty-one pairs of spinal nerves (8 cervical, 12 thoracic, 5 lumbar, 5 sacral and 1 coccygeal) attach to the spinal cord via anterior (motor) and posterior (sensory) roots through a series of rootlets. The spinal cord has two enlarged regions (cervical and lumbosacral), which correspond to the innervation of the limbs. Spinal roots arising from the lumbosacral enlargement and conus medullaris form bundles of nerve roots called the cauda equina (Figure 52.1). The cauda equina is located in a distended subarachnoid space called the lumbar cistern. Unlike the brain, the spinal cord has an inner core of grey matter with dorsal and ventral horns that unite through a grey commissure containing a small central canal (Figure 52.6). White matter surrounds the grey matter and can be divided into dorsal, ventral and lateral columns.

Vasculature of the spinal cord

The spinal cord is supplied by three longitudinal arteries (one anterior and two posterior) that are derived from branches of the vertebral, ascending cervical, deep cervical, intercostal, lumbar and lateral sacral arteries. Longitudinal spinal veins (three anterior and three posterior) drain the spinal cord in a similar distribution pattern to the arteries and have a direct continuity with the cranial sinuses.

Deborah Merrick

Table 53.1 Sensations mediated by the somatosensory system, with examples of corresponding receptors given

Tactile sensations (touch, pressure, vibration)	Proprioception		Pain
	Conscious	Non-conscious	
Cutaneous mechanoreceptors: Hair follicles (deformation) Meissner's corpuscles (touch, vibration) Merkel's receptors (pressure) Pacinian corpuscles (vibration) Ruffini's corpuscles (stretch)	Joint mechanoreceptors: Joint receptors(kinaesthesia)	Muscle mechano-receptors: Muscle spindles (limb proprioception) Golgi tendon organs (limb proprioception)	Nociceptors: Mechanical (sharp pricking pain) Thermal, mechano-thermal (slow, burning pain) Polymodal (mechanical stimuli, hot or cold burning sensation)

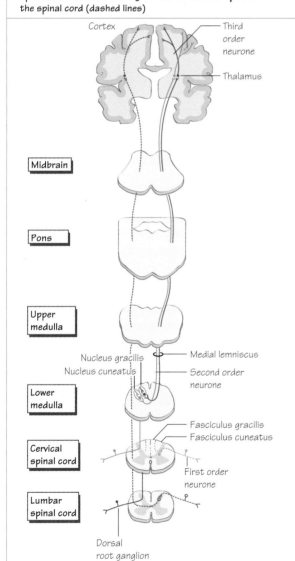

Figure 53.1 Sensory pathways, fasciculus gracilis and fasciculus cuneatus ascending in the dorsal column (bold lines) and spinothalamic fibres running in the anterolateral quadrant of the spinal cord (dashed lines)

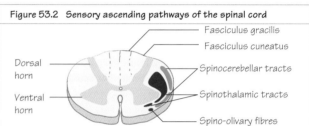

Figure 53.2 Sensory ascending pathways of the spinal cord

Figure 53.3 Visual cortex, as observed in an internal (medial) view of the brain

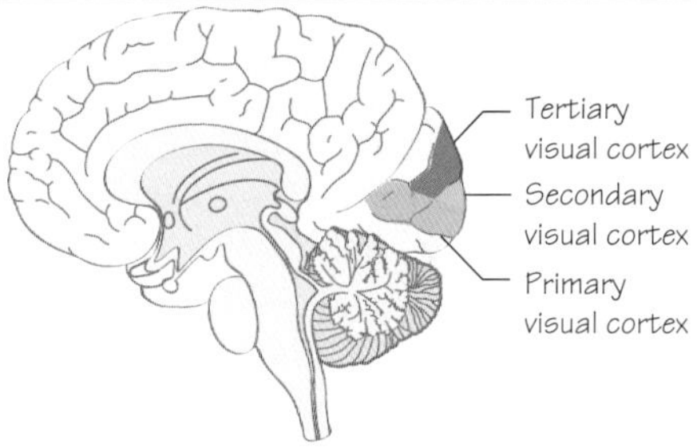

Figure 53.4 Auditory cortex, as observed in a lateral view of cerebral hemisphere

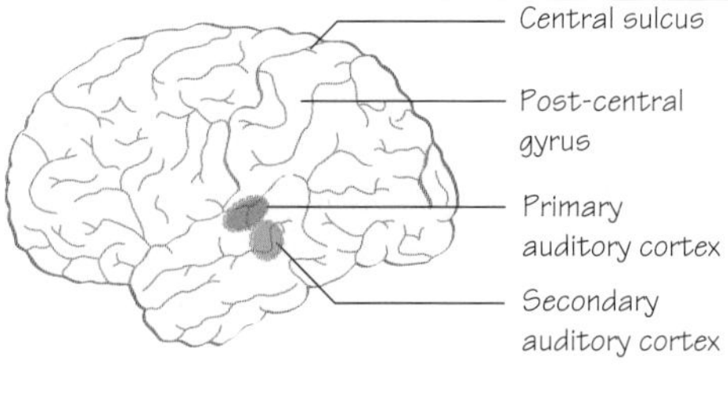

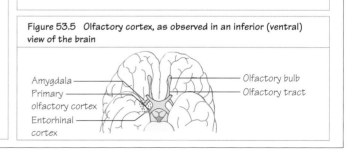

Figure 53.5 Olfactory cortex, as observed in an inferior (ventral) view of the brain

The sensory system monitors the body's internal and external environment. Sensory nerve endings (sensory receptors) respond to a stimulus, which is transmitted to the central nervous system for processing. The sensory system includes somatic, visual, auditory, vestibular, taste and olfactory (smell) systems. The sensory input can be divided into general (somatosensory) and special sensations.

Sensory receptors

These are specialised neuronal structures that make contact with our environment (Table 53.1). The afferents can be classified according to the type of stimulus they respond to. **Chemoreceptors** are sensory receptor that responds to certain chemical stimuli in the environment (e.g. olfactory neurones). **Mechanoreceptors** respond to mechanical pressure or distortion (e.g. hair cells of the cochlear), while **photoreceptors** react to light (e.g. rods and cones of the retina). **Thermoreceptors** respond to changes in temperature (e.g. cutaneous receptors) and **nociceptors** react to potentially damaging stimuli causing the perception of pain (e.g. cutaneous receptors). The sensory stimulus is converted into electrochemical energy of the nerve impulse, in a process called transduction.

Somatosensory system

This relays general sensory information such as touch, pressure and vibration (tactile sensations) through the nervous system via a series of neurones. In its simplest form, this comprises three neurones: first-order, second-order and third-order (Figure 53.1). Neurones segregate themselves into two main general sensory pathways: **spinothalamic** and **medial lemniscus** (dorsal column system).

Spinothalamic: sensory pathway conveying information of pain, temperature, light touch and pressure. The cell bodies of first-order neurones occupy the dorsal root ganglion of spinal nerves (Figure 53.1). Their axons pass into the spinal cord and synapse with cells of the dorsal horn. Second-order neuronal axons pass contralaterally before ascending in the anterolateral quadrant of the spinal cord (Figure 53.2). Most spinothalamic axons terminate in the **ventral posterolateral (VPL) nucleus** of the thalamus. Crude awareness of touch, pressure, pain and temperature are believed to be appreciated here. **Thalamocortical projections** (third-order neurones) pass from the thalamus via the internal capsule and corona radiata to the somatosensory area of the post-central gyrus. The size of the cortical area representative of a particular body region (**homunculus**) is proportional to the region's sensitivity. For example, the hands are disproportionally large due to their heightened sensitivity. The sensation of pain can be divided into 'fast pain' and 'slow pain' experiences approximately 0.1 and 1.0 s following a painful stimulus. Fast pain impulses travel directly to the VPL nucleus before passing to the cerebral cortex. Slow pain fibres end in the reticular formation, activating the entire nervous system.

Medial lemniscus: pathway involved in discriminative touch, conscious proprioception and sensing vibration. Axons from the posterior root ganglion pass into the dorsal columns of the spinal cord. The dorsal column contains two ascending tracts, the fasciculus gracilis and the fasciculus cuneatus. Unlike the spinothalamic system, these fibres remain ipsilateral until the medulla. Long ascending fibres from the sacral, lumbar and lower thoracic region are contained in the fasciculus gracilis. The fasciculus cuneatus comprises upper thoracic and cervical ascending fibres. Fibres synapse with second-order neurones in the nucleus gracilis or nucleus cuneatus of the medulla respectively (Figure 53.1). Axons of these neurones become contralateral, passing over to the opposite side of the spinal cord in the sensory decussation. They ascend (as the medial lemniscus) to synapse with third-order neurones in the VPL nucleus of the thalamus. Axons project to the cerebral cortex as previously described.

Spinocerebellar pathways: terminate in the cerebellar cortex, relaying non-conscious information about limb and joint position (proprioception).

Trigeminothalamic pathway: comparable to the spinothalamic and medial lemniscus pathways, although specific for the head region.

Cuneocerebellar tract: some fibres from the nucleus cuneatus pass to the cerebellum to relay non-conscious information on muscle-joint status related to the upper limb.

Spinotectal tract: sensory fibres ascend and synapse with neurones in the superior colliculus of the midbrain. This pathway is involved in bringing about movement of the eyes and head towards a source of stimulation (spinovisual reflex).

Spinoreticular tracts: pathway involved in influencing the level of consciousness, as second-order neurones synapse with neurones of the reticular formation.

Spino-olivary tract: pathway conveying information from cutaneous and proprioceptive organs to the cerebellum.

Special sensation

Specialised sensations are conducted directly to the brain. Sensory information is relayed via the **thalamus** (relay nuclei) to the cerebral cortex, with the exception of olfaction (smell). Information relating to olfaction is mainly transmitted to the cortex through pathways that do not synapse in the thalamus.

Visual: photoreceptors of the retina (rods and cones) convey visual information to ganglion cells. Axons of the ganglion cells project to the lateral geniculate body of the thalamus via the optic nerve and tract. The lateral geniculate nuclei pass information predominately to the visual cortex for interpretation (Figure 53.3).

Auditory: pressure waves cause vibrations of the basilar membrane that result in mechanical displacement of the cochlear hair cells. This leads to transduction, passing information via the vestibulocochlear nerve and medial geniculate nuclei to the primary auditory cortex (Figure 53.4).

Vestibular: vestibular hair cells, like cochlear hair cells, transduce minute displacements passing information via the vestibulocochlear nerve and vestibular nuclei to multiple brain regions (e.g. cerebellum).

Taste: first-order sensory neurones occupy most of the cell bodies of the geniculate ganglion. They project to the gustatory nuclei before terminating at the ventral posteromedial nucleus of the thalamus. Here projections pass to cortical areas for taste perception.

Olfactory: chemicals with odours are identified by specialised receptors (olfactory cells) located in the olfactory mucosa of the nasal cavity. The cells convey information of smell via the olfactory bulb and tract to several areas of the brain, including the primary olfactory cortex, amygdala and entorhinal cortex (Figure 53.5).

Deborah Merrick

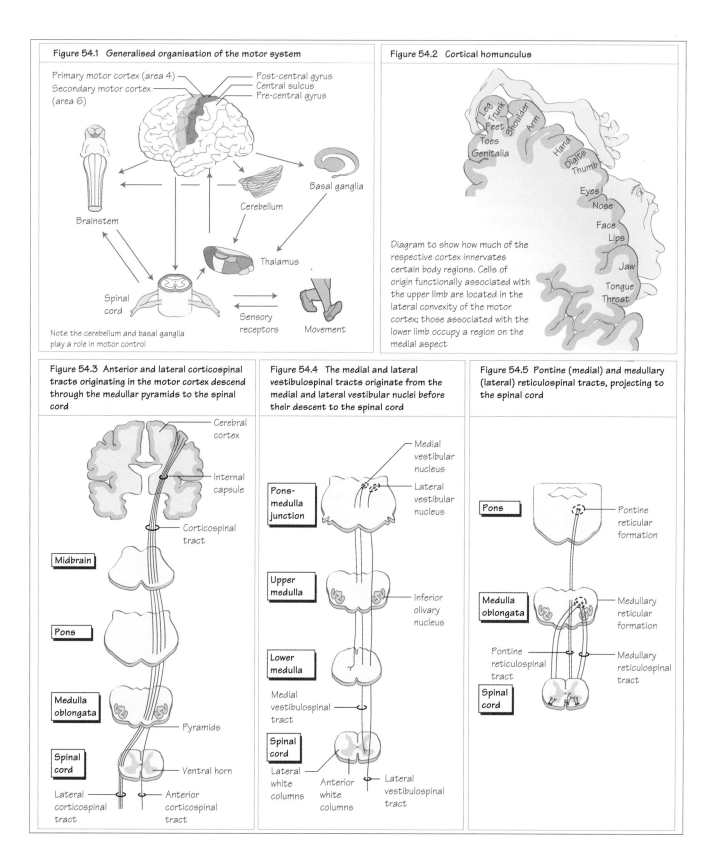

Figure 54.1 Generalised organisation of the motor system

Primary motor cortex (area 4)
Secondary motor cortex (area 6)
Post-central gyrus
Central sulcus
Pre-central gyrus

Basal ganglia

Cerebellum

Brainstem

Thalamus

Spinal cord

Sensory receptors

Movement

Note the cerebellum and basal ganglia play a role in motor control

Figure 54.2 Cortical homunculus

Leg
Trunk
Feet
Toes
Shoulder
Arm
Genitalia
Hand
Digits
Thumb
Eyes
Nose
Face
Lips
Jaw
Tongue
Throat

Diagram to show how much of the respective cortex innervates certain body regions. Cells of origin functionally associated with the upper limb are located in the lateral convexity of the motor cortex; those associated with the lower limb occupy a region on the medial aspect

Figure 54.3 Anterior and lateral corticospinal tracts originating in the motor cortex descend through the medullar pyramids to the spinal cord

Cerebral cortex

Internal capsule

Corticospinal tract

Midbrain

Pons

Medulla oblongata

Pyramids

Spinal cord

Ventral horn

Lateral corticospinal tract

Anterior corticospinal tract

Figure 54.4 The medial and lateral vestibulospinal tracts originate from the medial and lateral vestibular nuclei before their descent to the spinal cord

Medial vestibular nucleus

Lateral vestibular nucleus

Pons-medulla junction

Upper medulla

Inferior olivary nucleus

Lower medulla

Medial vestibulospinal tract

Spinal cord

Lateral white columns

Anterior white columns

Lateral vestibulospinal tract

Figure 54.5 Pontine (medial) and medullary (lateral) reticulospinal tracts, projecting to the spinal cord

Pons

Pontine reticular formation

Medulla oblongata

Medullary reticular formation

Pontine reticulospinal tract

Medullary reticulospinal tract

Spinal cord

The motor system is part of the central nervous system (CNS) and controls voluntary movements. Multiple brain regions work together to ensure coordinated motor control utilising a series of neurones called upper and lower motor neurones (Figure 54.1). Upper motor neurone is a term used to embrace all descending motor pathways from the brain (cerebral cortex and brainstem) which innervate lower motor neurones (of the spinal cord and brainstem). Lower motor neurones have cell bodies that lie in the CNS and function to innervate musculature. The major descending pathways include the corticospinal, vestibulospinal and reticulospinal tracts.

Corticospinal tracts

These are the primary motor pathway involved with voluntary, discrete and skilled movements. The tracts start in the cerebral cortex and terminate in the spinal cord. Approximately one-third of corticospinal fibres arise from the **pre-central gyrus** (area 4), referred to as the **primary motor cortex**. Another one-third of fibres arise from the **secondary motor cortex** (area 6), which is located rostral to the pre-central gyrus. The remaining fibres arise from the post-central gyrus, influencing sensory input to the nervous system.

Pre-central gyrus: site of origin of the fibres controlling motor activity (see Figure 54.1). The pre-central gyrus is organised somatotopically, where a body region corresponds to a particular point of the motor cortex (**homunculus**; Figure 54.2). The homunculus is a distorted image of the human body. Parts of the body that are responsible for fine movement (e.g. digits) occupy a much larger portion of the cortex, compared with body regions that are more coarsely controlled (e.g. trunk).

Corticospinal tracts: axons from pyramidal cells of the fifth layer of the cerebral cortex descend and converge in the corona radiata before passing to the posterior limb of the internal capsule. Fibres are grouped into those associated with the upper and lower extremities. The internal capsule continues into the basis pedunculi of the midbrain. On reaching the pons the tracts get broken up into fasciculi (bundles), which become grouped together to form the **pyramids** in the medulla oblongata (Figure 54.3). The pyramids are swellings that run down the ventral midline of the medulla oblongata. At the point where the medulla oblongata becomes continuous with the spinal cord, most of the fibres (~85%) have crossed the midline (pyramidal decussation). Decussated fibres enter the spinal cord running in the lateral white columns (**lateral corticospinal tracts**). These fibres descend in the spinal cord before terminating in the ventral horn at their target spinal cord level. Fibres that did not cross the midline (**anterior [ventral] corticospinal tract**) continue to descend in the ipsilateral spinal cord within the anterior white columns (Figure 54.3). Most of these fibres cross the midline within the cervical and upper thoracic spinal cord regions, to terminate in the contralateral ventral horn. Only the largest corticospinal fibres synapse directly with motor neurones. Most will synapse with interneurones, which in turn will synapse with alpha motor neurones and some gamma motor neurones. Early in the corticospinal tracts descend some fibres which return to the cortex to inhibit the activity of adjacent cortical regions. Other returning fibres pass to additional brain regions (e.g. reticular formation and olivary nuclei) to inform subcortical areas of the cortical motor activity, in case they are required to react to this via other descending pathways.

Corticobulbar tracts: fibres accompany the corticospinal tracts to the level of the brainstem where they synapse within the reticular formation (near cranial nerve nuclei) or on lower motor neurones associated with the cranial nerves.

Vestibulospinal tracts

These maintain upright posture and balance, resulting from action of the extensor muscles in opposing gravity. **Vestibular nuclei** located in the pons and medulla receive afferent fibres from the inner ear (**vestibular apparatus**) and from the **cerebellum**. Neurones from the lateral vestibular nucleus (**lateral vestibulospinal tract**) send axons uncrossed to the spinal cord where they descend in the anterior white column before terminating by synapsing with interneurones of the ventral horn (Figure 54.4). Neurones from ipsilateral and contralateral medial vestibular nuclei (**medial vestibulospinal tract**) descend in the anterior white column of the cervical spinal cord, terminating in the ventral horn.

Reticulospinal tracts

These mediate control over most movements that do not require dexterity or the maintenance of balance. Neurones derived from the reticular formation in the pons region project ipsilaterally to the spinal cord (pontine reticulospinal tract), descending through the anterior white column (Figure 54.5). Fibres arising from the medulla project contralaterally and ipsilaterally to the spinal cord (medullary reticulospinal tract) and descend in the lateral white column. Both sets of fibres terminate in the ventral horn, facilitating or inhibiting the alpha and gamma motor neurones.

Additional descending tracts: include tectospinal (reflex postural movements in response to visual and auditory stimuli) and rubrospinal tracts (facilitates activity of flexor muscles).

Motor neurones: located in the ventral horns of the spinal cord (and in motor nuclei of the cranial nerves), supplying the skeletal musculature. Collectively known as lower motor neurones, there are two types that supply muscles.

Alpha: large neurones that can innervate between fewer than 10 (where contraction is controlled precisely) to as many as several hundred (large, crude muscle movements) muscle fibres.

Gamma: less numerous in number than alpha, controlling the length and tension of the neuromuscular spindles (proprioceptive organs of skeletal muscle).

Execution of movement: descending pathways can be traced from motor areas of the cerebral cortex to lower motor neurones. However, other parts of the brain also play important roles in the motivation and planning phases, during the formulation of motor commands by the brain (e.g. prefrontal cortex and parietal lobe regions). The coordination of movement requires further input from varying brain regions, including: cerebral cortex, thalamus, subthalamic nucleus, substangia nigra, reticular formation, vestibular nuclei and the cerebellum (Figure 54.1).

Deborah Merrick

Figure 55.1 Relative position of the hypothalamus and thalamus

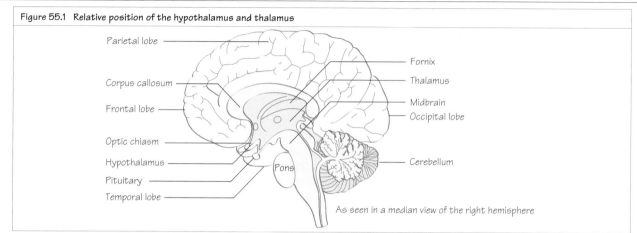

As seen in a median view of the right hemisphere

Figure 55.2 Location of the hypothalamic nuclei

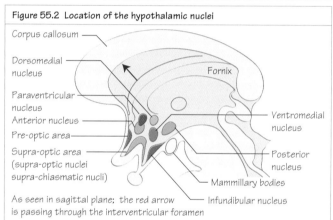

As seen in sagittal plane; the red arrow is passing through the interventricular foramen

Figure 55.3 Location of the main hypothalamic nuclei

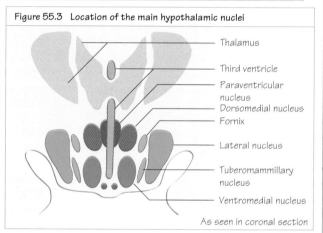

As seen in coronal section

Table 55.1

Nuclei	Function	Nuclei	Function
Anterior hypothalamic nuclei	Temperature regulation (response to heat)	Medial hypothalamic nuclei	Reduce food intake (satiety centre)
Posterior hypothalamic nuclei	Temperature regulation (response to cold)	Lateral hypothalamic nuclei	Increase food intake (hunger centre) and water consumption (thirst centre)

Figure 55.4 Arrangement of nuclei within the thalamus

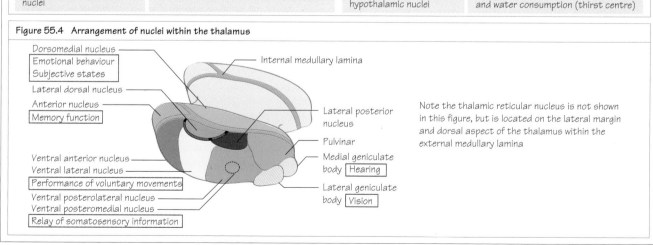

Note the thalamic reticular nucleus is not shown in this figure, but is located on the lateral margin and dorsal aspect of the thalamus within the external medullary lamina

The hypothalamus and thalamus form part of the **diencephalon**, which is located rostral to the brainstem and is divided by the midline third ventricle. The diencephalon is a forebrain derivative, known to function in maintaining **higher order cognition** and **homeostasis**.

Hypothalamus

The hypothalamus is a paired forebrain structure located below the thalamus, forming the floor and inferior walls of the third ventricle (Figure 55.1). It extends from the optic chiasm to the caudal border of the mammillary bodies. Anteriorly is the preoptic area, which is often described as part of the hypothalamus for functional reasons (Figure 55.2). The hypothalamus is bounded laterally by the internal capsule.

Subdivisions/nuclei: the multiple nuclei of the hypothalamus (Figures 55.2 and 55.3) can be divided into the following functional regions:
• anterior, middle and posterior (or);
• medial, lateral and paraventricular.
The nuclei have ill-defined boundaries and therefore some nuclei extend into neighbouring areas. The regions are arranged into regulatory and modulatory centres. For example, the medial hypothalamus contains most of the releasing hormones (which control pituitary function; Chapter 45) and is believed to act in modulating feeding, rage behaviour and control over autonomic functions (Figure 55.3 and Table 55.1). The lateral hypothalamus contains nuclei that are associated with a number of behavioural processes (e.g. drinking, predation).

Connections: located in the centre of the **limbic system**, the hypothalamus receives multiple inputs, including the cerebral cortex, viscera and limbic system. Efferent connections are also multiple and complex in nature. They include descending fibres to the brainstem/spinal cord, pathways of the **limbic system**, anterior nucleus of the thalamus and reticular formation in the tegmentum of midbrain. The hypothalamus communicates with the pituitary gland, which lies inferiorly (Figure 55.2). These two structures are connected via neuronal pathways that pass from the hypothalamic nuclei (supraoptic and paraventricular) to the posterior lobe of the pituitary and by blood vessels that allow communications to the anterior lobe of the pituitary (Figures 55.2 and 55.3). Through these pathways the hypothalamus can influence activities of the endocrine glands.

Function: the hypothalamus is able to influence the autonomic nervous system, and integrate this with the **neuroendocrine system**, ensuring homeostasis. Cells of the hypothalamic nuclei produce releasing factors and release-inhibiting factors that control hormone production of the pituitary gland (anterior lobe). The hypothalamus plays further important roles in temperature regulation, food intake, water balance, emotion and behaviour, and control of circadian rhythms (Figures 55.2 and 55.3).

Thalamus

The medial surfaces of the two midline walnut-shaped thalami form the lateral walls of the third ventricle. They often come into close contact and touch via the interthalamic adhesion (Figure 55.1). Anteriorly, the thalamus forms the posterior boundary of the interventricular foramen and posteriorly it expands to form the pulvinar.

Subdivisions/nuclei: strips of white matter (internal medullary lamina) divide the grey matter of the thalamus into anterior, medial and lateral divisions, each containing a group of nuclei with diverse functions (Figure 55.4). The anterior thalamic nucleus forms connections with the **cingulate gyrus, hippocampal** formation and **hypothalamus**. Its anatomical connections suggest a role in memory function. The nuclei located within the medial part of the thalamus include the large dorsomedial nucleus and several smaller nuclei. The dorsomedial nucleus is connected to the prefrontal cortex, hypothalamic and thalamic nuclei. This part of the thalamus integrates a variety of sensory information and functions in emotional behaviour. The lateral part of the thalamus is divided into a dorsal and ventral tier of nuclei. The former (lateral dorsal nucleus, the lateral posterior nucleus, pulvinar) are thought to connect to other thalamic nuclei, cerebral hemispheres and cingulate gyrus. The ventral tier of nuclei includes the ventral anterior nucleus and ventral lateral nucleus. Both nuclei are intimately involved in control of motor functions (Figure 55.4). The ventral tier also contains the ventral posterior nuclei, which comprise the ventral posteromedial and ventral posterolateral nuclei. The nuclei projections pass to the primary somatic sensory areas of the cortex. Additional thalamic nuclei are also present, including the **medial geniculate** (auditory) and **lateral geniculate** (visual) nuclei (see Figure 55.4).

Connections: these predominantly include those made between thalamic nuclei (excluding reticular nucleus) and the cerebral cortex. Reciprocal fibres pass back from the cerebral cortex to the thalamic nuclei. Thus it is likely that both the cortex and thalamus can modify each other's activities. The thalamus also acts a relay station for sensory-motor axonal loops between the cerebellum and basal nuclei (important for normal voluntary movements).

Function: the thalamus and cerebral cortex are integrally linked, which has resulted in the thalamus often being referred to as the gateway of the cortex. The thalamus acts as a relay for many subcortical areas and is particularly important in processing and relaying a variety of sensory and motor functions. For example, the visual system receives input from the retina, lateral geniculate nucleus (thalamus) and the visual cortex (occipital lobe). However, the thalamus does far more that just relay information; it integrates and regulates the transfer of information in a complex way. The thalamus is also believed to be involved in functions not considered to be sensory or motor related, such as regulating levels of consciousness.

Michael D Randall

The basis of neurophysiology, with the fundamentals of action potential propagation and synaptic transmission are covered in Chapters 19 and 20. The sheer complexity of the human brain is, in part, due to the vast number of synaptic connections made by each neurone and the considerable number of neurotransmitters with a range of actions, such as inhibition and excitation. Neural networks are immensely complex, with inhibitory and excitatory loops, and because a neurone may synapse with 10 000 other neurones and there are 10^{10} neurones in the human brain, this leads to the level of control and sophistication required of the CNS.

Physiological roles of the CNS

Integration of homeostasis as a neuroendocrine role (Chapters 45 and 55): responsible for the regulation of sex hormones (Chapter 50), metabolic hormones (Chapters 47 and 48), maturation (Chapter 45).

Regulation of physiological control of cardiovascular (Chapter 32), renal (Chapters 39 and 45) and respiratory (Chapter 26) systems and bladder control (Chapter 40) by neural mechanisms.

The regulation of appetite: this is a tightly regulated behavioural process that controls the intake of food in relation to metabolic needs. The hypothalamus plays a central role in the control of appetite and involves 5-hydroxytrytamine (inhibitory) and neuropeptide Y (stimulatory) as key transmitters. It is sensitive to a number of hormones such as leptin. Leptin is a peptide hormone produced by adipose tissue and its levels correlate with adiposity; as its levels increase appetite is suppressed. Dysregulation of this system is associated with the development of obesity. The gastrointestinal hormone cholecystokinin also provides a shorter-term inhibitory input.

The biological clock: the brain is the regulator of circadian rhythms. This is controlled via the suprachiasmatic nucleus (SCN) in the hypothalamus, which receives information about day length derived from the visual system. The SCN then regulates the pineal gland, which releases melatonin (levels increasing during dark periods).

Processing of sensory and somatosensory information, which underpins the awareness of the environment (e.g. pain, temperature, vision, hearing, taste balance) (Chapter 53). Perceiving sensory information such as pain leads to the awareness of pain.

Descending pathways, which modulate transmission in the spinal cord.

Spinal cord is responsible for motor output, sensory input and reflexes, which may be modulated via higher control.

Motor roles
• The motor cortex plans and initiations voluntary movements.
• The cerebellum is critical to positional coordination in response to somatosensory information from the spinal cord and other areas of the brain. The cerebellum contains highly sophisticated neural networks of Purkinje cells and granule cells, which carry out complex processing.
• Basal ganglia are deep in the cerebrum and are involved in motor control and dysfunction of this system occurs in Parkinson's disease (Chapter 57). The basal ganglia are also involved in cognitive and affective roles.

Higher functions

The real key to human brain is at the level of the higher functions that underpin the human, such as the ability to have emotions, thoughts, desires, fear, process visual images to lead to awareness of the environment, learning, and having both a short-term and long-term memory. The higher emotions are underpinned by the concept of consciousness.

The limbic system, which includes the hippocampus, amygdala, septal nucleus, cingulated gyrus and fornix, is involved in motivation, emotion, long-term memory and olfaction.

Long-term potentiation (LTP)

This is neuronal mechanism by which increased transmission at a synapse (Chapter 20) leads to an enhancement of activity or re-enforcement such that the effectiveness of the communication is increased. This may be via presynaptic mechanisms enhancing release and post-synaptic mechanisms via receptor and second-messenger upregulation. The excitatory neurotransmitter glutamate acting at NMDA receptors is associated with LTP. This ability to re-enforce communication is thought to underlie memory and the ability to learn.

In contrast to LTP, long-term depression (LTD) also occurs with reduced synaptic activity.

Neuronal plasticity

Both LTP and LTD are examples of neuronal plasticity in which neuronal function can adapt in relation to activity. Plasticity can also occur if neuronal pathways become damaged and adaptations can occur with new connections forming to compensate for any deficit.

Neurotransmitters and function

Our knowledge of the physiology of the CNS is still relatively limited and much of our current understanding comes for pathophysiology and altering function pharmacologically. For example, dopaminergic transmission is implicated in the nigostriatal pathway of the basal ganglia, as it is known that loss of dopaminergic function leads to Parkinson's disease. Conversely, treatment with precursors of dopamine or dopamine agonists provide effective treatments for Parkinson's disease, while dopamine receptor antagonists induce Parkinson-like symptoms. Table 56.1 summarises the actions and activities of some key neurotransmitters and modulators.

Table 56.1 Some key neurotransmitters together with their key sites of action, physiological roles and how their activity may be altered in neurological and psychiatric disorders and drug therapy
GPCR: G-protein coupled receptor

Neurotransmitter	Targets	Examples of neurological roles	Clinical relevance
Noradrenaline	α and β-adrenoceptors, which are all G-protein coupled	• Pre and post-synaptic actions • Involved in arousal and mood • Involved in cardiovascular control centres	• Inhibition of neuronal reuptake of noradrenaline is an effective antidepressant treatment • Stimulation of α_2-adrenoceptors leads to decreased sympathetic output and blood pressure lowering (Chapter 32)
Dopamine	D_1–D_5 dopamine receptors, which are all G-protein coupled	• Involved in mesocortical pathways • High concentrations in limbic system and hypothalamus • Transmitter in nigostriatal pathway in basal ganglia • Regulation of pituitary secretions • Involved in nausea and vomiting (chemoreceptor trigger zone) • Dopamine reward hypothesis: dopamine release is associated with pleasurable/addictive activities and may contribute towards addiction	• Loss of dopaminergic function leads to movement disorders in Parkinson's disease • Increased dopaminergic activity in the cerebral cortex is associated with schizophrenia • Dopamine receptor antagonists are anti-emetics • Attention deficit hyperactivity disorder responds to inhibition of dopamine reuptake
5-hydroxytryptamine (5-HT) also known as serotonin	5-HT_1–5-HT_7 receptors, which are all G-protein coupled, except 5-HT_3, which is ionotropic	• Raphe nucleus is main site of release and influences many areas • Involved in mood • Suppression of appetite • Involved in nausea and vomiting (chemoreceptor trigger zone)	• Inhibition of the reuptake of 5-HT is an effective antidepressant treatment • 5-HT_3 receptor antagonists are anti-emetics
Acetylcholine	• Muscarinic, are GPCRs. • Nicotinic, which are ionotropic	• Transmitter in cortex, midbrain and brainstem • Associated with memory	• Impairment of cholinergic function is associated with Alzheimer's disease
Histamine	Histamine H_1–H_3 receptors, which are all G-protein-coupled	• Associated with sedation/sleep • Hypothalamus • Vestibular nuclei	• H_1 receptor antagonists are sedating • H_1 receptor antagonists are effective in motion sickness
Melatonin	Melatonin receptors (MT_1–MT_3), which are all G-protein coupled	• Released by pineal gland • Released during darkness	• An effector of the biological clock • Melatonin is advocated for 'jet lag'
Adenosine	A_1–A_3 receptors, which are all G-protein coupled	• Inhibitory actions • Associated with sleep	• Caffeine is an adenosine receptor antagonist and has stimulatory effects
ATP	Purinoceptors • P_{2X} receptors, which are ionotropic • P_{2Y} receptors, are GPCRs.	• P_{2X} receptors are excitatory and may play a role in pain and mechanosensation	
Nitric oxide	Activation of guanylyl cyclase increasing cGMP	• May modulate long-term potentiation and depression	
Endogenous opioids, e.g. endorphins, dynorphin, enkephalins	μ, δ and κ receptors, which are all G-protein coupled and inhibit adenylyl cyclase	• These are peptides that mimic the action of morphine • They can suppression pain pathways and the perception of pain	• Opioids such as morphine are powerful analgesics by reducing pain transmission and its perception • Opioids also lead to euphoria and are highly addictive
Tachykinins, e.g. substance P and neurokinin	• Substance P: NK_1 receptors • Neurokinin A and B: NK_2 and NK_3 receptors • All GPCRs	• Neuropeptides • Substance P is involved in pain and inflammation	
Neuropetide Y	NPY receptors, which are all G-protein coupled	• Hypothalamus • Regulates appetite	
Endogenous cannabinoids, e.g. anandamide	CB_1 receptor and TRPV1 receptors on sensory nerves	• Widely distributed but poorly understood • Stimulates appetite	• Cannabinoid receptor antagonists reduce appetite
GABA	• $GABA_A$: associated with Cl⁻ channel • $GABA_B$: G-protein coupled leading to inhibition of adenylyl cyclase	• Principal inhibitory neurotransmitter.	• Enhancement of GABA activity at $GABA_A$ receptors by benzodiazepines leads to sedation, hypnotic and anxioloytic effects • General anaesthetics may enhance the actions of GABA • $GABA_B$ agonists are anti-spastic
Glycine	• Ligand-gated Cl⁻ channel	• Inhibitory transmitter in the brain and spinal cord	• Strychnine is an antagonist that causes convulsions by inhibiting the inhibitory effects of glycine
Glutamate	• NMDA/AMPA/kainate receptors: iontropic associated with Ca^{2+} influx • Metabotropic receptors: G-protein coupled	• Excitatory amino acid • Involved in long-term potentiation	

57 CNS disorders and treatments

Michael D Randall

Disorders of CNS can be broadly divided into **neurological** and **psychiatric** conditions. In neurological conditions, control and normal function of neurones is altered, for example there may be changes in neuronal excitability (e.g. epilepsy) or motor control (e.g. Parkinson's disease, multiple sclerosis). Psychiatric disorders involve changes in the 'mind' and may involve alterations in mood (e.g. depression), or perception and behaviour (e.g. schizophrenia).

Epilepsy

There are different forms of epilepsy, including:
- **absence epilepsy**: in which the patient is unaware of their surroundings appears to 'daydream'. This usually presents in childhood.
- **generalised tonic-clonic seizures**: these involve complete loss of consciousness with convulsions, involving uncontrolled movements of the body including the limbs.

Pathophysiology: in general, epilepsy is due to abnormal neuronal discharges, which may or may not spread across the brain. The cause may be due to a structural lesion, secondary to trauma, or due to some unidentified change.

   Treatment: drugs are used to prevent seizures and a primary target is to reduce neuronal excitability.
- *Carbamazepine*: thought to cause use-dependent inhibition of Na^+ channels and so reduce excitability.
- *Sodium valproate*: potentiates GABA and causes use-dependent blockade of Na^+ channels.
- *Lamotrigine*: causes use-dependent blockade of Na^+ channels and decreases the release of the excitatory neurotransmitter glutamate.

Parkinson's disease

Parkinson's disease is a relatively common neurodegenerative disease often associated with ageing. It is a disease of movement and is associated with tremor, rigidity and poverty of movement. There may be bradykinesia (slowness of movement), akinesia (lack of movement or rigidity) and dyskinesias (abnormal involuntary movements), and it may be associated with autonomic dysfunction.

   Pathophysiology: the disease is characterised by degeneration of dopaminergic neurones in the nigrostriatal pathway in the basal ganglia. Parkinson-like symptoms can be induced by drugs that block dopamine receptors, such as the antipsychotic drugs used in schizophrenia.

   Treatment: the aim is to replace dopaminergic neurotransmission.
- *Levodopa:* this is the precursor of dopamine and so will increase levels of dopamine and provide some relief from the symptoms. Administration of L-dopa is associated with widespread side effects due to the peripheral conversion of L-dopa to dopamine by dopa decarboxylase. To reduce these problems, L-dopa is given with an inhibitor of dopa decarboxylase, e.g. carbidopa.
- *Dopamine D_2 receptor agonists (e.g. rotigotine)*: increase dopaminergic activity in the basal ganglia and because the principal peripheral receptor is the dopamine D_1 receptor they have limited peripheral side effects. Their direct agonist activity circumvents the need for the nigrostriatal pathway to synthesis dopamine.

- *Monoamine oxidase B inhibitors (e.g. selegiline)*: MAO-B is involved in the metabolism of dopamine and so inhibition of this enzyme will increase the concentrations of dopamine.
- *Catechol-O-methyltransferase inhibitors*: COMT is also involved in the breakdown of dopamine, and inhibitors of this enzyme will increase levels of dopamine and so enhance dopaminergic function.

Multiple sclerosis (MS)

This is a long-term, debilitating condition that may run a course of relapse and remission.

   Pathophysiology: this is an autoimmune inflammatory condition in which the myelin surrounding neurones is damaged and this results in impaired nervous conduction. Common sites of demyelination include the optic nerve, brainstem, cerebellar connections and cervical spinal cord. MS may present with optic neuritis and weakness, and progress to severe disability with ataxia, spasticity and urinary incontinence.

   Treatment: current therapies have limited success. They include the following drugs.
- *Beta-interferon:* anti-inflammatory actions and is used in relapse and remitting disease.
- *Glatiramer*: immunomodulating drug.

Stroke

After heart disease and cancer, stroke is the third-biggest killer in the Western world. It is divided into:
- **ischaemic** or **thromboembolic stroke**: thrombus formation in the cerebral circulation leads to impaired blood flow and cerebral infarction. This constitutes about 85% of cases;
- **haemorrhagic stroke**: a burst blood vessel leads to bleeding within the brain. There may be swelling and impaired blood flow leading to infarction.

In both cases the death of brain cells leads to neurological deficits depending on which areas of the brain are affected.

   Treatment: ischaemic stroke is managed by restoring blood flow by dissolving the thrombus using thrombolytic drugs that activate plasminogen to plasmin, which digests fibrin. Prevention may involve control of blood pressure, statins and use of anti-platelet (e.g. low-dose aspirin, clopidogrel) drugs to prevent thrombosis. Haemorrhagic stroke may require surgical repair and/or conservative measures.

Pain

This is a normal physiological response to damage or adverse stimuli. It involves transmission of noxious stimuli via pain fibres to the brain, where pain is 'perceived'.

   Pathophysiology: tissue damage or inflammation involves a variety of mediators, which may enhance the stimulation of pain receptors. Prostaglandins derived from cyclooxygenase (Cox) enzymes are key mediators as they potentiate painful stimuli.

   Migraine is a specific condition associated with severe headaches, which may be unilateral and throbbing, and lasts for 4–72 h. There may also be vomiting, photophobia, phonophobia and sensitivity to movement. It is regarded as a neurovascular disease.

Neuropathic pain is a chronic condition where changes in neuronal function or the somatosensory system lead to innocuous stimuli leading to unpleasant sensations.

Treatment: pain management involves the use of analgesics as follows.
• *Non-steroidal anti-inflammatory drugs (NSAIDs)* (e.g. ibuprofen): these are Cox inhibitors that inhibit the production of prostaglandins.
• *Paracetamol*: is a simple analgesic with a poorly defined mode of action.
• *Opioids*: these are morphine-like substances which act at opioid receptors to hyperpolarise neurones and inhibit the transmission of pain in the spinal cord and act centrally to modify the perception of pain.
• *Local anaesthetics*: these block voltage-operated Na^+ channels in pain fibres and so inhibit action potential propagation and the conduction of pain (Chapter 19).
• *Migraine*: treated with analgesics and triptans (e.g sumatriptan). There are $5\text{-}HT_{1B/D}$ agonists that abort attacks by inhibiting the release of vasodilator neurotransmitters and constrict dilated arteries.
• *Neuropathic pain*: a number of anti-epileptic drugs and some anti-depressants are used.

Dementia

This is a broad area in which there is progressive impairment of cognitive function in which memory is primarily affected. There may also be behavioural changes.

Pathophysiology:
• **Alzheimer's disease** is the commonest form and involves a pathology of neurofibrillary tangles and neuronal loss.
• **Vascular dementia**: evidence of multiple infarcts.

Management: treatment of Alzheimer's disease has focused on attempting to improve cholinergic function, and acetylcholinesterase (AChE) inhibitors (e.g. galantamine) are used to prevent the breakdown of ACh and prolong its actions.

Depression

This is a common condition associated with low mood and negative thoughts.

Pathophysiology: this is poorly understood, but the commonest theory is the 'monoamine hypothesis', which states that depression is due to an alteration in central levels of noradrenaline and/or 5-hydroxytryptamine (5-HT) (serotonin).

Treatment: mild depression is thought to respond well to behavioural techniques such as cognitive behavioural therapy. Pharmacological treatment is used in more severe or refractory disease and aims to alter or restore brain chemistry. There is a time delay in pharmacological therapy (~2 weeks), which indicates that dug treatments have more complex effects that may be due to alterations in receptor functions and genomic effects. Commonly used antidepressants include the following.
• *Serotonin-selective reuptake inhibitors (SSRIs)* (e.g fluoxetine): these inhibit the cellular reuptake of 5-HT, leading to increased levels in the synaptic cleft. These increases in 5-HT levels are thought to lead to an alteration receptor populations and result in an improvement of symptoms.
• *Tricyclic antidepressants (TCAs)* (e.g. amitriptyline): these inhibit the neuronal uptake of both noradrenaline and 5-HT and are thought

to lead to an alteration receptor populations and result in an improvement of symptoms. They also have a number of pharmacological actions, including antagonism of muscarinic, histamine and 5-HT receptors. The antimuscarinic side effects lead to blurred vision, dry mouth, urinary retention and constipation, which limits their use.

Bipolar affective disorder

This is characterised by periods of low mood with manic episodes (which may involve grandiose behaviour, impatience, aggression, excessive enthusiasm, psychomotor agitation).

Treatment: drugs are used to stabilise mood.
• *Lithium*: used for both treatment and prevention. Its mode of action is uncertain but it may interfere with intracellular signalling via inositol triphosphate.
• *Carbamazepine and valproate*: prophylactic mood stabilisers in bipolar disorder and lack the extrapyramidal effects of the antipsychotic drugs.
• *Antipsychotics* such as haloperidol and chlorpromazine: used to control psychotic symptoms.

Anxiety

While a physiological response to stress is normal, when this becomes pathological or the response happens to an apparently innocuous signal, then this becomes anxiety. There may be a central component coupled with somatic symptoms (e.g. tachycardia, palpitations, sweating) due to increased sympathetic activity. Anxiety covers a range of conditions, including panic attacks (which may involve marked symptoms with a fear of impending death), general anxiety disorder and phobias (e.g. social phobias).

Management: this can be symptomatic to relieve the symptoms of increased sympathetic activity and involves the use of β-adrenoceptor antagonists. Other pharmacological approaches include the following.
• *Benzodiazepines* (e.g. diazepam): these enhance the actions of the inhibitory neurotransmitter GABA at $GABA_A$ receptors and are used in the short term as anxiolytics.
• *SSRIs*: some of these antidepressants are used to manage anxiety disorders in the longer term.

Schizophrenia

Schizophrenia presents with psychotic symptoms similar to the manic phase of bipolar affective disorder. The symptoms are grouped as positive (auditory hallucinations, delusions, thought disorder and disorganised communication) or negative (reduced activity with emotional flattening, withdrawal from society and cognitive deficit).

Pathophysiology: poorly understood but based on response to drug treatment, the commonly accepted theory is one of overactivity of dopaminergic neurones in the cortex.

Treatment: pharmacological management is aimed at reducing symptoms and this is achieved by use of antipsychotic drugs
• *Antipsychotics* (e.g. chlorpromazine, haloperidol): these act via antagonism of dopamine D_2 receptors in the cortex. As a side effect they also block dopaminergic transmission in the nigrostriatal pathway and may lead to Parkinson-like symptoms.
• *Atypical antipsychotics* (e.g. risepridone, olanzapine): in addition to D_2 receptor antagonism they also block 5-HT receptors and are associated with fewer movement disorders.

James Lazenby and Chien-Yi Chang

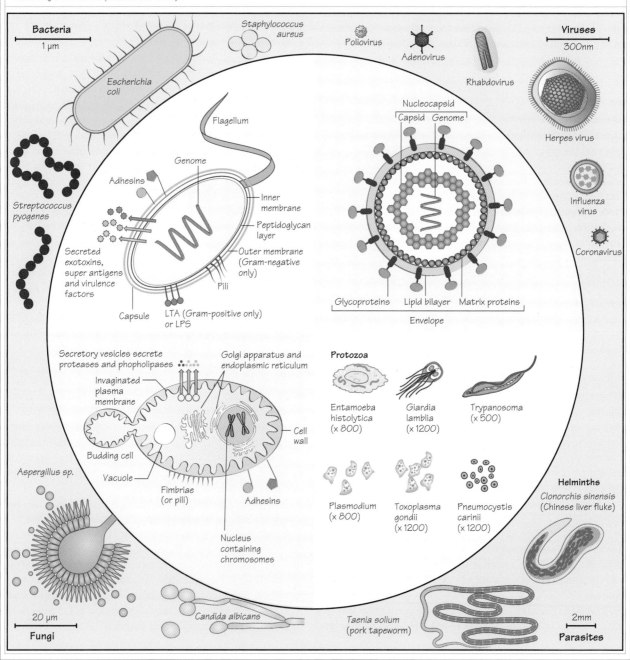

Figure 58.1 The defining features of the major types of pathogens: Bacteria, Viruses, Fungi and Parasites.
This figure depicts some common pathogens with the appropriate scale. In the centre circle a not to scale cartoon illustrates some of the key features of the different types of pathogens. All bacteria have a peptidoglycan layer surrounding an inner membrane, but Gram-negative bacteria also have an external membrane. Some bacteria also have a tough polysaccharide capsule for added protection from environmental stresses. Pili and flagella are used for attachment and motility. Bacteria make use of multiple secretion systems to release exotoxins, enzymes and other virulence factors. Lipoteichoic acid (LTA) and Lipopolysaccharide (LPS) are potent activators of innate immune responses. At their most basic, viruses are genetic material (DNA or RNA) surrounded by proteins arranged in regular structural repeating sub-units (the capsid). More complex viruses have an envelope made of a lipid bilayer supported by matrix proteins and studded with glycoproteins used for attachment and receptor mediated endocytosis. Fungi are highly varied but this simple schematic based on the *Candida* sp. illustrates the membrane bound organelles common to eukaryotic cells. *Candida* cells are able to reproduce by budding. Yeast cells possess fimbriae (or pili) for attachment and motility and adhesins that allow them to target specific host cells. They also possess secretory vesicles which can secrete virulence factors like proteases and phopholipases. Parasites can be divided into Protozoa (inside the circle) or the much larger Helminths (outside the circle).

Microbes are widespread in the environment (Figure 58.1). Most of them are free-living and obtain their energy from light and the oxidation of inorganic or dead organic matter. In contrast, a **parasite** lives in or on a living host from which it obtains nourishment. Most parasitic microbes are called **commensal** or **normal** flora and are generally harmless or beneficial to human health. A **pathogen**, however, is any microbial agent that can cause disease in a host. Some microbes are able to invade into the tissues, overcome the host defences and cause disease. They are termed **primary pathogens**. When host defences are impaired or compromised, such as breaking the skin, commensal flora may cause disease and are referred to as **opportunistic pathogens**. The process of invasion of the body is called **infection** and the mechanism of causing infection is called **pathogenesis**. There are five steps to establishing a successful infection.

1 *Attachment and entry*: pathogens attach to the host whereby they gain entry.

2 *Dissemination and multiplication*: once attached or inside the host, the pathogens replicate in number and move away from the initial site of colonisation.

3 *Evasion*: hosts possess mechanisms to protect against pathogens and pathogens have evolved ways to circumvent these defences.

4 *Exit*: in order to continue their life cycle, pathogens also need to leave the original host and spread to fresh hosts. This is often in the normal secretions of the host such as saliva, mucus, or faeces.

5 *Damage*: damage to the host, either directly from the pathogen or as collateral damage from the host response to the pathogen, is often a consequence of pathogen infection.

To identify the organisms causing specific diseases Robert Koch, in 1890, set out criteria known as Koch's postulates.

1 The organism must be present in every case of the disease.

2 The organism must be isolated from diseased host and grown in pure culture.

3 The pure culture must be shown to induce the disease in an experimentally infected host.

4 The organism must be recoverable from the experimentally infected host.

These criteria were well established for living bacterial pathogens but their applicability to pathogens, such as viruses and prions, is problematic.

Bacteria

Bacteria are **prokaryotes** that possess **virulence determinants** for facilitating pathogenesis. For many pathogenic bacteria, colonisation of the host tissues is the initial step of infection and involves interaction between specific receptors on the host cell and different **adhesins** on the bacterial surface. For example, pili (or fimbriae) and flagella provide motility and adhesion in *Vibrio cholerae* and *Campylobacter jejuni*, while *Streptococcus mutans* produces an exopolysaccharide allowing it to adhere to teeth.

Pathogenic bacteria possess several mechanisms to avoid or neutralise host defence systems. For example, to avoid phagocytosis by macrophages *Neisseria meningitis* produces a thick extracellular polysaccharide capsule. *N. meningitidis* also avoids antibody-mediated immune responses by altering of the surface antigens which allows longer survival within a host and makes vaccine development difficult for these organisms.

Many bacteria cause tissue damages by producing toxins. **Endotoxin**, or **lipopolysaccharide** (LPS), a component of the outer membrane of **Gram-negative bacteria**, and **lipoteichoic acid** (LTA), a component of the cell wall of **Gram-positive** bacteria, are potent activators of immune and inflammatory responses. In contrast, **exotoxins** are secreted by pathogenic bacteria and have diverse effects on the host. Shiga toxin produced by *Shigella* inhibits the protein synthesis of host cell while *Staphylococcal* haemolysin forms lytic pores in blood cells.

James Lazenby and Chien-Yi Chang

Viruses

Viruses are **obligate intracellular parasites** and as such cannot make energy or proteins independently. Viruses exist in a latent state until interaction with the appropriate receptor on the host cell whereby they become incorporated. Once inside the cell the biochemical processes of the cell become co-opted to make more viral particles (the **virion**).

Viruses vary widely in size and complexity: at the most basic the virion is essentially the **genome** (either single- or double-stranded DNA or RNA) surrounded by structural proteins, enzymes and nuclear binding proteins (the **capsid**). This is referred to as the **nucleocapsid** and is released from the host cell when the cell lyses. The capsid protects the genetic material of the virus from many environmental challenges and allows these viruses to exist for a long time in the environment and pass through the gastrointestinal tract. Some viruses escape the cell by budding from the cell membrane. In this process, the virus particle is encapsulated in a protein matrix and a lipid bilayer studded with glycoproteins (the **envelope**). These glycoproteins have a variety of roles, such as aiding in attachment to the host cell (e.g. GP120 and GP41 in human immunodeficiency virus [HIV]) or as virulence factors (e.g. haemagglutinin and neuraminidase in influenza). Enveloped virions are very sensitive to inactivation and as such are generally passed from person to person by the exchange of fluids.

Viruses have many virulence mechanisms, mainly to evade host detection and eradication:

- sequestration
- blockade of antigen presentation
- cytokine evasion
- inhibition of apoptosis
- antibody evasion.

Viruses cause damage to the host by disruption of the host cell processes, or lysis of the host cells, or as a result of damage from a persistent and ongoing engagement of host inflammatory or immune responses. For example, HIV causes immunosuppression because its host cells are immune cells, which, when lysed or destroyed, leads to acquired immune deficiency syndrome (AIDS).

Fungi

Fungi are **eukaryotic** organisms, including yeasts and moulds, which occupy a diverse range of environmental niches, but only a small percentage are routinely associated with human disease. Most fungal pathogens are opportunistic and acquired from the environment (with the main exceptions being **dermatophytes** and *Candida albicans*). **Mycoses** (fungal infections) are separated according to the tissue depth of the initial colonisation. Systemic mycoses can affect many different tissues and are often internal, being inhaled into the lungs or spreading through mucosal sites on the body such as the female genital tract. In most cases, there needs to be some depletion of the host defences, such as disruption of the normal microbial flora, or immunosuppression or depletion (for example, pneumonia from *Aspergillus* sp. in chemotherapy patients, or *Pneumocystis jiroveci* pneumonia in those with AIDS). Pathogenic fungi can avoid clearance by killing the engulfing immune cell (e.g. *Candida albicans* can escape clearance by producing long hyphae, which skewer the engulfing macrophage), or avoiding

phagocytosis (e.g. *Cryptococcus neoformans* produces a polysaccharide capsule). Damage to the host comes from the breakdown of host tissues by secreted proteases and lipases as well as the secretion of metabolites, such as alkaloids, which can cause acute organ damage.

Parasites

Medical parasitology relates specifically to invertebrate animals capable of causing disease.

- **Protozoa**: protozoa are simple unicellular microorganisms that range in size from 2 to 100 μm. They include amoebae, flagellates and ciliates. Included in this group are the agents responsible for malaria (*Plasmodium sp.*), toxoplasmosis (*Toxoplasmia gondii*) and leishmaniasis (*Leishmania sp.*).
- **Helminths**: metazoa are multicellular macroscopic parasites that include the helminths and arthropods. Helminths can be divided into nematodes (cylindrical-bodied worms such as hook worm or pin worm) and the platyhelminths (flat-bodied worms such as flukes and tapeworms).

Protozoan and helminth infections are virtually always acquired from an exogenous source and can enter the host in a myriad of ways, including oral ingestion (e.g. *Giardia lamblia*, which causes diarrhoea) and penetration though the skin, often via an arthropod vector (e.g. malaria is transmitted by female mosquitoes). The mechanisms by which these parasites attach are also highly varied, with some using adhesins and receptor-mediated attachment like many bacteria and viruses (e.g. *Leishmania mexicana* attaches via CR2 on host cells) and others using mechanical means (e.g. *G. lamblia* attaches using a ventrical disk that clamps on to the host intestinal epithelium). The mechanisms that cause the symptoms of disease are also different. While many protozoan pathogens secrete molecules such as phospholipases and proteases that directly damage the host cell membranes, pathologies from helminth infections are generally the result of the size and longevity of the parasite, which can disrupt host physiological functions, such as blocking bile ducts or compressing parts of the central nervous system. Many parasites utilise mechanisms common to bacterial species to avoid host immune responses, for example, the *Plasmodium* sp. can vary surface antigens, mimic host antigens, directly suppress immune responses and reside intracellularly within the host.

Prions

Prions are transmissible aberrant proteins. Prions are thought to cause a variety of spongiform encephalopathies in mammals, notably **Creutzfeldt-Jakob disease** (CJD) and Kuru in humans. It is thought that the normal cellular prion protein (PrP^c) exists in mammalian tissues and when it comes into contact with the misfolded isoform (PrP^{sc}), the normal version converts and thereby becomes resistant to degradation by proteases, leading to a build up of the aberrant protein, resulting in disease. While prions can be isolated from other tissues, only the brain shows evidence of pathology. It is thought that prions spread by ingestion or injection of brain tissue from contaminated individuals, although there is also a genetic mutation that leads to cases of familial prion disease. Because the prion protein is a host protein, no immune response is initiated and lack of an inflammatory response is a characteristic of prion disease.

Antimicrobial chemotherapy

Bacterial, fungal and viral infections pose significant morbidity and mortality to man and there are a number of drugs that are used to manage infections. Bacterial infections are managed by antibacterial drugs, which include antibiotics. These agents exploit differences between eukaryotic host cells and the prokaryotic bacteria. For example, penicillins target the formation of the bacterial cell wall (by inhibiting the transpeptidases responsible for cross-linking peptidoglycans) and macrolides target the bacterial ribosomes. Viral infections are more difficult to manage by targeting differences in biochemistry, but targets include viral DNA polymerases, neuramidases and HIV reverse transcriptases. Tables 58.1 and 58.2 contain some examples of antimicrobial agents, their modes of action and common usages.

Table 58.1 Commonly used antibacterial agents and their modes of action and uses

Antibacterial agents	Mode of action	Uses
Penicillins, e.g. amoxicillin, phenoxymethyl penicillin, flucloxacillin	Inhibition of cross-linking of peptide side chains	Phenoxymethyl penicillin: tonsillitis. Flucloxacillin: impetigo, cellulitis. Amoxicillin: chest infections, otitis media, UTIs
Cephalosporins, e.g. cefalexin, cefotaxime, cefaclor	Binding to beta-lactam-binding sites and inhibiting cell wall synthesis	Septicaemia, pneumonia, meningitis, biliary tract infections, peritonitis, UTIs
Tetracylines, e.g. tetracycline, doxycycline	Inhibition of protein synthesis, through interfering with tRNA binding	*Chlamydia*, exacerbation of chronic bronchitis (*Haemophilus influenzae*), periodontal disease, acne, respiratory and genital *Mycoplasma* infections. Doxycycline in malaria prophylaxis
Macrolides, e.g erythromycin, clarithromycin	Prevent the translocation movement of the bacterial ribosome along the mRNA and prevent protein synthesis	Suitable alternative in patients who are allergic to penicillin. Respiratory infections, whooping cough, Legionnaires' disease, *Campylobacter* enteritis
Aminoglycosides, e.g gentamicin	Irreversibly bind to the bacterial ribosomes leading to an inhibition of protein synthesis	Gentamicin is used in various infections such as septicaemia, meningitis, acute pyelonephritis and endocarditis
Sulphonamides and trimethoprim	Inhibition of folate synthesis and reduces the precursors of DNA and RNA	Pneumonia in AIDS patients, toxoplasmosis and nocardosis. Acute exacerbation of chronic bronchitis, otitis media and UTIs
Quinolones, e.g. ciprofloxacin, ofloxacin	Inhibition of bacterial DNA gyrase	*Pseudomonas aeruginosa, Haemophilus influenzae, Campylobacter*

Table 58.2 Commonly used antiviral and antifungal agents and their modes of action and uses

Anti-infective agent	Mode of action	Uses
Antiviral, e.g. aciclovir, famciclovir, zanamivir.	Aciclovir: inhibition of herpes virus DNA polymerase. Zanamivir: a neuramidase inhibitor that prevents the entry and release of the viral particles from the host cells	Aciclovir: herpes simplex and herpes varicella. Zanamivir: influenza
Imidazoles, e.g. clotrimazole	Inhibition of P450-dependent demethylase, which converts lanosterol to ergosterol; the accumulation of lanosterol disrupts fungal membrane	Fungal infections
Triazoles, e.g. itraconazole, fluconazole	As for imidazoles	Fungal infections
Other antifungal agents: griseofulvin, terbinafine	Terbinafine inhibits the conversion of squalene to lanosterol, with the accumulation of squalene causing cell death. Griseofulvin: interferes with fungal microtubules and nucleic acid synthesis	Griseofulvin: suitable for tinea infections but not candidiasis

59 Recognition of pathogens

Lucy Fairclough and Ian Todd

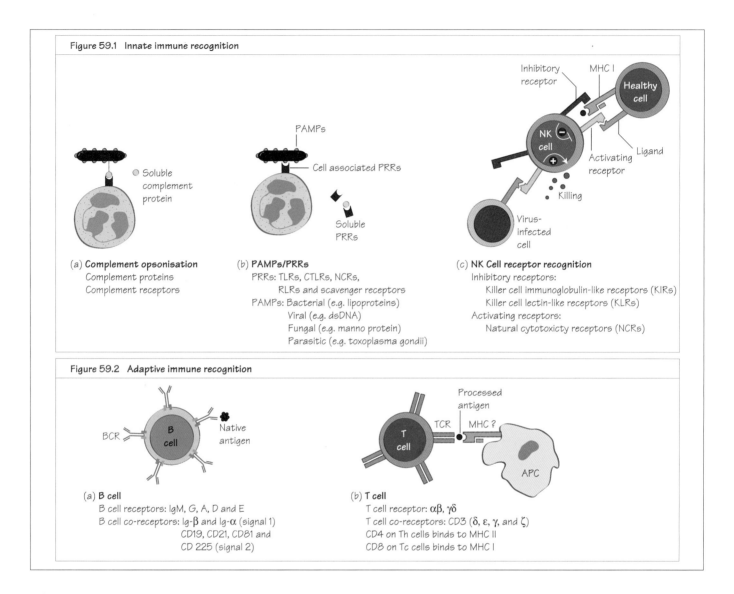

Figure 59.1 Innate immune recognition

(a) **Complement opsonisation**
Complement proteins
Complement receptors

(b) **PAMPs/PRRs**
PRRs: TLRs, CTLRs, NCRs,
        RLRs and scavenger receptors
PAMPs: Bacterial (e.g. lipoproteins)
           Viral (e.g. dsDNA)
           Fungal (e.g. manno protein)
           Parasitic (e.g. toxoplasma gondii)

(c) **NK Cell receptor recognition**
Inhibitory receptors:
        Killer cell immunoglobulin-like receptors (KIRs)
        Killer cell lectin-like receptors (KLRs)
Activating receptors:
        Natural cytotoxicty receptors (NCRs)

Figure 59.2 Adaptive immune recognition

(a) **B cell**
B cell receptors: IgM, G, A, D and E
B cell co-receptors: Ig-β and Ig-α (signal 1)
                    CD19, CD21, CD81 and
                    CD 225 (signal 2)

(b) **T cell**
T cell receptor: αβ, γδ
T cell co-receptors: CD3 (δ, ε, γ, and ζ)
CD4 on Th cells binds to MHC II
CD8 on Tc cells binds to MHC I

The major functions of the immune system are the recognition of pathogens by interacting with microbes and their components, and defence of the body by the elimination of microbes and their components. **Immune recognition** and **defence** are achieved in two ways: by components of the immune system that generate **innate immunity**, and others that generate **adaptive immunity**.

The main features of innate immunity are that it is quickly activated when infection occurs; it remains the same on repeated exposure to the same microbe and is moderately efficient. The main features of adaptive (also known as acquired) immunity are that it is more slowly activated, but its efficacy improves on repeated exposure to the same

microbe. Once activated, adaptive immunity is highly efficient and provides specific responses tailored to each individual type of microbe.

Innate recognition

Innate immunity provides a general response to categories of microbe and is triggered by the recognition of both **complement proteins** that have **opsonised** the pathogen, and chemical structures that are characteristic of microbes (termed **pathogen-associated molecular patterns** [PAMPs]). Further recognition is achieved by receptors expressed on **natural killer** (NK) cells.

Complement opsonisation (Figure 59.1(a))

Complement is the name for a collection of about 30 proteins found in the circulation and in tissue fluids that were initially described by their ability to 'complement' the effects of antibodies. Various complement proteins act as activation enzymes, defence molecules and regulatory proteins. Activation of complement proteins is triggered by infection by pathogens and immune activation, and occurs as a cascade or chain reaction with amplification built in. Once activated, fragments of complement bind to the surface of the pathogen, effectively '**opsonising**' the pathogen so it can be seen by cells of the immune system expressing complement receptors (such as macrophages).

Pathogen-associated molecular patterns (PAMPs) and pathogen recognition receptors (PRRs) (Figure 59.1(b))

Chemical structures that are characteristic of microbes are often termed pathogen-associated molecular patterns (PAMPs), e.g. bacterial lipopolysaccharide and viral double-stranded RNA. These PAMPs interact with pattern recognition receptors (PRRs) expressed by cells (e.g. **toll-like receptors [TLRs]**, **C-type lectin receptors [CTLRs]**, **NOD-like receptors [NLRs]**, **RIG-like helicase receptors [RLRs]** and scavenger receptors) or soluble PRRs. Cell-associated PRRs enable phagocytosis of PAMPs and associated microbes, activation of cells and consequent release of inflammatory mediators to amplify the immune response. Soluble PRRs can directly attack the microbe and enhance phagocytosis of PRR bound PAMPs, as well as activating the proteolytic cascade resulting in lysis of the microbe.

Cell receptor recognition (Figure 59.1(c))

NK cells recognise target cells via a large repertoire of activating and inhibitory receptors in an antigen non-specific manner and are therefore able to act quickly. There are three main classes of receptor on NK cells: **killer cell immunoglobulin-like receptors** (**KIRs**) and **killer cell lectin-like receptors** (**KLRs**) that are largely inhibitory and detect levels of HLA class I, and **natural cytotoxicity receptors** (NCRs) that are exclusively activating receptors. Healthy cells constitutively express HLA class I molecules that bind to inhibitory receptors on the NK cell surface, thereby blocking any stimulatory receptor signalling. However, if HLA class I expression is reduced, when a virus is attempting to avoid detection, this inhibitory signalling is absent and the cell will be killed. Equally, if a cell is under stress and up-regulates the expression of HLA class IB-like molecules such as MIC-A and MIC-B, activating signals, via the NKG2D receptor for example, override inhibitory signalling in the NK cell and the target cell will be killed.

Adaptive recognition

Adaptive immunity involves recognition of **antigens** specific to each type of microbe that are recognised by antigen receptors that are clonally expressed by **lymphocytes**. Thus lymphocytes are the cell type responsible for the properties of adaptive immune recognition.

B cell receptor (BCR) (Figure 59.2(a))

The antigen recognition receptors expressed by B cells are surface immunoglobulins (sIg) that specifically bind native antigens to the B cell surface. All the sIg molecules expressed by a single B cell have identical antigen-combining sites, i.e. a single B cell is specific for a single antigen epitope. When a B cell binds an antigen to its sIg and becomes activated, it differentiates into a plasma cell that secretes antibodies (soluble immunoglobulins) with the same combining sites

(i.e. the same antigenic specificity) as the sIg: thus a B cell produces antibodies that recognise the antigen it originally bound.

The body contains millions of families or **clones** of B cells, each expressing Ig with a different antigen-combining site. Thus an antigen will interact with those clones whose sIg bind it with highest affinity (**clonal selection**). Activation of the B cells that bind antigen results in their proliferation, thus increasing the number of B cells of the specific clones, and some of these are maintained in the body as **memory cells**. However, sIg only has a tail region of three amino acids so cannot signal into the cell. For this reason the BCR does not just contain sIg but also Igβ (CD79b) and Igα (CD79a), which enables signalling. For a B cell to become fully activated, probably as a safeguard mechanism, they require a second signal. One such form of co-stimulation is the BCR co-receptor complex that can engage with molecules such as complement that may be on the same target surface (i.e. a bacterium). The BCR co-receptor consists of CD19, CD21 (CR2), CD81 and CD225.

If the same antigen enters the body again, it will interact specifically with these memory cells, which are reactivated more rapidly and in larger numbers than in the primary response, hence giving the faster and bigger response that characterises adaptive immunity.

T cell receptor (Figure 59.2(b))

The antigen recognition receptors expressed by T cells are called **T cell receptors** (**TCRs**) and are composed of two polypeptide chains (α and β chains or occasionally γ and δ chains). There is no secreted form of the TCR, i.e. T cells do not produce an equivalent to antibodies secreted by B cells.

Both the α and β chains of the TCR are anchored in the surface membrane. Each chain is about the same size as an immunoglobulin light chain. Indeed, the TCR α and β chains are each composed of two immunoglobulin-like domains with strong structural homologies with immunoglobulin domains; for this reason, the TCR is said to be a member of the immunoglobulin superfamily. In each chain, the domain proximal to the membrane is constant in structure between T cells (C_α and C_β), whereas the domains distal to the membrane are variable in structure between T cells (V_α and V_β) and form a single antigen-combining site; thus the TCR has one antigen-combining site, whereas sIg on B cells has two.

The main function of T cells is to do things to other cells of the body in the context of an immune response. Some T cells, called **T helper** (**Th**) cells, help other cells of the immune system to fulfil their functions, e.g. Th cells activate B cells to produce antibodies, and stimulate the phagocytic and killing activity of macrophages. Other T cells, called **T cytotoxic** (**Tc**) cells, kill tissue cells that have become infected by microbes.

The TCR of T cells cannot interact directly with microbes and their antigens, but bind only to fragments of antigenic proteins (i.e. antigen peptides) associated with tissue cells, thereby targeting the T cells to mediate their helper or cytotoxic activities against these cells. Cells that present antigen peptides that T cells can bind to are termed **antigen presenting cells** (**APC**). In the cytoplasm of APCs, microbial proteins are broken down into peptides, and some of these antigen peptides than associate with specialised peptide-binding proteins that hold the peptides on the APC surface where they are available to interact with the TCR of T cells. In humans, the antigen-binding proteins are called **HLA** proteins (**human leucocyte antigens**); more generally, in humans and other species, they are termed **MHC** proteins (**proteins of the major histocompatibility complex**).

Lucy Fairclough and Ian Todd

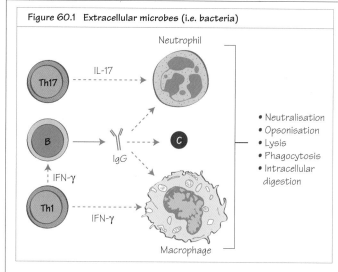

Figure 60.1 Extracellular microbes (i.e. bacteria)

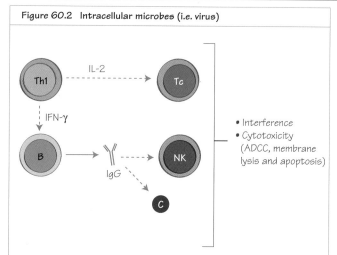

Figure 60.2 Intracellular microbes (i.e. virus)

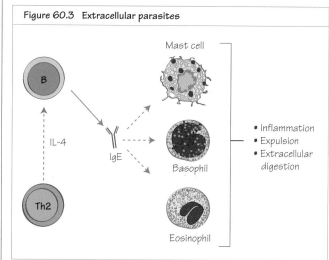

Figure 60.3 Extracellular parasites

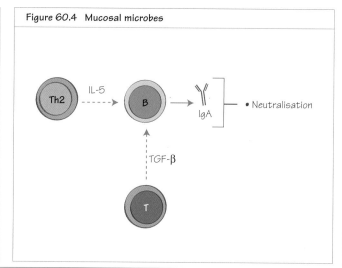

Figure 60.4 Mucosal microbes

Immune defence is achieved by components of the immune system that generate innate immunity, and others that generate adaptive immunity. The body is exposed to numerous classes of microbes and the immune system has to manage these different threats to the body. Furthermore, differences in nature, mode of entry, mechanisms of replication and spread in the body of different infective agents mean that a range of defensive mechanisms is necessary.

Extracellular microbes (e.g. bacteria)
(Figure 60.1)
Innate immune defence is mediated by various cell types, including **leucocytes** (e.g. neutrophils) and epithelial cells. These cells produce

antimicrobial peptides called **defensins** that are directly damaging to certain microbes.

With regard to the adaptive immune response, B cells secrete antibodies (mainly IgG) that may have defensive effects simply by binding to antigens, e.g. neutralising the activities of bacterial toxins or viruses. Antibodies can also act as intermediaries to activate other defensive components that interact with the **Fc** regions of antibodies. Thus IgM and IgG antibodies can activate the complement system of proteins and virtually all cells of the immune system express Fc receptors (FcR).

Macrophages and neutrophils are phagocytes that engulf microbes and digest them intracellularly. Macrophages are tissue-resident cells derived from blood monocytes; neutrophils circulate in the blood and are recruited into sites of infection and inflammation. The acute phase proteins **C-reactive protein** and **mannose-binding lectin** can opsonise bacteria for uptake by macrophages and neutrophils, and also activate complement.

Macrophages and neutrophils recognise microbes using either pattern recognition receptors (PRRs), or receptors for complement (CR) or antibodies (FcR). This interaction triggers phagocytosis, with the microbe being internalised into a membrane-bound vesicle called a phagosome. Cytoplasmic lysosomes that contain digestive enzymes then fuse with the phagosome, releasing the digestive enzymes on to the surface of the microbe and bringing about its degradation. In addition, the phagocyte produces reactive oxygen species that enter the phagosomes, helping in the degradation and producing a pH appropriate for the activity of the digestive enzymes.

T cells, specifically CD4 T helper cells, play an important role in coordinating and driving the most appropriate immune response. Th17 cells, characterised by secretion of interleukin-17, support neutrophil function, CD4 Th1 cells secrete interferon-gamma supporting macrophage function, whereas.

Intracellular microbes (e.g. viruses)
(Figure 60.2)
Viruses do not have the metabolic machinery for self-replication and so must infect cells in order to replicate. Some defensive strategies of the immune system are directed against free virus particles, destroying them directly or neutralising their ability to infect cells. Other strategies are directed at the infected cells, either blocking virus replication or killing the infected cells.

Strategies directed at intracellular viruses include a combination of mechanisms that target the intracellular phases of virus infection. The early innate response by **interferons** and natural killer (NK) cells limits the growth and spread of the infection. The adaptive response by CD8 cytotoxic T cells takes longer to activate, but its high efficiency may be sufficient to clear the infection.

Virus infection triggers the infected cells to produce and secrete type 1 **interferons** (IFN-α and IFN-β). These bind to receptors on neighbouring cells and trigger an antiviral state in which these cells are resistant to virus replication. This is because interferons induce enzymes that degrade viral mRNA and inhibit protein synthesis. Type 1 interferons also enhance expression of HLA class I, thereby making cells better targets for CD8 cytotoxic T cells, and activate natural killer cells.

NK cells have two mechanisms of recognising cells as targets for killing. The first involves a large repertoire of activating and inhibitory receptors (Chapter 59). The other involves IgG antibodies binding to native viral antigens expressed on the surface of infected cells; NK cells express Fc receptors for IgG that can then bind to the antibodies, thus attaching them to the surface of the infected cells, which they can then kill – this is termed antibody-dependent cellular cytotoxicity (ADCC).

Although NK cells and Tc cells employ different mechanisms to identify virus-infected cells as targets for killing (Tc cells recognise HLA class I-associated peptides (Chapter 59), these two types of killer cell use similar mechanisms to bring about target cell destruction. There are two types of killing mechanism that the killer cells employ,

both of which result in the induction of target cell apoptosis. The killer cells possess granules that contain two types of protein, which are released on to the target cell surface: the **perforins** are similar to the C9 complement protein of the membrane attack complex. They are inserted into the target cell's surface membrane and facilitate uptake of the **granzymes**, which gain entry to the target cell cytoplasm where they activate **caspase** enzymes that initiate the apoptosis pathways. The Tc cells also express a surface protein called Fas-ligand that interacts with Fas protein on the target cell surface; this interaction also activates the apoptosis pathways.

Extracellular parasites (e.g. helminths)
(Figure 60.3)
Extracellular parasites are too large to be engulfed by phagocytes or killed by CD8 cytotoxic T cells and NK cells. They are removed by generating an inflammatory response through the actions of eosinophils, mast cells and basophils. This removal is mediated by IgE, an immunoglobulin isotype produced by B cells.

Eosinophils can mediate extracellular digestion. They express FcR that bind IgG or IgE, and they also express complement receptors. Thus opsonisation of a parasitic worm by antibodies and C3b facilitates binding of numerous eosinophils to the parasite surface. Eosinophils have cytoplasmic granules containing a range of digestive proteins, e.g. major basic protein and eosinophil cationic protein; these are released on to the surface of the parasite to bring about extracellular digestion.

Mast cells are tissue cells that express high affinity-FcR that bind IgE antibodies from surrounding tissue fluid. Thus mast cells become coated with IgE antibodies and therefore acquire the antigenic specificities of these antibodies. When an antigen specifically binds simultaneously to two or more IgE antibodies on a mast cell surface (i.e. the antigen cross-links or bridges the IgE), this triggers the release of inflammatory mediators. Release of inflammatory mediators by mast cells can be similarly triggered by the complement activation peptides C3a and C5a (these peptides also attract and activate neutrophils at sites of inflammation).

Mast cells contain numerous granules in which are stored preformed inflammatory mediators (e.g. histamine, heparin, tryptase); these are released immediately upon mast cell triggering. Mast cell activation also induces the synthesis of newly formed mediators that are released over a longer period of time, e.g. leukotrienes and prostaglandins derived from arachidonic acid, and cytokines.

Mucosal microbes
Mucosal microbes are neutralised by the actions of IgA, an immunoglobulin isotype produced by B cells. IgA is present in blood and internal tissue fluids as a monomer. The dimeric IgA is transported across mucosal epithelium into the mucosal secretions of the gastrointestinal, respiratory and genitourinary tracts. This occurs because of an IgA-binding receptor (the poly-Ig receptor) expressed by mucosal epithelial cells; part of this receptor remains attached to the secreted IgA dimer and is called secretory piece. IgA is also secreted by the mammary gland into milk, and so mother's IgA is transferred to confer protection in the gut of suckling infants. B cells produce IgA under stimulation by IL-5 (produced by CD4 T helper type 2 cells) or TGF-β (produced by CD4 T regulatory cells).

Lucy Fairclough and Ian Todd

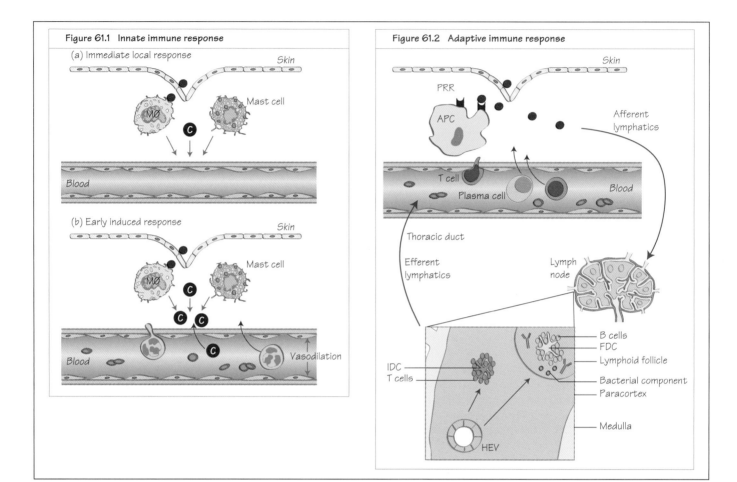

Figure 61.1 Innate immune response
(a) Immediate local response
(b) Early induced response

Figure 61.2 Adaptive immune response

The immune system works to generate appropriate responses for removal of pathogens that invade the body. Innate immunity is quickly activated when infection occurs but remains the same on repeated exposure to the same pathogen and is only moderately efficient. Adaptive immunity is more slowly activated due to the requirement for information about the invading pathogen to be taken to naïve T and B lymphocytes in the local secondary lymphoid tissues (e.g. lymph nodes). However, once activated it provides specific responses tailored to each individual type of pathogen.

Innate immunity (Figure 61.1)
Immediate local response (Figure 61.1a)
The first infection by a particular microbe generates a primary immune response. This normally requires pathogens to penetrate surface epi-

thelial barriers of the body, e.g. the epidermis. An immediate local innate response in the infected tissues is generated by components of the immune system resident in those tissues (e.g. macrophages, mast cells and complement proteins). This also generates inflammatory mediators (augmented by the activation of mast cells) that attract further leucocytes and serum proteins into the infected tissues from the bloodstream.

Macrophages are phagocytes that engulf (phagocytose) microbes and digest them intracellularly. Macrophages are tissue-resident cells derived from blood monocytes that phagocytose bacteria using pathogen recognition receptors (PRRs) and after opsonisation with the acute phase proteins: C-reactive protein and mannose-binding lectin. These acute phase proteins can also activate complement, causing generation of the complement peptides C3a and C5a (see below).

Mast cells contain numerous granules in which are stored pre-formed inflammatory mediators. Mast cell activation also induces the synthesis of newly formed mediators that are released over a longer period of time, e.g. leukotrienes and prostaglandins derived from arachidonic acid, and cytokines. Release of these inflammatory mediators can be triggered by the complement activation peptides C3a and C5a, which can also attract and activate neutrophils at sites of inflammation.

Early induced response (Figure 61.1b)

Activation of mast cells (as above) causes release of inflammatory mediators that attract further leucocytes and serum proteins into the infected tissues from the bloodstream. These inflammatory mediators cause vasodilatation that increases the volume of blood reaching the tissues and reduces the rate of blood flow so that leucocytes, especially neutrophils, move more slowly through the blood. In conjunction, there is increased **vascular permeability** that facilitates the movement of neutrophils and complement proteins into the infected tissues. Movement of neutrophils through the tissue to the site of infection is achieved by chemotaxis, with immobilisation and activation when the site of infection is reached.

Chemotaxis involves the directional movement of cells in response to chemical signals (chemoattractants). For example, chemokines produced by activated cells (e.g. macrophages) at the site of infection diffuse through the tissue and bind to receptors, where they impinge on the 'leading edge' of neutrophils. This stimulates new integrin expression at the leading edge of the cell so that it forms new contacts with tissue cells or connective tissue components. Old integrin contacts at the trailing edge of the cell are gradually lost, so the cell moves up the concentration gradient of chemokine towards the site of infection.

Neutrophils, like macrophages, are phagocytes that engulf microbes and digest them intracellularly. However, unlike macrophages they circulate in the blood and are only recruited into tissues during infection and inflammation.

Adaptive immunity (Figure 61.2)

While the above innate response is being generated, antigens are carried from the site of infection to local secondary lymphoid tissues (e.g. **lymph nodes**) in order to generate an adaptive immune response. Some antigens are carried free in the lymph, and some are captured by specialised cells called **antigen-presenting cell**s (**APCs**), which are present in most tissues of the body. These APCs migrate to the lymphoid tissues carrying the antigens with them via the afferent lymphatics. In the lymphoid tissues, the antigens activate naïve T and B lymphocytes that specifically recognise them (which will be only a few of all the lymphocytes in these tissues). The specifically activated lymphocytes and antibodies (produced by the B lymphocytes) can then recirculate back to the site of infection. In the tissues, APCs' main function is antigen capture, and in lymphoid tissues, it is antigen presentation.

During the process described above, antigen in the form of immune complexes preferentially localises to **follicular dendritic cells** (**FDCs**) in the B cell-containing follicles or germinal centres. Antigen transported by APCs is presented to CD4 T helper cells in the paracortex which come into close contact with the APCs that become interdigitating dendritic cells (IDC). These T cells then assist in the generation of B lymphoblasts, which then migrate in to the follicle (together with some T cells), where they undergo further maturation and selection through interaction with FDCs in germinal centres. Specific T and B lymphocytes then leave the lymph nodes via the medulla and efferent lymphatics to enter the blood via the thoracic duct.

Once in the blood the effector T and B lymphocytes traffic around the body to the site of infection. Within inflamed tissues, the endothelial cells lining blood vessels are activated by inflammatory mediators to express adhesion molecules that facilitate the adhesion of leucocytes to the blood vessel walls and their migration across the walls. The initial interactions (called capture and rolling) are mediated by selectins (E-selectin and P-selectin expressed by the endothelium, and L-selectin expressed by leucocytes) that bind to highly glycosylated proteins (mucins). This facilitates the interaction of the leucocytes with chemokines on the surface of the endothelium that trigger activation of adhesion molecules called integrins expressed by leucocytes. The integrins form strong interactions with the endothelial cells by binding to ligands called intercellular and vascular cell adhesion molecules (ICAM and VCAM); this is called the activation and flattening stage.

Leucocytes bound to the endothelium pass between adjacent endothelial cells (facilitated by the loss of tight junctions between endothelial cells), again using integrin interactions; this is termed extravasation. As discussed above, the cells move through the tissue by chemotaxis (the directional movement of cells in response to chemical signals) where they assist in removal of the pathogen.

If re-infection with the same type of pathogen occurs soon after the response above, then pre-formed antibodies and effector B and T lymphocytes will be available immediately. A later re-infection will generate a secondary immune response by memory lymphocytes formed during the primary response; these give a faster and bigger response than occurred in the primary response, hence the term adaptive immunity.

In addition to the local inflammatory effects at the site of infection, a body-wide response to infection also occurs, termed the **acute phase response**. This is mediated primarily by systemic effects of the cytokines **interleukin-1**, **interleukin-6** and **tumour necrosis factor**, that are variously produced by activated macrophages, lymphocytes, mast cells and other activated cells. They affect various tissues around the body when released into the bloodstream at significant concentrations. Collectively, these cytokines induce fever by effects on the hypothalamus, promote increased levels of circulating leucocytes (leucocytosis) by release from the bone marrow, and stimulate the liver to produce antimicrobial acute phase proteins such as **C-reactive protein** and **mannose-binding lectin**.

62 Immunopathology

Ian Todd and Lucy Fairclough

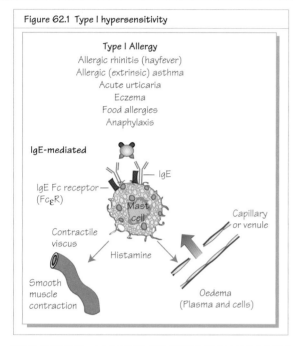

Figure 62.1 Type I hypersensitivity

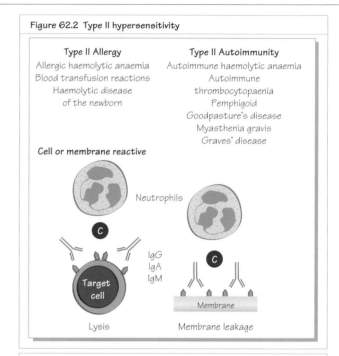

Figure 62.2 Type II hypersensitivity

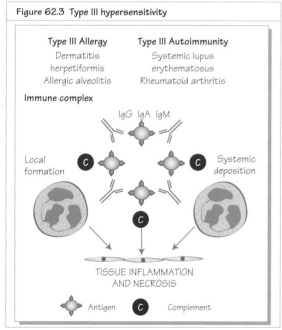

Figure 62.3 Type III hypersensitivity

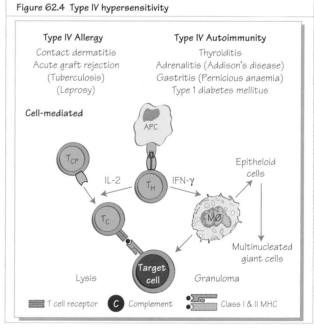

Figure 62.4 Type IV hypersensitivity

Diseases that involve tissue damage as a consequence of inappropriate adaptive immune responses can be categorised on the basis of either the source of the stimulating antigens (allergy or autoimmunity) or the consequent mechanisms of tissue damage involved (hypersensitivity mechanisms types I–IV).

Adaptive immunity to infection involves recognition of foreign (microbial) antigens and damage to the foreign microbes. **Allergy** is a consequence of inappropriate activation of adaptive immunity by non-infective foreign antigens (allergens) resulting in damage to tissues. In **autoimmunity**, tissue damage results from activation of autoreactive lymphocytes that recognise self-tissue components as autoantigens.

Type I hypersensitivity – atopic allergy
(Figure 62.1)

This involves IgE antibodies and mast cells: 'atopy' refers to a propensity for production of high levels of IgE. Allergen-specific IgE molecules, bound to Fcε receptors on mast cells, are cross-linked by specific allergens, triggering release of preformed inflammatory mediators by degranulation (e.g. histamine) and synthesis of newly formed mediators (e.g. leukotrienes and prostaglandins). These mediators induce inflammation and smooth muscle contraction.

T_H2 cells play a central role in the induction type I hypersensitivity, e.g. by secretion of IL-4 that stimulates IgE production by B cells, and IL-5 that stimulates eosinophils. The immediate elicitation phase of a type I hypersensitivity response is generated by mast cell activation, whereas T_H2 cells and eosinophils can be implicated in the late phase reaction that can result in chronic tissue damage.

Different types of atopic disorder are induced by different types of allergen and routes of exposure.
• Allergic rhinitis is commonly triggered by pollen allergens that activate mast cells in the upper respiratory tract – hence the name 'hay fever'.
• Wheezing associated with allergic asthma involves bronchial constriction in the lower respiratory tract, often caused by an allergic response to house dust mite constituents.
• Food allergens may cause local symptoms in the gut (e.g. vomiting, diarrhoea), but once absorbed into the bloodstream may have wider effects, e.g. skin reactions (urticaria, eczema) or potentially life-threatening systemic effects (anaphylaxis) as exemplified in severe nut allergies.
• There are no clear examples of autoimmune diseases that involve type I hypersensitivity.

Type II hypersensitivity – cell or membrane reactive (Figure 62.2)

This involves IgG, IgA, or IgM antibodies that bind to cell surface membranes or connective tissue components. These induce damage by activating complement and/or triggering neutrophils to release digestive products and reactive oxygen species.

Allergic haemolytic anaemia can be induced by drugs that bind to erythrocytes and if antibodies are generated against these drugs, then erythrocyte lysis can result; similarly, autoimmune haemolytic anaemia involves autoantibodies specific for erythrocyte surface autoantigens, and autoimmune thrombocytopaenia involves autoantibody-induced platelet destruction. Naturally occurring antibodies to blood group antigens expressed by erythrocytes (e.g. anti-A and anti-B antibodies) can cause life-threatening reactions to incompatible blood transfusions. The main cause of haemolytic disease of the newborn is maternal IgG antibodies to the rhesus D antigen expressed by the erythrocytes of a D-positive fetus developing in a D-negative woman; these IgG antibodies cross the placenta from the mother to the fetus and cause destruction of fetal erythrocytes.

Autoantibodies to basement membranes cause tissue damage to the skin in pemphigoid (skin epidermal basement membrane) and Goodpasture's disease (kidney glomerular basement membrane).

A special case of type II hypersensitivity (sometimes called type V) involves autoantibodies to membrane-associated receptor proteins.

Myasthenia gravis can involve autoantibodies specific for the acetylcholine (ACh) receptors expressed on muscle cells at the neuromuscular junction (Chapter 22). These autoantibodies block binding of ACh released from nerve endings, and also induce internalisation and degradation of receptors. This results in extreme muscle weakness due to a lack of nerve stimulation of muscle contraction. In Graves' disease, autoantibodies specifically bind to the TSH receptor expressed by thyroid follicular cells and stimulate thyroid hormone production. The action of these 'thyroid-stimulating antibodies' is not regulated (as is TSH itself), leading the overproduction of thyroid hormones and hyperthyroidism (Chapter 47).

Type III hypersensitivity – immune complex disease (Figure 62.3)

This involves numerous soluble antigens and antibodies cross-linking to form a lattice structure known as an immune complex (IC) that may precipitate out of solution and/or become lodged in tissues. Immune complexes can activate complement and neutrophils leading to tissue damage.

An example is allergic alveolitis caused by production of antibodies to inhaled fungal spores. Immune complex formation in the walls of the alveoli leads to inflammation and fibrosis. This results in breathlessness due to poor gas exchange across the alveolar walls (as distinct from the wheezing in asthma that is due to constriction of the bronchi). Dermatitis herpetiformis is a skin condition associated with gluten-sensitive gut inflammation (coeliac disease) and involves IgA antibody-containing immune complex deposition.

In the autoimmune disease systemic lupus erythematosus (SLE), autoantibodies are produced to a range of ubiquitous cellular constituents, particularly nuclear components. Among these antinuclear antibodies (ANA) are autoantibodies specific for DNA. Autoantigen/autoantibody immune complexes form in SLE (e.g. DNA/anti-DNA). These deposit in various tissues, causing tissue damage, e.g. in kidney glomeruli, in the skin, joints and central nervous system.

In rheumatoid arthritis much of the damage occurs in joints. Some of this damage is due to immune complexes formed by rheumatoid factors, which are IgM and IgG autoantibodies that are themselves specific for IgG.

Type IV hypersensitivity – cell-mediated hypersensitivity (Figure 62.4)

This involves activation of helper T cells (principally T_H1 cells) by their interaction with antigen-presenting cells. The activated T_H1 cells secrete cytokines, e.g. interleukin-2 that can activates T_C cells and interferon-gamma that can activate macrophages (and possibly lead to their dedifferentiation into epithelioid cells and fusion to form multinucleate giant cells). Reactions of this type are seen in the chronic phases of the mycobacterial infections that cause tuberculosis and leprosy.

Contact allergens that induce a type IV hypersensitivity reaction seen clinically as contact dermatitis include metals (e.g. nickel, chromium) and plant products (e.g. poison ivy).

In a number of autoimmune diseases the target cells are destroyed principally through the activity of autoreactive T cells.
• Hashimoto's thyroiditis (Chapter 47).
• Addison's disease (adrenalitis) (Chapter 48).
• Pernicious anaemia (Chapter 33).
• Type 1 diabetes mellitus (Chapter 46).

63 Immunodeficiency disorders

Ian Todd and Lucy Fairclough

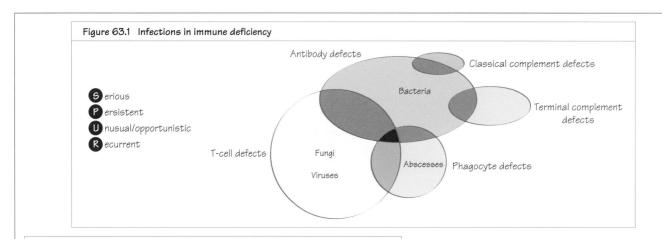

Figure 63.1 Infections in immune deficiency

- **S**erious
- **P**ersistent
- **U**nusual/opportunistic
- **R**ecurrent

Antibody defects

Classical complement defects

Bacteria

Terminal complement defects

T-cell defects

Fungi

Viruses

Abscesses

Phagocyte defects

Figure 63.2 Neutrophil functional defects

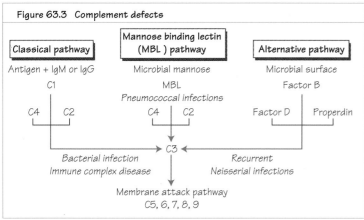

Leucocyte adhesion deficiency

Killing

Respiratory burst

Chemotaxis

Bacteria

Phagocytosis

Chronic granulomatous disease

Figure 63.3 Complement defects

Classical pathway	Mannose binding lectin (MBL) pathway	Alternative pathway
Antigen + IgM or IgG	Microbial mannose	Microbial surface
C1	MBL	Factor B
	Pneumococcal infections	
C4 C2	C4 C2	Factor D Properdin

C3

Bacterial infection
Immune complex disease

Recurrent
Neisserial infections

Membrane attack pathway
C5, 6, 7, 8, 9

Figure 63.4 Lymphocyte defects

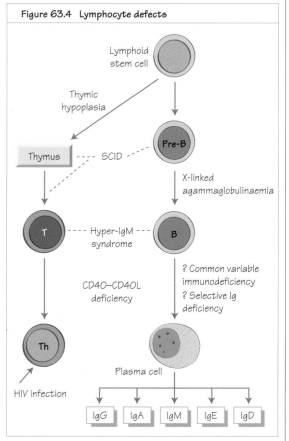

Lymphoid stem cell

Thymic hypoplasia

Pre-B

Thymus - - - SCID - - -

X-linked agammaglobulinaemia

T

Hyper-IgM syndrome

B

CD40–CD40L deficiency

? Common variable immunodeficiency
? Selective Ig deficiency

Th

Plasma cell

HIV infection

IgG   IgA   IgM   IgE   IgD

The nature of immunodeficiency disorders (Figure 63.1)

Immunodeficiency refers to defective immune function that leads to increased susceptibility to infection. These disorders are categorised as primary or secondary.

Primary immunodeficiencies are usually due to inherited mutations in genes with immunological functions. They are mainly very rare conditions. **Secondary immunodeficiencies** are acquired as a consequence of environmental insults and/or as a consequence of other disease processes.

Immunodeficiencies are characterised by infections that tend to be serious, persistent, unusual (opportunisitic), recurrent – giving the acronym **SPUR** (Figure 63.1).

The types of infection that occur often reflect the nature of the defects in immune components (Figure 63.1). Thus, bacterial infections are often associated with deficiencies in antibodies, complement, or phagocytes (the latter also leads to abscess formation); T cell defects often involve viral or fungal infections.

Phagocyte defects (Figure 63.2)

Primary deficiencies can affect phagocytes (particularly neutrophils) at various levels, e.g. production, adhesion, chemotaxis and killing activity (intracellular digestion).

Neutrophils are the most plentiful type of white blood cell (50–70% of leucocytes), but are short-lived (about 5 days, but only 1–2 days when activated), and produced in the bone marrow in enormous numbers (about one million per second). Thus any suppression of neutrophil production can have a dramatic effect with greatly increased risk of infection. Defects in neutrophil production can be primary (e.g. Kostmann's disease; cyclic neutropenia), or secondary to other disease processes (e.g. leukaemia, infection) or treatment with antiproliferative cancer chemotherapy.

Two examples of rare primary defects in the function of mature neutrophils are:

• **leucocyte adhesion deficiency** – lack of expression of leucocyte integrins that are necessary for the adhesion of leucocytes (including neutrophils) to activated endothelial cells at sites of infection/inflammation; thus neutrophils cannot migrate from the circulation into infected tissues;

• **chronic granulomatous disease**, which involves defects in enzymes involved in the generation of reactive oxygen species. In this case, neutrophils can migrate to sites of infection but are inefficient at killing pathogens; this generates sites of indolent infection and neutrophil accumulation (known as granulomas).

Complement deficiencies (Figure 63.3)

The complement system of proteins (Chapters 62 and 63) can be activated by three different pathways that coalesce at the activation of the C3 protein. The **Classical Pathway** is activated when C1 protein binds to complexes of antigen with IgG or IgM antibodies. Defects of the Classical Pathway and C3 are also associated with immune complex disease. This is because immune complexes (see type III hypersensitivity in Chapter 62) activate the classical pathway (by binding C1q), leading to C3b association with the complexes. This facilitates binding of immune complexes to complement receptors on erythrocytes and removal of the complexes by liver macrophages. This immune complex clearance cannot happen if there are defects in C1, C2, C3, or C4 resulting in a tendency for immune complexes to accumulate.

Mannose-binding lectin (MBL) is an acute phase protein that can activate the complement system when it binds to microbial polysaccharides. MBL deficiency is particularly common (3% of the population) and is associated with pneumococcal, and other bacterial, infections.

The **Alternative Pathway** is activated when C3b (derived from C3) binds to microbial surfaces and associates with factor B. All three pathways of complement activation result in cleavage of C3 and activation of the Membrane Attack Pathway; the membrane attack complexes (generated from C5–9) damage the lipid membranes of microbes. Neisserial infections are associated especially with defects in the Alternative and Membrane Attack Pathways.

B lymphocyte and antibody deficiencies

Some primary antibody deficiencies inhibit the generation of mature B cells, e.g. X-linked agammaglobulinaemia due to mutations affecting Bruton's tyrosine kinase enzyme. Other primary antibody deficiencies are due to defects in B cell activation and maturation and/or B cell interaction with helper T cells; some become manifest in adults rather than children (e.g. common variable immunodeficiency); they are under diagnosed with the possibility of irreversible tissue damage due to repeated chronic infections (e.g. bronchiectasis) if untreated (e.g. by immunoglobulin replacement).

Selective immunoglobulin deficiencies include IgA deficiency, which is the most common primary immunodeficiency, affecting about 1/600 of the population. Hyper-IgM syndrome is due to defects in immunoglobulin class switching, and includes deficiency of CD40 or CD40-ligand expression, which is required for effective interaction between helper T cells and B cells.

There are several secondary causes of antibody deficiency, including **lymphoproliferative disease**, renal/gut loss of IgG, malnutrition and immunosuppressive drugs.

T cell defects and severe combined immunodeficiencies (SCID) (Figure 63.4)

A number of immunodeficiency disorders affect mainly T cells. A rare primary T cell deficiency occurs in DiGeorge syndrome, which involves impaired development of the thymus and other tissues in the face/neck/chest due to a defect in fetal development.

Adaptive immunity is broadly affected in SCID, leading to generalised susceptibility to infection (bacterial, viral, fungal), essentially from birth. There are many types of primary defect associated with SCID; the most common mutation affects expression of the receptors for the cytokines interleukin-2, 4, 7, 9, 15 and 21. Other types of defect include mutations in genes required for generating T cell and B cell antigen receptors, and in expression of HLA proteins. SCID is often only treatable by bone marrow transplantation (and gene therapy in some cases).

Acquired immunodeficiency syndrome (AIDS) is a well-known secondary T cell immunodeficiency caused by infection with human immunodeficiency virus (HIV). The virus can be transmitted by sexual intercourse; sharing infected needles; infected blood or blood products; from mother to baby at birth or via breast milk.

HIV infects T cells, dendritic cells and macrophages because the surface glycoprotein (gp120) of the virus binds to the **CD4 protein** expressed by these cell types. Dendritic cells pick up the virus in epithelia and transfer it to T cells in lymphoid tissues; CD4 T cells are then the major source of HIV throughout infection.

HIV replicates in activated CD4 T cells and, consequently, lymphoid tissue is the major reservoir of HIV. Infected dendritic cells and macrophages can spread the infection to other tissues (e.g. brain). After the acute phase of infection an immune response by CD8 T cells, CD4 T cells and NK cells contains (but does not clear) the infection; the infection becomes chronic and virus mutation leads to escape from immunological recognition and gradual depletion of the body's CD4 T cells. AIDS develops as CD4 T cells numbers fall below 200/μL of blood (less than 20% of normal levels) and susceptibility to multiple opportunistic infections ensues.

Although a vaccine against HIV is not yet available, **highly active antiretroviral therapy** (HAART) of infected individuals with combinations of reverse transcriptase and protease inhibitors can be very effective in reducing viral loads to undetectable levels, with dramatic improvements in life expectancy.

64 Cancer

Stuart Brown

Figure 64.1 The cell cycle

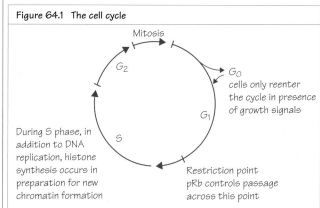

During S phase, in addition to DNA replication, histone synthesis occurs in preparation for new chromatin formation

Restriction point pRb controls passage across this point

G_0 cells only reenter the cycle in presence of growth signals

The stages of the cell cycle are shown. The length of the arrows in each phase gives an approximation of the time taken by each stage i.e if the cell divides in 24 hours S phase is approximately 8 hours and M phase 1–1.5 hours. In addition to pRB control of passage through G_1, p53 is responsible for controlling passage through G_1, G_2 and M phases

Figure 64.3 Function of oncogene products

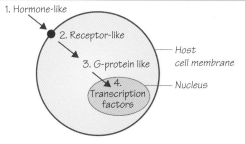

1. Hormone-like
2. Receptor-like
3. G-protein like
4. Transcription factors
Host cell membrane
Nucleus

Think! What could stimulate cell division?
Oncogene products mimic the various factors which can cause cell division. They can be (1) hormone-like (e.g. the v-sis oncogene codes for platelet-derived growth factor, (2) receptor-like (e.g. the v-erb B product mimics a modified epidermal growth factor receptor which behaves as if the ligand is always attached, (3) G protein-like (the ras oncogene product mimics the alpha subunit of a trimeric G protein. Point mutations in the ras gene can lead to loss of the GTPase activity necessary to switch the signal off following activation and (4) transcription factors (e.g. the c-myc gene codes for a transcription factor)

Figure 64.2 Cell transformation by RNA tumour virus

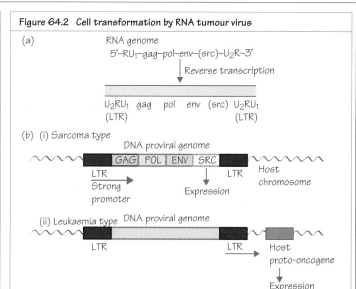

(a) RNA genome
5'-RU$_1$-gag-pol-env-(src)-U$_2$R-3'
Reverse transcription
U$_2$RU$_1$ gag pol env (src) U$_2$RU$_1$
(LTR) (LTR)

(b) (i) Sarcoma type
DNA proviral genome
GAG POL ENV SRC
LTR Strong promoter
Expression
LTR
Host chromosome

(ii) Leukaemia type DNA proviral genome
LTR LTR
Host proto-oncogene
Expression

(a) Following RNA tumour virus infection the RNA genome is reverse transcribed into a double stranded DNA copy. During this process the ends of the genome are modified to produce long terminal repeat sequences which contain all the elements necessary for promoting transcription

(b) The proviral DNA copy of an RNA virus integrates at random into a host chromosome.
(i) The strong promoter activity in the leftward LTR guarantees the viral genes, including the sarcoma gene in the sarcoma viruses, will be transcribed. (ii) Leukaemia virus do not contain an oncogene. However, the rightward LTR will cause over expression of genes close to the viral insert. If a previously silent host proto-oncogene is in that location it will be over-expressed

Figure 64.4 Sequential changes to oncogenes and tumour suppressor genes during the formation of colon cancer

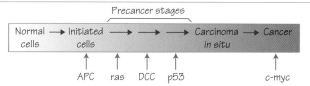

Precancer stages

Normal cells → Initiated cells → → → Carcinoma in situ → Cancer

APC ras DCC p53 c-myc

Although the order of the events can vary the first event is usually loss of the APC (apoptosis poyposis coli) tumour suppressor gene on chromosome 5 (5q21). Loss of this controlling gene can trigger polyp formation. Cells in each polyp will contain the abnormal gene. Thus there is a much larger population of 'initiated' cells and hence a much greater chance that one of these cells will undergo further mutagenic events

Normal cell growth is controlled by the cell cycle. A series of events ensures a cell grows and divides to produce two identical daughter cells when necessary. Cells enter the cell cycle when instructed by extracellular growth signals. In the absence of these signals cells can enter a special phase known as G_0. Cells in this stage are often referred to as being differentiated and will often be synthesising proteins specific to their cell type. Cells in G_0 may be instructed to enter cell division by extracellular signals.

Tumour cells are derived from normal cells. Genetic changes in normal cells can alter the behaviour of those cells. Thus cancer is a genetic disease. It is very common in the Western world. Approximately 1 in 4 people will be diagnosed with cancer in their lifetimes. One thousand people a day are diagnosed with cancer; that's one every 2 minutes.

The cell cycle (Figure 64.1)
When a cell is instructed to divide by an extracellular growth signal it enters into the cell cycle. The events are divided into four phases.
• *G1 phase:* cells will check the environment to ensure sufficient nutrients are available to sustain growth. They also check the integrity of the DNA molecules for any damage. There is a specific point, the **restriction point** or R point, through which a cell will not pass if DNA damage is detected.
• *S phase:* the DNA present in the chromosomes is replicated.
• *G2 phase:* the integrity of the replicated DNA is checked and the cell prepares for mitosis.
• *M phase:* in the **mitotic phase** chromosomes condense and the cell divides to produce two daughter cells each containing a faithful copy of the parental DNA.

Oncogenes
RNA tumour viruses can cause cancer in humans. Two broad classes of RNA tumour virus exist: acute acting, originally called sarcoma viruses, and those that act in a chronic manner, called leukaemia viruses. They have an RNA genome that is reverse transcribed by **RNA-dependent DNA polymerase** (Figure 64.2a) into a proviral double-stranded DNA molecule that integrates into a host chromosome after the virus infects a host cell. New virus components are synthesised and new virus particles assemble at the cell membrane and bud from the host cell, thus the host cell is not lysed by new viral growth.

The RNA virus genome contains genes essential for growth. The genes are called **gag, pol**, and **env genes** (Figure 64.2b). The gag gene codes for the core viral proteins ('gag' actually stands for 'group-specific antigen'. The viruses were identified using antibodies to detect the core proteins and divided into groups according to which antibodies detected them). The 'pol' gene codes for the viral-specific reverse transcriptase enzyme and the 'env' gene codes for the viral envelope proteins. Sarcoma viruses were also found to contain another gene, called 'src' for sarcoma gene. This gene is known as an **oncogene** as it can be responsible for initiating the cell transformation process.

Different viral oncogenes are present in different sarcoma viruses. Surprisingly, genes similar to these are found in our human genome. They are termed **proto-oncogenes** and are usually silent in differentiated cells. Cells infected by sarcoma virus produce viral oncoproteins that initiate cancer cell formation. However, cell transformation can also be initiated by the presence of a leukaemia-type RNA tumour virus. If the replicated DNA copy of an RNA viral genome integrates next to a silent host oncogene it can cause it to be overexpressed. The reverse transcription process generates identical sequences at both ends of the proviral DNA not originally present in the viral RNA, called long terminal repeats (LTRs). These sequences contain elements that promote transcription, i.e. strong promoter regions and enhancer regions.

There are many different types of oncogene now known, coding for a variety of different gene products; they can activate cell division or inhibit apoptosis (Figure 64.3). The different types of gene product can be divided into five major groups.
• *extracellular growth signals*, e.g. v-sis gene product from the Simian sarcoma virus mimics platelet-derived growth factor;
• *growth factor receptors*, e.g. the v-erb B gene product from the erythroblastosis virus mimics the epidermal growth factor receptor, except that it acts as if a ligand is constantly bound;
• *G protein-like*, e.g. ras (**rat s**arcoma) oncogene product. One of the first oncogenes to be discovered in humans. When stimulated, G proteins become active by binding GTP. This is immediately broken down by a GTPase activity, present in the protein, to limit the signal. Point mutations in many oncogene products of this type result in the loss of GTPase and hence the growth signal is always on;
• *transcription factors*, several oncogene products mimic transcription factors and switch on growth genes;
• *cancer may result from the absence of cell death*. Alteration of gene expression involved in programmed cell death, apoptosis, will lead to excess cell mass, e.g. overexpression of bcl-2 or mutation of bax genes can alter apoptosis.

Tumour suppressor genes (TSG)
Originally termed antioncogenes as they oppose the action of oncogenes, tumour suppressor genes have two primary functions: they act to regulate passage through the cell cycle (hence the term 'gatekeeper genes') and they can help maintain DNA integrity (hence the term 'caretaker genes'). These genes are usually recessive, i.e. inactivation or loss of both alleles is necessary to lose their function. The retinoblastoma gene (pRB, 13q14) was identified from studies on families with children who developed retinoblastoma. From this the **'2-hit' hypothesis** was developed, which stated that children may develop the disease in two ways: either they lose both pRb genes early in life or they may have inherited only one normal pRb gene and hence only have to lose the function of that gene in one cell. The latter group develop the tumours earlier in life and often in both eyes. These properties are mimicked in other common tumours such as breast cancer. Women who inherit an abnormal breast cancer gene, BRCA1 or 2, will develop the disease earlier in life and often in both breasts. Clearly it is far more likely to lose one normal gene from a population of cells containing one normal gene than two normal genes in the same cell.

The pRB gene product controls passage through the restriction point in G_1 (Figure 64.1). It is crucial for normal cell cycle control, and in its absence cells will cycle inappropriately. In the presence of appropriate extracellular growth signals, pRb is gradually hyperphosphorylated during the G_1 phase and this initiates events leading to S phase.

TSG activity may be lost by loss of the protein product rather than loss of gene expression. DNA tumour viruses produce proteins which can interact with TSG proteins and prevent their action. This explains how cervical carcinoma can be caused by a papilloma viral infection (HPV). Two early gene products produced by the virus not only bind to the pRB protein, but degrade it. Hence the cell behaves as if it has lost the pRb gene and loses cell cycle control.

p53 (17p13) is a TSG that has a major impact on the incidence of human cancer. p53 genes are mutated or deleted in more than 70% of all human tumours. p53 displays both gatekeeper and caretaker activities. It is responsible for monitoring cell cycle restriction points and is also involved in monitoring DNA integrity and regulating DNA repair when necessary. It is responsible for halting passage through G_1 if DNA is damaged, for example (Figure 64.1). Levels of p53 are strictly maintained in normal cells.

Cancer formation

Cancer is a genetic disease but it is not caused by a single gene defect. Normal cells accumulate mutations and deletions in oncogenes and TSGs until they are sufficient to transform the cell. Cancer cells may contain tens of mutations when fully developed. TSGs such as p53 are responsible for maintaining DNA integrity and repair. A cell that cannot repair DNA will accumulate many more mutations than one with a normal DNA repair system.

Cancer is not caused by a single gene defect. Colon cancer has been extensively studied with regard to the types of mutation that occur during cancer development and is representative of many other tumours. The stages that the normal cells undergo are (Figure 64.4):
• **hyperplasia**: increase in normal cell number;
• **metaplasia**: transformation of one cell type into another that would not normally be in that tissue;
• **dysplasia**: alteration of the size, shape and organisation of the cells;
• **pre-invasive cell formation**: polyp formation;
• **neoplasia**: literally new growth. Neoplasia is used to mean abnormal new growth or cancer.

The cells that develop into a primary tumour as a result of mutations will continue to accumulate more mutations. As a result, individual cells in the primary tumour may develop properties that allow them to leave the primary site and invade through a basement membrane into lymph and blood vessels (intravasation). They then travel through the bloodstream until they find a new site to colonise (extravasation). This is the process of metastasis. The formation of secondary tumours at distant sites from the primary is probably responsible for approximately 90% of cancer deaths.

65 Chemotherapy

Michael D Randall

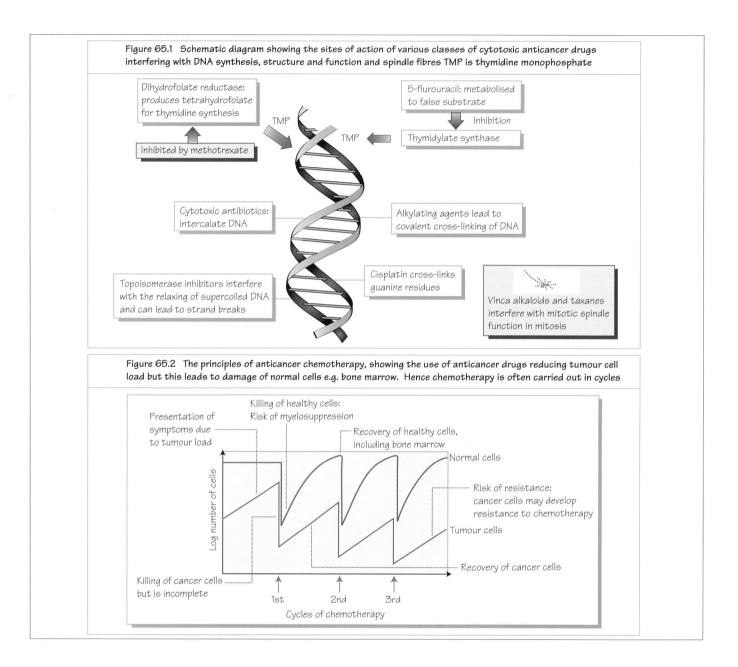

Figure 65.1 Schematic diagram showing the sites of action of various classes of cytotoxic anticancer drugs interfering with DNA synthesis, structure and function and spindle fibres TMP is thymidine monophosphate

Dihydrofolate reductase: produces tetrahydrofolate for thymidine synthesis

Inhibited by methotrexate

TMP

TMP

5-flurouracil: metabolised to false substrate

Inhibition

Thymidylate synthase

Cytotoxic antibiotics: intercalate DNA

Alkylating agents lead to covalent cross-linking of DNA

Topoisomerase inhibitors interfere with the relaxing of supercoiled DNA and can lead to strand breaks

Cisplatin cross-links guanine residues

Vinca alkaloids and taxanes interfere with mitotic spindle function in mitosis

Figure 65.2 The principles of anticancer chemotherapy, showing the use of anticancer drugs reducing tumour cell load but this leads to damage of normal cells e.g. bone marrow. Hence chemotherapy is often carried out in cycles

Killing of healthy cells: Risk of myelosuppression

Presentation of symptoms due to tumour load

Recovery of healthy cells, including bone marrow

Normal cells

Risk of resistance: cancer cells may develop resistance to chemotherapy

Tumour cells

Recovery of cancer cells

Killing of cancer cells but is incomplete

Log number of cells

1st   2nd   3rd

Cycles of chemotherapy

Anticancer chemotherapy is used to manage a range of cancers and may be used to reduce the size of a tumour or prevent the spread of cancer via **metastasis**. In the case of haematological cancers, anticancer chemotherapy may be used to reduce the cancerous cell load prior to bone transplantation (in certain leukaemias) or eradicate the disease (in certain lymphomas).

Chemotherapy works on the principle of **cytotoxicity**, in which chemicals are used to kill cells, and many of the agents target rapidly dividing cells by attacking the biochemical processes associ-

ated with DNA replication and cell division (Figure 65.1). Therapeutically, this leads to the killing of **rapidly dividing cells**, which is often a characteristic of cancer cells. However, this also results in damage to rapidly dividing 'normal' cells such as epithelial cells and bone marrow cells. The latter adverse effect leads to **myelosuppression** and results in anaemia, reduced platelet counts (risk of bleeding) and reduced white cells counts (risk of infection). Myelosuppression is usually the key limiting factor and so chemotherapy is often carried out in cycles, in which the patient receives a dose of chemotherapy to kill the cancer cells and there is then a delay of typically 3 weeks before the next dose, as this allows the bone marrow time to recover (Figure 65.2). By carrying out the treatment in cycles there is a substantial reduction in cancer cell load, followed by a period to allow recovery of the bone marrow. During this time the cancer cells remaining can proliferate, but the next cycle brings about another substantial reduce in cancer cell load and this is repeated. Anticancer drugs are classed by the site and mode of action.

Antimetabolites

These interfere with the synthesis of purines and /or pyrimidines.
• **Dihydrofolate reductase (DHFR) inhibitors** (e.g. methotrexate): act by inhibition of DHFR, which is the enzyme that catalyses the conversion of dihydrofolate to tetrahydrofolate. This results in the inhibition of synthesis of the nucleoside thymidine, which is essential for DNA synthesis. These are regarded as antifolate agents.
• **Pyrimidine analogues** (e.g. 5-flurouracil): 5-flurouracil is metabolised to fluorodeoxyuridine monophosphate, which is a false substrate that inhibits thymidylate synthase and so prevents the conversion of dUMP to thymidine monophosphate TMP required for DNA synthesis.
• **Purine analogues** (e.g. 6-mercaptopurine) are activated by hypoxanthine phosphoribosyltransferase to toxic metabolites and inhibit the synthesis of purines essential for DNA and RNA.

Chemical modification of DNA

• **Alkylating agents** (e.g. cyclophosphamide): these are highly reactive agents that chemically modify DNA by alkylation, which leads to the covalent cross-linking of DNA and so interferes with DNA replication, transcription and repair.
• **Platinum compounds** (e.g. cisplatin): cause cross-linking of guanine residues, resulting in DNA damage.
• **Cytotoxic antibiotics**: these chemically interact with DNA via intercalation.
   • In the case of doxorubicin the intercalation between DNA bases prevents the actions of topoisomerase II (which normally relaxes DNA supercoils) and so prevents transcription. This also leads to DNA fragmentation and inhibition of repair.
   • Mitomycin is a bifunctional alkylating agent that cross-links DNA and causes damage.

Topoisomerase inhibitors (e.g. etoposide)

• Topoisomerases are a group of enzymes that 'relax' supercoiled DNA, an essential step in DNA replication. Topoisomerase inhibitors complex with topoisomerase II and DNA, leading to a break in the DNA strand. This leads to inhibition of DNA replication and RNA transcription.

Mitotic inhibitors

These are important for the process of cell division and may be targeted by:
• **vinca alkaloids** (e.g. vincristine): these inhibit mitotic spindle formation by inhibition of tubulin polymerisation;
• **taxanes** (paclitaxel): these stabilise the spindles by inhibiting depolymerisation and so prevent mitosis.

Clinically, the above anticancer drugs are often used in combination, such that drugs with different sites of action are used. This means that lower doses can be used to limit toxicity and also reduce the risk of resistance, which can complicate the use of anticancer chemotherapy.

Targeted therapy

Recent advances in our understanding of cancer have led to newer, more selective approaches.
• **Oestrogen receptor antagonists** (e.g. tamoxifen): some breast cancer cells are sensitive to oestrogen and in patients with oestrogen-sensitive cancers tamoxifen is used to inhibit the oestrogen-dependent activation of these cells.
• **Aromatase inhibitors**: these prevent the conversion of androgens to oestrogen via aromatase and so have anti-oestrogenic effects. Once again these are beneficial in oestrogen-sensitive breast cancers.
• **Trastuzumab**: a monoclonal antibody that targets the human growth factor receptor-2 (HER2) and is used in metastatic breast cancers that express the HER2.
• **VEGF antibodies** (e.g. bevacizumab): these target vascular endothelial growth factor that is associated with angiogenesis, which leads to neovascularisation (and therefore nutrient supply) to tumours. Therefore agents interfere with the formation of blood supply to tumours.
• **Rituximab**: this is a monoclonal antibody against CD-20, which is a cell surface marker on leukocytes associated with non-Hodgkin's lymphoma.
• **Tyrosine kinase inhibitors** (e.g. imatinib): chronic myeloid leukaemia (CML) is associated with the abnormal Philadelphia chromosome codes for the *bcr-abl* protein. This protein has tyrosine kinase activity and so promotes cell proliferation. Therefore tyrosine kinase inhibitors selectively interfere with proliferation in the mutant cells. Imatinib is used in the chronic phase of CML and leads to better patient outcomes compared with the use of conventional chemotherapy and bone marrow transplantation.
• **Epidermal growth factor (EGF) tyrosine kinase inhibitors** (e.g. erlotinib): these interfere with signalling associated with cell activation. Therefore these agents target mutant cells expressing this specific tyrosine kinase activity, e.g. erlotinib is used in some lung and pancreatic cancers.

Adverse effects

Many of the anticancer drugs have severe toxic effects. As described above, meylosuppression is inevitable with cytotoxic agents and this can be overcome by using colony-stimulating factors (CSFs), which can promote the synthesis of certain white cell lines in haemopoiesis (Chapter 33). Nausea and vomiting is also a very common adverse effect and is associated with certain agents. This may be managed with anti-emetic drugs that target either peripheral afferent nerves or the central effects of toxins in the chemoreceptor trigger zone in the brain. Such anti-emetic drugs include histamine H_1 receptor antagonists, dopamine receptor antagonists and 5-HT_3 receptor antagonists.

Resistance to chemotherapy

Anticancer chemotherapy may fail due to the development of resistance. Modes of resistance include:
• increased efflux of drug from the cells through increased expression of multidrug resistance 1 (MDR1);
• increased DNA repair, especially for alkylating agents and cisplatin;
• loss of hormone-dependent cell growth.

Appendix 1: Cross references to *Medicine at a Glance (Davey)*

Chapter in *Medical Sciences at a Glance*	Clinical relevance and significant chapters in *Medicine at a Glance*	
Medical Sciences at a Glance, 1st edition (Randall, 2014)	*Medicine at a Glance*, 3rd edition (Davey, 2010)	*Medicine at a Glance*, 4th edition (Davey, 2014)
Part 1 Cellular structure and function		
Chapter 1 Cells		
Chapter 2 Organisation of cell membranes		
Chapter 3 Cell organelles		
Chapter 4 Protein biochemistry	Alzheimer's disease (Chapter 197) Prion diseases (Chapter 197)	Alzheimer's disease (Chapter 204) Prion diseases (Chapter 204)
Chapter 5 Lipid biochemistry	Hyperlipidaemia (Chapter 80)	Hyperlipidaemia (Chapter 82)
Chapter 6 Carbohydrate biochemistry	Glycation (Chapters 151 and 152)	Glycation (Chapters 156 and 157)
Chapter 7 Basic mechanism of drug action	Adverse drug reactions (Chapter 231)	Adverse drug reactions (Chapter 243)
Part 2 Cellular metabolism		
Chapter 8 General principles of cellular metabolism		
Chapter 9 Enzymes		
Chapter 10 Central metabolic pathways		
Chapter 11 Fat metabolism	Ketoacidosis (Chapters 138 and 152)	Ketoacidosis (Chapters 143 and 157)
Chapter 12 Glucose metabolism	Type 1 diabetes mellitus (Chapters 151 and 152) Type 2 diabetes mellitus (Chapters 151 and 152)	Type 1 diabetes mellitus (Chapters 156 and 157) Type 2 diabetes mellitus (Chapters 156 and 157)
Chapter 13 Amino acid metabolism		
Part 3 Molecular and medical genetics		
Chapter 14 Principles of molecular genetics		
Chapter 15 DNA and RNA		
Chapter 16 Gene expression		
Chapter 17 Medical genetics		
Part 4 Nerve and muscle		
Chapter 18 Cell excitability	Hyperkalaemia (Chapter 136) Hypokalaemia (Chapter 136)	Hyperkalaemia (Chapter 141) Hypokalaemia (Chapter 141)
Chapter 19 Nervous conduction		
Chapter 20 Synaptic transmission		
Chapter 21 Autonomic nervous system		
Chapter 22 Neuromuscular transmission	Myasthenia gravis (Chapter 203)	Myasthenia gravis (Chapter 210)
Part 5 Respiratory system		
Chapter 23 Structure of the respiratory system		
Chapter 24 Respiratory physiology	Chest X-ray (Chapter 99)	Chest X-ray (Chapter 102)
Chapter 25 Gas transport		
Chapter 26 Control of breathing		
Chapter 27 Acid-base physiology	Arterial blood gases (Chapter 98) Disorders of acid-base balance (Chapter 138)	Arterial blood gases (Chapter 100) Disorders of acid-base balance (Chapter 143)

Chapter 28 Respiratory Pathophysiology	Asthma (Chapter 104) Chronic obstructive pulmonary disease (Chapter 105) Fibrosis (Chapter 110) Lung function tests (Chapter 95) Lung infections (Chapters 102 and 103) Respiratory failure (Chapter 97)	Asthma (Chapter 109) Chronic obstructive pulmonary disease (Chapter 110) Fibrosis (Chapter 115) Lung function tests (Chapter 97) Lung infections (Chapters 107 and 108) Respiratory failure (Chapter 99)
Part 6 Cardiovascular systems		
Chapter 29 Structure of the cardiovascular system		
Chapter 30 Cardiac physiology	Arrhythmias (Chapters 92 and 93) Heart murmurs (Chapter 17) Valve disease (Chapters 86 and 87)	Arrhythmias (Chapters 94 and 95) Heart murmurs (Chapter 17) Valve disease (Chapters 88 and 89)
Chapter 31 Cardiovascular physiology	Oedema (Chapter 14)	Oedema (Chapter 14)
Chapter 32 Blood pressure	Hypertension (Chapter 79)	Hypertension (Chapter 81)
Chapter 33 Blood: 1	Anaemias (Chapters 50, 171 and 172) Aplastic anaemias (Chapter 174) Blood counts (Chapter 181) Haemolytic anaemias (Chapter 172) Iron deficiency anaemia (Chapters 121 and 171) Megaloblastic anaemia (Chapters 171 and 181) Sickle cell (Chapter 173) Thalassaemias (Chapter 173)	Anaemias (Chapters 50, 176 and 177) Aplastic anaemias (Chapter 179) Blood counts (Chapter 186) Haemolytic anaemias (Chapter 177) Iron deficiency anaemia (Chapters 126 and 182) Megaloblastic anaemia (Chapters 176 and 186) Sickle cell (Chapter 178) Thalassaemias (Chapter 178)
Chapter 34 Blood: 2	Anticoagulants (Chapter 184) Antiplatelet drugs (Chapter 184) Disseminated intravascular coagulation (Chapter 183) Leukaemias (Chapters 175 and 176) Lymphomas (Chapter 177)	Anticoagulants (Chapter 189) Antiplatelet drugs (Chapter 189) Disseminated intravascular coagulation (Chapter 188) Leukaemias (Chapters 180 and 181) Lymphomas (Chapter 182)
Chapter 35 Cardiovascular pathophysiology	Acute coronary syndrome (Chapter 81) Atherosclerosis (Chapter 80) Chronic heart failure (Chapter 85) Ischaemic heart disease (Chapters 13 and 82) Stroke (Chapter 194)	Acute coronary syndrome (Chapter 83) Atherosclerosis (Chapter 82) Chronic heart failure (Chapter 87) Ischaemic heart disease (Chapters 13 and 84) Stroke (Chapter 201)
Part 7 Renal system		
Chapter 36 Structure of the renal system		
Chapter 37 Renal physiology: filtration and tubular function	Renal function (Chapter 135)	Renal function (Chapter 140)
Chapter 38 Renal physiology: loop of Henle		
Chapter 39 Regulation of body fluids	Acute renal failure (Chapter 145) Chronic renal failure (Chapter 146)	Acute renal failure (Chapter 150) Chronic renal failure (Chapter 151)
Chapter 40 Bladder function and dysfunction	Benign prostatic hypertrophy (Chapter 149) Dysuria (Chapter 35) Urinary tract infections (Chapter 150)	Benign prostatic hypertrophy (Chapter 154) Dysuria (Chapter 35) Urinary tract infections (Chapter 155)
Part 8 Digestive system		
Chapter 41 Structure of the gastrointestinal system		
Chapter 42 Upper gastrointestinal physiology	Dyspepsia (Chapter 30) Dysphagia (Chapter 29) Gastro-oesophageal reflux disease (Chapter 118) Peptic ulceration (Chapter 119)	Dyspepsia (Chapter 30) Dysphagia (Chapter 29) Gastro-oesophageal reflux disease (Chapter 123) Peptic ulceration (Chapter 124)
Chapter 43 Lower gastrointestinal physiology	Constipation (Chapters 24 and 133) Crohn's disease (Chapter 123) Diarrhoea (Chapters 25 and 133) Inflammatory bowel disease (Chapter 123) Irritable bowel syndrome (Chapter 133)	Constipation (Chapters 24 and 138) Crohn's disease (Chapter 128) Diarrhoea (Chapters 25 and 138) Inflammatory bowel disease (Chapter 128) Irritable bowel syndrome (Chapter 138)

Chapter 44 The liver	Alcoholic liver disease (Chapter 129) Ascites (Chapter 33) Cholestasis (Chapter 126) Hepatitis (Chapter 127) Jaundice (Chapter 30) Liver failure (Chapter 128) Liver function tests (Chapter 122)	Alcoholic liver disease (Chapter 134) Ascites (Chapter 33) Cholestasis (Chapter 131) Hepatitis (Chapter 132) Jaundice (Chapter 30) Liver failure (Chapter 133) Liver function tests (Chapter 127)
Part 9 Endocrine system		
Chapter 45 Hypothalamus and pituitary	Acromegaly (Chapter 154) Pituitary tumours (Chapter 159)	Acromegaly (Chapter 159) Pituitary tumours (Chapter 164)
Chapter 46 Endocrine pancreas	Type 1 diabetes mellitus (Chapters 151 and 152) Type 2 diabetes mellitus (Chapters 151 and 152)	Type 1 diabetes mellitus (Chapters 156 and 157) Type 2 diabetes mellitus (Chapters 156 and 157)
Chapter 47 Thyroid gland	Calcium balance (Chapter 157) Hyperthyroidism (Chapter 156) Hypothyroidism (Chapter 155)	Calcium balance (Chapter 162) Hyperthyroidism (Chapter 161) Hypothyroidism (Chapter 160)
Chapter 48 Adrenal glands and steroid hormones	Addison's disease (Chapter 158) Conn's syndrome (Chapter 158) Cushing's syndrome (Chapter 136)	Addison's disease (Chapter 163) Conn's syndrome (Chapter 163) Cushing's syndrome (Chapter 141)
Part 10 Reproductive function		
Chapter 49 The genital system		
Chapter 50 Reproductive physiology	Hypogonadism (Chapter 160)	Hypogonadism (Chapter 165)
Chapter 51 Human embryology		
Part 11 Central nervous system		
Chapter 52 Structure of the central nervous system		
Chapter 53 The sensory system	Sensory pathways (Chapter 56)	Sensory pathways (Chapter 56)
Chapter 54 The motor system	Motor pathways (Chapter 56)	Motor pathways (Chapter 56)
Chapter 55 Hypothalamus and thalamus		
Chapter 56 Central nervous system function		
Chapter 57 Disorders and treatments	Anxiety (Chapter 228) Bipolar affective disorder (Chapter 228) Dementia (Chapter 197) Depression (Chapter 228) Epilepsy (Chapter 198) Multiple sclerosis (Chapter 199) Parkinson's disease (Chapter 205) Schizophrenia (Chapter 228)	Anxiety (Chapter 240) Bipolar affective disorder (Chapter 240) Dementia (Chapter 204) Depression (Chapter 240) Epilepsy (Chapter 205) Multiple sclerosis (Chapter 206) Parkinson's disease (Chapter 212) Schizophrenia (Chapter 240)
Part 12 Infections and immunity		
Chapter 58 Pathogens	Bacteraemia (Chapter 161) Bacterial infections (Chapter 165) Fungal infections (Chapter 164) Infections (Chapter 41) Malaria (Chapter 166) Prion diseases (Chapter 197) Tuberculosis (Chapter 167) Viral infections (Chapter 162)	Bacteraemia (Chapter 166) Bacterial infections (Chapter 170) Fungal infections (Chapter 169) Infections (Chapter 41) Malaria (Chapter 171) Prion diseases (Chapter 204) Tuberculosis (Chapter 172) Viral infections (Chapter 167)
Chapter 59 Recognition of pathogens		
Chapter 60 Defence against pathogens		
Chapter 61 Integration of the immune response		

Chapter 62 Immunopathology	Allergy (Chapter 75) Alveolitis (Chapter 109) Anaphylaxis (Chapter 74) Eczema (Chapter 216) Systemic lupus erythematosus (Chapter 214)	Allergy (Chapter 77) Alveolitis (Chapter 114) Anaphylaxis (Chapter 76) Eczema (Chapter 223) Systemic lupus erythematosus (Chapter 221)
Chapter 63 Immunodeficiency disorders	HIV infections (Chapter 163) Immunodeficiency (Chapter 170)	HIV infections (Chapter 168) Immunodeficiency (Chapter 175)
Part 13 Cancer		
Chapter 64 Cancer biology	Aetiology (Chapter 186) Breast cancer (Chapter 189) Cancer with unknown primary (Chapter 191) Colorectal cancers (Chapter 131) Lung cancers (Chapter 116) Pancreatic cancer (Chapter 125) Prostate cancer (Chapter 190) Upper GI cancers (Chapter 130)	Aetiology (Chapter 191) Breast cancer (Chapter 194) Cancer with unknown primary (Chapter 196) Colorectal cancers (Chapter 136) Lung cancers (Chapter 121) Pancreatic cancer (Chapter 130) Prostate cancer (Chapter 195) Upper GI cancers (Chapter 135)
Chapter 65 Chemotherapy	Cancer management (Chapter 187)	Cancer management (Chapter 192)

Index